Welfare Medicine in America

Welfare Medicine in America

A Case Study of Medicaid

Robert Stevens
Rosemary Stevens

With a new introduction by
Rosemary Stevens

Routledge
Taylor & Francis Group
LONDON AND NEW YORK

Originally published in 1974 by The Free Press

Published 2003 by Transaction Publishers

Published 2017 by Routledge
2 Park Square, Milton Park, Abingdon, Oxon OX14 4RN
711 Third Avenue, New York, NY 10017, USA

First issued in hardback 2017

Routledge is an imprint of the Taylor & Francis Group, an informa business

Library of Congress Catalog Number: 2002068461

Library of Congress Cataloging-in-Publication Data

Stevens, Robert Bocking.
Welfare medicine in America : a case study of Medicaid / Robert Stevens and Rosemary Stevens.
p. cm.
"With a new introduction by Rosemary Stevens."
"Originally published in 1974 by the Free Press"—T.p. verso.
Includes bibliographical references and index.
ISBN 0-7658-0957-5 (paper : alk. paper)
1. Medicaid. 2. Medical policy—United States. I. Stevens, Rosemary, 1935- II. Title.

RA412.4 .S746 2003
368.4'2'00973—dc21 2002068461

ISBN 13: 978-1-138-54041-5 (hbk)
ISBN 13: 978-0-7658-0957-5 (pbk)

For Carey and Richard

Contents

PART II: THE EUPHORIC DEMISE *July 1965 – January 1968*

PART III: THE STORM *January 1968 – July 1970*

PART IV: BENIGN NEGLECT *July 1970 – June 1973*

Introduction to the Transaction Edition

Health and the State before the Mid-1970s: Structure, Power, and Rhetoric in England and the United States

In July 1946, the British government passed landmark legislation to create the National Health Service (NHS), which was implemented in 1948. In July 1965, almost twenty years later, President Lyndon Baines Johnson signed far-reaching legislation in the United States that is the basis for the present Medicare and Medicaid programs. Looking back from the early twenty-first century, both actions were successful in extending health services to previously underserved populations. Each country crafted legislation that drew on preexisting organizational patterns in medicine, on proposals for health reform formulated in earlier years, and on prevailing assumptions about the purposes and limits of government. In Great Britain, the NHS guaranteed health services that were largely free at the time of use, nationalized the hospitals, and built a top-down command and control health care system. In the United States, Medicare provided government-sponsored health insurance limited to the older generations (sixty-five-plus years of age) irrespective of income—individuals whom the private insurance sector demonstrably could not serve. Medicaid provided subsidy to the states to provide additional health benefits to elderly residents whose incomes fell below specified levels, as well as to disabled, blind, and deaf individuals, and to needy families with children.[1]

Nevertheless, in these, as in other countries, no one has been satisfied with the results. Massive organizational changes, problems, and expenses have accompanied the rise of each nation's version of the "health care state."[2] There is considerable unease on both sides of the Atlantic about how much medical care, and of what quality, should be accessible to all members of the population; which services should be subsidized by government; how best to stimulate private initiative and meet consumer preferences; whether co-payments and means testing are prudent or unfair social mechanisms; and how much tax money should be allocated to health care in light of competing social goods, such as national defense, public education, and controlling the overall rate of taxation. The recent history of the NHS has been aptly described as one of "continuous revolution,"[3] or, more gently perhaps, of "perpetual evolution."[4] The same can be said of health care in the United States, where "creative chaos"[5] is the kindest comment on the turmoil of the present. This is a good time to reconsider the historical baggage carried into each national health care system, and to take a new look at these huge national experiments in comparative perspective. It is in this spirit that *Medical Practice in Modern England* and *Welfare Medicine in America* are here offered to a new generation of readers and critics.

It is an honor and a privilege to see books one has written and that were published many years ago reissued. As an illustration of the time that has gone by since, my talented research assistant for *Medical Practice* is now the Rt. Hon. Michael Meacher, M.P., Minister for the Environment in the U.K. government. Why should anyone read these books today? Taken together, the two books describe English and American health care, their similarities and differences in providing health care to their respective populations, in an important period for health policy in both countries, between World War II and the early 1970s. Combined, they serve to emphasize how social legislation reflects past cultural practices rather than future expectations. In Rudolf Klein's apt phrase, this is the "politics of the second best."[6] The books show the impact of legislative action on powerful and potential players in health care organization and financing (often with unexpected consequences); illustrate the inertia and resilience of the social organizations involved in change; and emphasize the importance of implementation as a policymaking vehicle. All are useful messages for the present. "In any democratic system," writes Mark Peterson," a policy decision is always a beginning rather than an end."[7]

These books may also carry different meanings to today's readers than to their counterparts of, respectively, 1966 and 1974. They will, first, I hope, help to emphasize the importance of social/organizational history as a central explanatory technique for policy studies. The books were written at a time when historical studies with a wide sweep of subject matter and complex themes were thought unfashionable within the mainstream of the social sciences. Now, thankfully, the pendulum has swung. A new audience of social scientists in historical sociology and other fields may find these studies enlightening and helpful.

With the passage of time, these books have also become historical artifacts in their own right, contemporary documents of a rich, earlier period. It is a truism worth repeating that history reflects the ideas of the time in which it was written. Each of these books offers a unique view of the political, social, economic, organizational, and ideological issues influencing medical practice and health services as one informed observer (myself for the first book) and two (Robert Stevens and myself for the second) then saw them. Though they were not initially planned for this purpose, *Medical Practice in Modern England* and *Welfare Medicine in America* present today's readers with comparative historical case studies of the role of government in the two countries, the relationship between public and private sectors, and the relative choices made in bringing health services to the population. Old questions can be asked anew; specifically, how was the welfare state in medicine negotiated for health care in England, and with what results for the providers of care?; and, how did the implementation and reception of Medicaid shape America's version of a welfare state, and again, with what effects on the organization of care?

Medicaid provides an important window on health policy in the United States for at least two reasons. It demonstrates America's commitment to serve those in need, despite deep divisions about how best to serve the population as a whole; and it serves as a backstop and support of the private sector (insurance companies, for-profit and not-for-profit hospitals, medical practice corporations, etc.), through which it channels funds. As we showed in *Welfare Medicine in America*, Medicaid has also served, politically, to preempt broader proposals for national health insurance. Medicaid (like Medicare) poured money into privately run hospitals, making the old public hospitals seem marginal or irrelevant, though some great public hospitals survive to this day.[8] In contrast, both private and public hospitals were nationalized in Great Britain. Understanding the arguments, problems, and successes of those times does much to explain where the two systems find themselves today.

I look forward to bringing *Medical Practice* and *Welfare Medicine* to the attention of readers like my students, who were not born when these books were written but who live with the consequences of the policies and politics they describe. There is a new audience of historians and social scientists who are interested in the 1960s and 1970s, and indeed of the twentieth century as a whole. Younger readers also have a vested interest in the future of health policy. Current students in England who reach my present age will experience a very different NHS than the one originally designed, perhaps even different from what it is at present. American students will be Medicare and perhaps Medicaid recipients in the 2060s, one hundred years after the Medicare and Medicaid legislation—assuming those programs survive until then.

Author and Authors

Before considering the two books, comparatively and as scholarly studies, warts and all, some autobiographical comments may be helpful to set the stage. Like others who remember the 1960s, we are not the same persons, with the same thoughts, environment, or experiences, as we were then—young scholars probing the messiness, antecedents, and immediacy of what was then the present.

Medical Practice in Modern England was my first book, published when I was thirty-one years of age, and I have a special affection for and pride in it. Several of the British reviewers assumed I was American, though fortunately not holding this against me in their reviews of the book. I am a native Briton who became a U.S. citizen in 1968. Between 1957 and 1961 I was a graduate student in applied social science at the University of Manchester, trained for health care management in Sheffield and London, and worked in the NHS as a trainee and administrator. In 1961-62, while planning for the research that would lead to *Medical Practice*, I was a full-time public health student at Yale. All of my work, now as then, reflects the comparative perspectives that come from the shock of discovery. Through my English eyes, the American health system of the 1960s seemed illogical, contested, and impenetrable. Yet I was learning about the American system and its history with a cohort of American graduate students who seemed remarkably unfazed by its peculiarities, as indeed was I, at the time, about the NHS. Two pertinent understandings were thus made clear early on, equally relevant today. First, it is easy to accept familiar social structures without adequately questioning their rationale or roots; hence the importance of comparative perspectives. Second, the way in which any health system is organized and paid for can best (perhaps only) be understood through studying its own idiosyncratic history. In returning to England in the shadow of the Medicare debates of the early 1960s, I saw more clearly than before the anomalies, inconsistencies, and conflicts embedded in the NHS. Similarly, I turned to the research for *Welfare Medicine in America* in the early 1970s with the ability to dwell intellectually in both cultural systems.

I was then married to Robert B. Stevens, a distinguished historian/lawyer at the Yale Law School, who was also a critical and valued mentor for the English book. Robert Stevens has focused most of his scholarly attention on the history of legal institutions. However, in 1970 he published an edited volume on the statutory history of social legislation in the United States.[9] We decided to join forces to work on Medicaid, aided by work done by graduate students in courses we were both teaching. I was then on the faculty of the Yale Medical School. *Welfare Medicine in America*, authored jointly and seamlessly, benefited from the mix of social science, public health, and legal perspectives that we brought to the project. The legal perspective was particularly important in the absence of strong national policy direction because, as is evident in the book, policymaking for Medicaid has been enmeshed in legal decisions, clarifications, wrangling, and rulings.

The Books in Comparative Perspective

I will present my own reactions to rereading these books in 2002 after a brief description and comparison, so as to place them in the environment in which they were written. *Medical Practice in Modern England: The Impact of Specialization and State Medicine*, first published in 1966, describes the invention and implementation of the National Health Service in England with special focus on the role of the national organizations of medicine and the implications of the NHS for the medical profession. My goal was to trace the history of specialization in medicine as a major trend after World War II, which affected, in turn, medical practice, the availability of health care, and the organization and costs of health services. Inevitably this meant analyzing the NHS as well as the formal organization and behavior of the medical profession. This book thus attempts to do two things: to provide a balanced historical analysis of the NHS as a central element in Britain's welfare state (as seen from the early 1960s), and to explore the role of medical organizations in shaping it and being shaped by it. I tried to avoid the divisive political rhetoric over "socialized medicine" that then distinguished health care debates on both sides of the Atlantic, in order to describe the practical realities that lay beneath; that is, the shaping of the health care system and power relations in it. As the book shows, the organization of the NHS solidified preexisting professional divisions in British medicine, between specialists and primary care doctors, and between primary care and hospitals.

In the United States, during the same period, the rapid specialization of medicine after World War II led to all-out competition among specialists for patients who could pay for their services in a largely private market. Private health insurance for the working population fueled increased demand for hospital and medical services. The quiet, American version of government aid for population coverage was tax relief, to encourage employers to organize and subsidize health insurance for employees. Federal funds were also made directly available in the 1940s and 1950s to help build a hospital and specialist infrastructure, through grants to states for building hospitals and the rapid expansion of biomedical research in increasingly specialized medical schools.[10]

While the NHS recognized general practitioners as having an essential structural role in England, with formalized relationships to both specialists and patients, there were no such protections for family doctors in the United States, where primary doctors and specialists competed for patients. At the very time the NHS was controlling the supply of medical specialists through salaried service and limited positions, the American system encouraged doctors to specialize. Indeed the proliferation of specialists, specialties, and subspecialties engendered professional and political concern about the decline of primary care, particularly evident in the 1960s.

In theory, Medicare and Medicaid could have required patients to have a primary care doctor with a gatekeeper role in the United States. By that time, though, the private market system was entrenched as a model of nonintervention by government agents. Thus Medicaid, as we showed in *Welfare Medicine*, introduced a huge system of government subsidy of services for the poor in the private sector in the late 1960s. The combined result of

Medicare and Medicaid, implemented at the same time and along similar lines, was to pour additional money into the preexisting medical system, flaws and all. In stimulating demand for services (and paying for them), the two programs also encouraged additional private investment, notably in the nursing home industry.

Medical Practice in Modern England was published the same year Medicare and Medicaid were implemented. Both books have a strong comparative perspective. *Medical Practice* drew on my awareness of contemporary concerns about health and medicine in the United States and reflected my desire to bring the English experience to American readers, as well as to those in Britain and elsewhere. This strategy worked. *Medical Practice* was well reviewed in Britain, Canada, and the United States. Americans of the time tended to ignore or dismiss the NHS as an irrelevant, unacceptable aspect of a "socialized" state, or as the progeny of a poor, backward relative. "American physicians have been at once frightened of and fascinated by the British national health scheme," erroneously assuming that British traditions were similar to those in the United States, wrote a leading American commentator on the book.[11] Britons were equally toplofty about American health policy. It was easy to take the moral high ground, dismissing the American system for its lack of universal health coverage and its reliance on the crassness of the private market.

Yet even in the 1960s the two systems had much in common. For example, both countries had problems accommodating to the growing importance of hospitals as centers of medical treatment after World War II. In both there was concern about how to link an array of medical and community services to best serve those with chronic conditions. In both countries the future of primary care was on the national agenda. In both, too, there was surprisingly little information about the way medicine was actually practiced, and little was known about the quality of care. Consumers were not much in evidence as any form of driving force for change—as marked by their notable absence in each of these books. In both countries the high prestige of the medical profession was assumed to mirror uniformly high standards of clinical practice and behavior, without scrutiny from the public or the health care system.

At root these were organizational and managerial problems rather than strictly political issues, as later developments in both countries made clear. However, this sense of the commonality of organization and management across nations took a long time to become central to health care debates among academics and policymakers. The commonalities were obscured in politically-couched debates for and against state socialism, while comparative models tended to explain a nation's health services according to its place on a public-private continuum, with Britain and the Soviet Union at one end of the spectrum (the most socialist) and the United States at the other (the most market-oriented). I recall a talk I gave to an international audience of social scientists in Berlin in the early 1980s on comparative management of health care systems, without making reference to Marxism or any other ism, and this was received as a novel approach, even then. *Medical Practice* takes a pragmatic rather than an ideological position about the implementation of the NHS; even more so perhaps than does *Welfare Medicine*. Perhaps there were (and still are) things each country could learn from the other. The NHS of the 1960s might even be a possible harbinger of things to come in the United States, however horrifying or welcome that might be. Today many Europeans feel a rather similar fascination in contemplating health care in the United States as a model of privatization, managed and non-managed competition, and tolerance (however reluctantly) of 41 million uninsured residents.

Medical Practice in Modern England examines the antecedents and passage of the NHS Act in 1946, emphasizing concurrent developments in medical practice and the political roles of the profession; the emerging problems affecting administrative and medical hierarchies, ranging from determining medical incomes to planning for the future of family practice; and the interactions between the medical profession and the NHS in the early 1960s. The book shows how preexisting patterns of medical practice, already outmoded in the 1930s, were grafted into the NHS as a political compromise to ensure its passage and gain support from the medical profession in the 1940s, and beyond. Medical organizations were influential in shaping the service, particularly the institutional representatives of powerful specialties.

Not only was the division in British medicine between general practitioners and consultants (specialists) strengthened, with implications up to the present, professional leadership was also divided into two sets of institutions with separate goals. The British Medical Association largely represented general practitioners, who sought practice autonomy and private status in the new service. The Royal Colleges represented the consultants, who had no problem with salaried employment in the NHS hospital service, coupled as it was with their control of specified hospital beds and little or no regulation over their activities. In this critical implementation period, the specialists monopolized the hospitals, while general practitioners monopolized patients through controlling primary care. The NHS reinforced primary care as specialization was threatening it, and curbed the more general move toward specialism, as was happening in the United States in the 1950s and 1960s. Since there was no similarly (bi-modal) divided profession in the United States, the representative structures for medicine were different. In the 1960s, the American Medical Association represented the American medical profession writ large. However, a myriad of specialty associations were already rising to power. In the 1970s, as we note in *Welfare Medicine*, the AMA was losing members, again with ramifications to the present.

By the mid-1960s, the NHS had achieved its goal of providing a comprehensive, universal health service to the population, within overall budgetary constraints. The service was given virtually free at the time of delivery, was government-operated, and largely supported by general taxation. The administrative structures, though, were creaking. However good state medicine might be, the NHS was a vast bureaucratic system based on traditional institutions, whose virtue (at least then) was organizational stability rather than nimbleness in the face of change. Yet both the epidemiology of disease and the scientific and technological potential of medicine were changing fast on both sides of the Atlantic. General, specialist, and hospital practice were transformed after World War II with the advent of antibiotics and other powerful pharmaceuticals, together with new diagnostic and therapeutic techniques.[12] The population was aging, and the focus of health was shifting from acute to chronic conditions. Lasting themes were evident: how best to organize primary care; how to coordinate different aspects of health services; how to balance generalist and specialist care; and how to encourage teamwork, evaluation, up-to-date professional education, and medical efficiency. The medical profession had considerable authority within the service, but also had to negotiate with the NHS (and exerted pressure on government) in order to further the income of its own separate sectors. The book raises significant questions about power and authority in medical care, demonstrates that professional leadership may be *enhanced* rather than reduced under government programs (a still novel view in the United States), and stands as an early case study for asking a central question about the NHS: how (if at all) can any state (or perhaps any huge private corporation) own, operate, fund, and manage a health service, negotiate the power structures and economic tradeoffs inherent in each of these functions, and satisfy taxpayers, patients, physicians, and other health care stakeholders?

Welfare Medicine in America: A Case Study of Medicaid remains the only scholarly study to date of the implementation of the Medicaid program, from the enabling legislation in 1965 through self-evident problems by the early 1970s. The contested quest for national health insurance runs as a continuing background theme for the rapidly moving changes in Medicaid's program and direction, as does Medicaid's signal role in the late 1960s and early 1970s as an expression of the American welfare state. We were fortunate that this book, too, was welcomed at the time by reviewers in terms of its apparent objectivity, synthesis of social, economic, and organizational approaches, its ability to raise fundamental questions about the state and health care provision, and not least, its wealth of detail.

Welfare Medicine focuses more strongly on philosophical questions about the state's role in guaranteeing medical care than does *Medical Practice*, reflecting the fact that I regarded the NHS, not unreasonably, as a done deal philosophically in the 1960s. Its policy of universal, comprehensive services was established and, to American eyes, remarkably non-controversial. In contrast, American health care lurched along, sustained by the rhetoric of government-supported private enterprise but without clear policy definition. A central theme of *Welfare Medicine* is that Medicaid had no clear goals; hence the ease with which, on the one hand, it was heralded as the "sleeper" in the Medicare/Medicaid legislation, which might turn into socialized medicine for all in the United States, while on the other hand it was rapidly cut back to a traditional welfare program as costs rose. "What is the human good which medicine serves?" asked one reviewer, provoked to such questions by the book; "In what sense do the needs of some constitute rights which impose duties on others?" We describe "a social policy unable to settle on a distinct concept of welfare or of rights, wavering between a Rawlsian advantaging of the most disadvantaged and the reluctance of Nozick's minimal state to interfere with the liberty of individuals."[13]

Medicaid was (and is) a national program of federal grants to states to pay for medical services to needy families with children and to individuals who are elderly, blind, or disabled. Introduced into a culture of health care provision that assumed a central role for private enterprise in health insurance but recognized that government should support that market and act responsibly when the market fails, Medicaid stemmed from a long history of welfare policies and politics in the United States. The book begins with a brief history of the alternative and competing (if simplistic) philosophies for justifying the provision of health care to those who demonstrably need it—and who can be identified as "needy" through bureaucratic rules. These basic views were represented in the politics of "social insurance" versus "public assistance" approaches to social legislation in the 1960s. The former characterizes Medicare, which provides national health insurance with limited benefits to those sixty-five years of age and over, to disabled individuals, and to those who would otherwise die from kidney failure. Medicaid was built on American public assistance principles, and thus includes a means test as condition for entry, state rather than federal administration, and an eligibility structure that followed preexisting welfare provisions. Initially, as we show, it was not clear whether Medicaid was a "right" for potentially qualified beneficiaries or merely a state-dominated, churlish privilege. Medical benefits for those within the program could (and can) be quite generous, more so than for Medicare.

It was evident in the early 1970s that more needed to be known about the actual workings of the Medicaid program as implemented in the states. How, otherwise, was anyone to interpret the sometimes heady, sometimes alarmed expectations of Medicaid critics who saw the program as the "thin end of the wedge of socialized medicine?" Sociologist Michael M. Davis's much earlier comment on the importance of applied social research in health care in the United States bears repeating to this day, as a continuing refrain: "[W]here many people take sides and where more than two sides exist analysis is needed *more than pronouncement*."[14] We show, through state case studies, that implementation in the states demonstrated distinctive initial preferences, based on prior state experiences. Notably, California expressed a strong service commitment for those covered but put strict limits on Medicaid eligibility, while New York announced generous eligibility standards in a less organized service system. However, disillusion soon set in across the board as it became evident that costs were escalating far beyond expectation. The book traces the "euphoric demise" of Medicaid by early 1968, with the beginning of a period of political storm in Washington and the states, including finger-pointing, retrenchments, Congressional reappraisals, and new (though largely unimplemented) proposals from the Nixon administration.

The last five chapters cover the period July 1970-June 1973; that is, contemporary to the writing of the book. Federal administration was strengthened, but Medicaid costs continued to climb rapidly in the states. While the English system was reorganized in 1974 (largely unsuccessfully) around consensus management at the community level, Medicaid providers were being charged with fraud. From the 1970s to the present there has been continuing tension about Medicaid's role as a national program rather than as a diverse collection of State programs operating under federal rules; and there has been further tension as to whether, in any event, those rules should be tight or loose. Federalism remains a question central to American policymaking. At the same time, the hidden nature of the American welfare state, marked by opposition to a strong central governmental role for health care, threw many decisions to the courts. In retrospect, both lawyers and the legal system are remarkably absent as players in the NHS, as *Medical Practice in Modern England* demonstrates (though during the past ten years the courts have been more willing to intervene in the U.K.). Legal issues were sufficiently important in Medicaid implementation that we devoted a chapter of *Welfare Medicine* to the important role of the legal system (the courts) in crafting Medicaid as American social policy, in efforts to clarify its goals, eligibility, and basic rules.

Whether Medicaid was a "health" or a "welfare" program was an important issue in 1973. Today Medicaid is characterized as a right for state-specified health services for those individuals who are admitted to the program.[15] In the early 1970s, the question was open as to whether Medicaid was a stopgap alternative to universal national health insurance or a necessary piece of welfare reform. Today, after the failure of the ambitious Clinton Administration health reform proposals of 1993-94, and with the job-oriented, welfare reform movement trimming the welfare rolls since 1996, that question is no longer relevant. Medicaid, supplemented by a new federal-state program for extending health services to children, has its own established niche. It is a huge program of government purchase of health services for large segments of the population, paying the costs for a third of all births, a fourth of all health care for children under the age of five, and half of all nursing home care in the United States.[16]

Managing a system of public purchase of care in the private sector, problematic throughout the early years of Medicaid, remains a central challenge—

not just for Medicaid, but for Medicare as well, and indeed for any proposals for extending the public role in health care in the United States. At a core level *Welfare Medicine* raises fundamental questions as to what a much-sought single-payer insurance system might entail and what it might look like in the United States, at least as applying to those most in need of care. Today's practice is moving toward enrolling Medicaid beneficiaries in managed care, through contracts for specified services between the states and private insurers, which then contract with competing health care providers. The early days of Medicaid implementation, designed to bring the poor into the "mainstream" of middle-class medicine through paying middle-class fees, now seem naively optimistic—and have long since passed away. As the power of setting fees for privately insured patients moved from health care providers to the insurance purchasers in the 1990s, power relationships changed in American medicine. Today Medicaid managed care contracts often bring fiscal hardship to the private providers. Indeed, payment levels are so low for some hospital outpatient services that they are reportedly not worth collecting, taking into account the cost of billing for such services and the ever-present threat of a fine-tooth comb audit.

Both books vividly demonstrate the difficulty of implementing a single-payer system, even under the best of circumstances. Medicaid, like the NHS, exaggerated the weaknesses of the health care system, contributed to increased costs, and imposed new constraints on hospitals and physicians. Both books highlight the unintended consequences of legislative and regulatory action, and show how far health care policy has been made, and by extension continues to be made, through actions taken to correct problems generated at a previous stage of implementation. Hence the continuing reforms, slogans for mobilizing change, and new approaches that have marked health service provision in both countries to the present.

The basic attributes of each health service were in place at the time each book was written: England with its commitment to the whole population and seemingly intractable problems of organizing services; the United States committed to private health insurance for as many people as possible, based on the workplace, with some major gaps in coverage filled by government, and with the organization of services largely left to the private sector. In theory, either was a workable system. Why neither worked as well as expected is explored in these books, filtered through the times in which each book was written.

Reappraisals in 2002

If filtered through our own times, how might these books be written today? As dwellers in the present, we are irretrievably affected by the experiences of health care, more general aspects of the social, political, and economic environment, and the ever-changing language of debate since the 1970s. It would be impossible to write about the NHS up to 1966 or Medicaid up to 1974 without taking the wisdom of hindsight into account; or perhaps, more accurately, a rather different set of cultural (temporal) biases. This more recent past includes debates about the failure of government action in health care in both countries in the 1970s, followed by reactive shifts toward private market solutions, including the virtues of competition and belief in better management in the 1980s; and then reaction in turn against such shifts in the 1990s and beyond—leading in England to the present upheavals of the NHS around consumerism, building primary care groups, and bringing private investment and management into the NHS; and in the United States to critiques and regulation of managed care corporations, and efforts to mobilize action around the quality of care. Doctors are dissatisfied in both countries, threatened by a perceived loss of clinical autonomy and increased surveillance of professional work through the move toward clinical governance in England and through practice guidelines and medical audits in the United States.

Today's language of debate is more attuned to business terms than to those of social service. Even though both books focus on structures, institutions, and management of health care, they assume that health services are different from other major economic enterprises; indeed, that as social services they are more akin to education than to (say) the banking industry. This was indeed a general view in the 1960s and early 1970s. Administrators were not educated for "management" in business schools, but for "administration" in schools of public health, public welfare, or (in England) social administration. Today in the United States, there is an army of health analysts in academia, banking, accounting, stock market analysis, business consulting, law, lobbying, think tanks, and elsewhere, drawn from many disciplines, each with vested interests in the system. Such roles existed thirty or forty years ago (we can see them in *Welfare Medicine*), but in nothing like today's profusion. The language of business has become ingrained as a vehicle for thinking about health care, infusing health policy in both countries—from the idea of internal markets in England to managed care in the United States. By the late 1980s it was natural for me, writing about the history of American hospitals, to frame my study in terms of their long, interweaving roles as charities and businesses.[17] Today I might say of the two books: In England, the good feelings engendered by the politics of egalitarianism overrode considerations of efficiency; while in the United States, belief in the efficacy of the market produced enormous social inefficiencies.

Today's policy questions focus more overtly than before on the role of government in the economy and in public budgets (of which health care is now a significant part), and as a manager of individual and social risk; on the future of professions as social institutions; on the impact of health systems on patients (and vice versa), and on consumerism more generally; on the moral value of a one-class system of health care (more like the NHS) versus a more stratified set of choices dependent on income and individual choice (more like the United States); on federalism and the relative authority of (and division of taxes between) the nation and states in domestic policy in the United States, a major theme for the future of Medicaid; on devolution and decentralization of authority for health care in Great Britain; and on the relationships between markets, professions, and states. While we touch on many of these questions in the books, there is now a large scholarly literature that would have to be taken into account in any new appraisal. On the other hand, because there was relatively little relevant secondary analysis (the work of other scholars) to draw on while we were doing the research for the books, we had the advantage of working in, and thinking across, relatively clear fields. We also had the privilege of doing contemporary fieldwork and conducting interviews with leading participants.

When the books were written, the literature of feminism was still quite young. It is disconcerting to read the then-common stylistic use of "he" to stand for an undifferentiated individual, including a doctor or a patient. Writing about these topics now, I would include a discussion of the role of health services for women and the role of women workers as a matter of course. Medicaid, for example, has a disproportionate effect on women, because of its primary role in serving mothers with young children at one end of the life course, and the elderly (predominantly female) at the other. On both sides of the Atlantic, too, increased cultural diversity has raised new themes. None of these comments changes the intrinsic value of the books as creatures of their time. But it is instructive, looking back, to see the embedded values they present.

For example, both books are remarkably, even quaintly, optimistic about the potential role of government to create better health care systems—too optimistic in the light of subsequent events. At the very least, I would now be much more critical of the NHS and the problems of a government service in England, and much less sanguine about the potential of the federal government to effect social change in the United States. I think I would also be more charitable toward those attempting to implement Medicaid in its early years, recognizing more clearly with the advantage of distance the complexities and uncertainties of those years. Moreover, national health insurance was demonstrably *not* just around the corner, as we sometimes seem to suggest.

My younger self accepted the nationalization of hospitals and the centralization of services in the NHS far more readily than I would now. Partly that was because it was a fait accompli, and seemed a natural parallel to other forms of nationalization after World War II, including that of energy corporations and the railways. Nevertheless, I could have been more critical. Most interesting, I think, from today's perspective is that the NHS centralized in one organization the means of production of health services (hospitals, specialists, family practitioners, and so on) *and* the means of paying for them. While the NHS could be seen as an incremental extension of the older national health insurance scheme, the combination of the functions of provider and guarantor of services (what we would now think of as seller and buyer) was actually quite radical. In theory, the NHS could have become a contractual service, with government buying services in the private sector, not unlike the health insurance systems of countries like Germany or France, or for the more limited sectors of the population covered by Medicare and Medicaid in the United States. Efforts by the Conservative government to create "internal markets" failed as one redesign of the NHS. In any event, the British government has been bedeviled by having to act as proprietor of a vast array of services and as employer of often obstreperous, disaffected groups, while also representing patients and fighting for budgets in Parliament. The sheer magnitude of the administrative tasks deserves scrutiny as a business proposition. Going the rounds in England in 2001 was the jest that the British NHS, with about one million employees, is the largest (public) organization in the world, with the exception of the Chinese army.[18]

The recent history of the NHS has been a saga of how to reorganize and reintegrate the organizations that were taken over on the "appointed day" for implementation of the NHS in 1948 into a more effective delivery system at the local level—and how far to go in separating the roles of buyer and seller. In recent years the pendulum has swung toward consumer satisfaction (a theme that was remarkably absent in the more paternalistic health service of 1966). Would this focus have come earlier if the health system had not been nationalized in the first place? Would the old public (local government) hospitals, taken into the NHS, have been abandoned in a more private system, like some formerly distinguished American public hospitals, or privatized like the California hospitals after Medicaid? Would previously charitable (voluntary) hospitals now behave more overtly as businesses, as in the United States? The answer to all of these questions is, perhaps. My purpose in raising such questions is merely to observe that these are the kinds of questions that would now infuse reexamination of the materials of *Medical Practice*.

Similarly, in *Welfare Medicine*, we would now, I think, give more emphasis to the management theme underlying the Medicaid program; that is, the problems inherent in any system of public purchase of health care from independent providers or through private insurers. These themes are now critical and current. We might also give less emphasis to the "philosophical"—actually, the rhetorical—bases for distinguishing public assistance and social insurance. Medicaid has taken on a new currency in the last five or six years, as efforts have been made simultaneously to get individuals of working age off welfare, but also to include health coverage to additional children (and sometimes immediate family members) through extended federal-state programs known as child health insurance programs, or CHIP.[19] Significantly, given the history of the negative rhetoric of "assistance," both Medicaid and the new programs are now called "insurance." Meanwhile, Medicare, like Social Security income payments, has been tarred with the new negative rhetoric of "entitlements." The basic dichotomy of insurance versus assistance is not a currently fashionable organizing theme, though it may reappear, of course, in the future.

It may still be possible to depict the history of American social policy for health services as one of intermittent efforts to extend medical technology to the masses. How to insure low-income workers who, through no fault of their own, are without health insurance is currently a vexing political question. So is extending out-of-hospital pharmaceutical benefits as an additional benefit for Medicare beneficiaries. Perhaps the United States will eventually attain universal health insurance coverage in some way or another, and for some or other level of service. However, it is not currently realistic to see Medicaid or Medicare as a step toward a universal national health insurance program, to be built in either of their images. We are older and possibly wiser through experience than when *Welfare Medicine* was written.

Future generations will bring their own, probably very different, perspectives to the history presented in *Medical Practice* and *Welfare Medicine*. The language of debate may well change again, and the research questions will reflect the predilections and experiences of that present. I hope these two books will be read with interest into the future, both for their materials and themes, and as a window into their times; and that they will provoke thought and stimulate original research by others.

The broad questions with which we began remain for exploration by younger scholars. Why do we have the patterns of organization, the health benefits, and the problems that we do? Why have we not been able or willing to design financing and organizational systems to bring the uncontroversial benefits of medicine efficiently to all members of the population, whether through government, the private sector, or a public-private mix? Why is there unease on both sides of the Atlantic about how much medical care, and of what quality, should be accessible to all members of the population? Given the very different cultural histories of each health system—a clear message of these books—how far are the systems actually converging? Which services are best subsidized by government, and why? What are the best ways to stimulate private sector initiative and meet consumer preferences? How much tax money should be allocated to health care in light of competing social goods, such as national defense, public education, or controlling the overall rate of taxation? And on what grounds do we judge any national system a success or a failure?

Rosemary A. Stevens
Philadelphia, 2002

NOTES

1. A primary characteristic of the U.S. health care system, then as now, is the multiplicity of ways in which the federal government funds and otherwise affects health services. One ramification of this has been to avoid strong central control; another has been to disguise the extent of government involvement. The latest figures show 10 percent of the U.S. population covered by Medicaid in 1999, 11 percent by Medicare, 64 percent by private health insurance (typically via place of employment), and 16 percent uninsured. Medicaid, with its 40 million enrollees, is now a larger program in terms of costs than Medicare. Medicaid is also the single largest source of federal funds flowing to the states. For state data see Kaiser Family Foundation, State Health Facts Online. www.statehealthfacts.kff.org. For general information on Medicaid see Kaiser Commission on Medicaid and the Uninsured, www.kff.org, as well as ongoing work by the Urban Institute, www.urban.org and the Commonwealth Fund, www.cmwf.org.

Official statistics generally credit government expenses as representing 45 percent of all health expenditures in the United States. However, these figures include government employees, whose health insurance is purchased in the private sector, under the heading of private rather than public expenditures. If included as public expenses instead, actual government expenditures rise to about 60 percent in the United States (Daniel M. Fox, Milbank Memorial Fund, personal communication). Better comparative statistics, based on common definitions, are needed for more precise cross-national analysis of the relative weight of government spending across different nations.

2. The useful term "health care state" has come into currency as a term to describe the contributions and the effects of public mechanisms to subsidize, provide, and regulate health services—in part as a successor term for the outdated term "welfare state" as applied to health care. See Michael Moran, *Governing the Health Care State: A Comparative Study of the United Kingdom, the United States and Germany* (Manchester and New York: Manchester University Press, 1999); Richard Freeman, *The Politics of Health in Europe* (Manchester and New York: Manchester University Press, 2000); European University Institute, European Forum, Centre for Advanced Studies, Conference, Opening Statement by the organizers, Maurizio Ferrera, Anna Guillen, and August Osterle, *Beyond the Health Care State: Institutional Innovations and New Priorities in Access, Coverage and Provision of Health Services,* Florence, Italy, February 20-27, 1999, www.iue.it, accessed March 9, 2002.

3. Charles Webster, *The National Health Service: A Political History* (Oxford and New York: Oxford University Press, 1998), 140.

4. Stephen Gillam, "Perpetual Evolution: A Stocktake," in *What Has New Labour Done for Primary Care? A Balance Sheet*, ed. Stephen Gillam (London: King's Fund, 2001), 1-29.

5. James C. Robinson, *The Corporate Practice of Medicine: Competition and Innovation in Health Care* (Berkeley: University of California Press, 1999), xii. A widely used term reflecting the often-perceived turbulence of health care as a negative movement is "destabilization." See Eli Ginzberg, "The Destabilization of Health Care," *New England Journal of Medicine* 315 (1986):757-61.

6. *Only Dissect: Rudolf Klein on Politics and Society,* ed. Patricia Day (Cambridge: Blackwell, 1996):319.

7. Mark A. Peterson, "Editor's Note," *Health Politics and Policy in a Federal System,* special edition of *Journal of Health Politics, Policy and Law* 26 (2001):1221.

8. See Harry F. Dowling, *City Hospitals: The Undercare of the Underprivileged* (Cambridge: Harvard University Press, 1982); Charles Brecher and Sheila Spiezo, *Privatization and Public Hospitals* (New York: Twentieth Century Fund, 1995); and Sandra Opdycke, *No One Was Turned Away: The Role of Public Hospitals in New York City Since 1900* (New York: Oxford University Press, 2000).

9. *Statutory History of the United States: Income Security,* ed. Robert B. Stevens (New York: Chelsea House Publishers in association with McGraw Hill, 1970).

10. I deal with these themes in *American Medicine and the Public Interest* (New Haven: Yale University Press, 1971; reissued with a new introduction, Berkeley: University of California Press, 1998).

11. Richard Magraw, book review, *Annals of Internal Medicine* 66 (1967):451.

12. I pay too little attention to these changes in the book, perhaps being too close to them at the time. For a more integrated (science/practice/organization) approach, see Irvine Loudon, John Horder, and Charles Webster, *General Practice Under the National Health Service, 1948-1997* (Oxford: Oxford University Press, 1998). On the relationship between health policy and the shift to chronic conditions in the United States, see Daniel M. Fox, *Power and Illness: The Failure and Future of American Health Policy* (Berkeley: University of California Press, 1993).

13. Albert R. Jonsen, book review, *Journal of Medicine and Philosophy* 1 (1976):283. The references are to John Rawls, *A Theory of Justice* (Cambridge: Belknap Press of Harvard University Press, 1971) and Robert Nozick, *Anarchy, State and Utopia* (New York: Basic Books, 1974).

14. Quoted by George Rosen, "Michael M. Davis (November 19, 1879-August 19, 1971): Pioneer in Medical Care," editorial, *American Journal of Public Health* 62 (1972):322.

15. Sara Rosenbaum, "Medicaid," *New England Journal of Medicine* 346 (February 21, 2002), 635-640.

16. ibid., 635.

17. Rosemary Stevens, *In Sickness and in Wealth: American Hospitals in the Twentieth Century* (New York: Basic Books, 1989; reissued with a new introduction, Baltimore: Johns Hopkins University Press, 1999).

18. This includes a notable exchange between Philip Hammond, M.P. and Alan Milburn, the Secretary of State for Health, during debate on the Health and Social Care Bill in the House of Commons. Hammond criticized the "hands-on control" and "micro-management" of the NHS and asked if the Secretary of State "can point to a single successful productive enterprise on this scale...organized on a centralized basis..." Milburn replies, "The Chinese army." Hammond was not impressed. House of Commons Hansard Debates for 10 Jan 2001 (pts 29-30). www.parliament.the-stationery-office.co.uk/pa/cm200001/cmhansard/, accessed March 11, 2002.

19. Over time, Medicaid has diverged from its ties to cash assistance, allowing more individuals to be included for health benefits alone. In 1996 Medicaid was formally "delinked" from cash assistance. The descriptive rhetoric

also changed. The federal-state programs formally known as Aid to Families with Dependent Children (AFDC) were renamed Temporary Aid for Needy Families (TANF). In 1998, of the almost 21 million children enrolled in Medicaid, about 8 million were "welfare related" and 13 million "poverty related" or "other." Congress enacted the State Children's Health Insurance Program (CHIP) under the Balanced Budget Act of 1997. The new program was designed to pay the costs of care for children under nineteen years of age who are not eligible for Medicaid and whose family incomes fall below 200 percent of the poverty line. Kaiser Commission on Medicaid and the Uninsured, "Health Coverage for Low Income Children," March 2001. www.kff.org, accessed December 20, 2001.

Acknowledgments

Clearly a book such as this has been dependent on the generosity and goodwill of many persons.

First, we must thank our many students at the Yale Law School, the Yale Medical School, and Yale College. They have not only generated much of the data on which we have relied but, more importantly, they have forced us to refine and rethink our ideas about health-care policy in general and Medicaid in particular. We have indicated in footnotes our reliance on their papers, but we appreciate that this recognition is an inadequate token of appreciation for the excitement and insights these students have brought to the subject. We must also thank especially Charles Bryan, B.A. Virginia 1970, Yale Law School Class of 1974, who worked as our research assistant during the summer of 1972. His humor and diligence were of inestimable value.

Second, we are deeply in debt to many officials in both federal and state government. At the National Center for Health Services Research and Development, we must thank Sherman Williams, Jere Wysong, David Fitch, and Winston Dean for encouraging us to turn our earlier work into a book. The staff of the Medical Services Administration could not have been more encouraging and helpful, although they frequently disagreed with us vigorously; none of the opinions offered in this volume should be attributed to them. We should also like to include the various officials in state government who have helped us, especially those in California, Connecticut, Illinois, Massachusetts, New York, Rhode Island, Vermont, and Virginia. Providers and recipients in these states were also generous in giving information and opinions.

Third, we should like to thank various colleagues and friends for their generosity in reading the manuscript. In particular, we are grateful to Sam Bloom at New York University, David Mechanic at Wisconsin, Lee Albert and Anne-Marie Foltz at Yale, Herbert Kaufman at the Brookings Institution, and Richard Danzig and Lawrence Friedman at the Stanford Law School. They have selflessly read large parts of this manuscript and made innumerable helpful comments. If we have failed to benefit the fault is ours, not theirs.

Finally, we must thank those who made the project possible financially. The original work on Medicaid was undertaken by the first author under a grant from the Russell Sage Foundation to study the development of social policies in the 89th and 90th Congresses. The second author's early work was supported by grant number HS-00374 from the National Center for Health Services Research and Development.[1] We built on this work in a series of seminars we offered in "Medical Care and the Law" and "Health Care Policy." Support for these seminars has come from the Ford Foundation Urban Studies Grant to the Yale Law School and the Health Services Research Center of the Institution for Social and Policy Studies at Yale. We were able to bring our work up to date, primarily during the summer of 1972, with funds provided by the National Center for Health Services Research and Development.[2] Funds for source checking and final research were provided by the Yale Law School out of the Commonwealth Fund's grant for Law, Science and Medicine.

For typing innumerable drafts of this book we should like to thank Stephanie Remiszewski and Marcia Richardson. They were both superb in their efforts. For the gruelling job of checking our footnotes and sources we willingly thank Thomas Fitzpatrick, B.A. Yale, 1973, and Robert Mann, J.D. Yale, 1973; and in connection with this chore we should especially like to thank the staff of the Government Documents room at Yale. Finally we must thank Linda Mattison for her editorial assistance.

As this is the first time either of us has dedicated a book, we should perhaps explain that because we have managed to produce a book together we think it is appropriate to thank our third grader and our first grader for letting us get on with our "homework."

Robert Stevens
Rosemary Stevens

Green River, Vermont
September 1, 1973

NOTES

1. This earlier research appears in Rosemary Stevens and Robert Stevens, "Medicaid: Anatomy of a Dilemma," *Law and Contemporary Problems*, Spring 1970, p. 348.

2. In connection with these funds, we have been asked to include the following acknowledgment:

Part of the research on which this volume is based was performed under Contract No. HSM–110–72–265 with the National Center for Health Services Research and Development, Department of Health, Education and Welfare. The work was commissioned as part of the National Center's program of stimulating independent studies of different areas of health care policies. It should be emphasized, however, that the opinions, conclusions and recommendations expressed in this volume are those of the authors.

Prologue

We undertook this study for three major reasons. First, Medicaid is a vital program. During Fiscal Year 1973 it provided care for twenty-three million Americans, more than one tenth of the population. Second, Medicaid is a huge program. During that same period, it consumed over nine billion dollars of public funds, some five billion coming from federal revenues. Third, Medicaid is in many ways the most direct involvement with the provision of medical care undertaken by either the federal government or the states. If the future does hold massive new participation by the government in the field of health, the experience of Medicaid could well determine its shape. Despite Medicaid's coverage, its cost, and its implications, however, it has not been studied in depth at any level or in any systematic way. It therefore offers a near-perfect opportunity to analyze the governmental role in shaping medical-care policy through the detailed study of one particular program.

The massive program of welfare medical care that is Medicaid was designed to bring substantial federal subsidies to states to provide comprehensive health services to needy persons, "needy" being defined by each state. Implementation diluted the original goals; nevertheless, the scope of the program is impressive. Services are provided to welfare recipients (the so-called "categorically needy") and also, in a number of states, to other specified low-income persons (the "medically needy"). The services are made available through private and public hospitals, by profit-making and nonprofit nursing homes, by private physicians, and by a host of other professionals and health agencies, which are then reimbursed for these services by the state. Medicaid, together with its sister program Medicare (which provides specified health-insurance benefits for the elderly), is a public program whose success relies on cooperation from the private sector. It is a classic example of the "public-private mix." By also involving different levels of government, Medicaid is also perhaps the most "pluralistic" of health programs at a time when pluralism has become a password in medical-care politics. Medicaid's problems thus have far more than a parochial significance. From its successes and failures lessons are to be learned for the future development of the American health system.

In some ways, the Medicaid program has been phenomenally successful. It now exists in every state except Arizona and, at some time or other, it may have helped every sixth American. Yet Medicaid has come under increasing fire from various quarters. Its cost increases, coupled with persistent budget overruns, have focused Congressional attention on rising medical-care prices, on inefficient program management, and on waste and sometimes deceit on the part of both medical-care providers and recipients. In eight short years, Medicaid has moved from a glittering symbol of the "Great Society" to a problem to be tackled by the "New Federalism." The earlier optimism that poverty could be overcome through federal initiative has been followed by a period of legislative concern, fiscal retrenchment, and general skepticism.

Why is this? Medicaid, as we shall see, represented no entirely new philosophy or administrative approach. Nevertheless, it offered two potentially important new concepts. It contained, first, an important extension of principle in the concept of medical indigence, which before 1965 had been applied only to a limited number of the needy, notably the elderly. Second, the 1965 legislation promised to extend the concept of vendor payments (direct payments from the state to providers of medical care in the private as well as the public sector) to a system much more like that of private insurance. Indeed, there was considerable discussion at the time of Medicaid's passage emphasizing that the poor would receive the same care, from the same sources, as the rich: this was known as bringing Medicaid recipients into the "mainstream" of medicine.

From the beginning, there were to be built-in tensions between the concept of private medicine for the needy implicit in the legislation and the prevailing attitudes and machinery of the welfare system. Moreover, the cash-assistance programs on which Medicaid relied reflected their own problems and social ambivalence. If anything, "welfare" was premised on the assumption, drawn from the Elizabethan poor laws, that the poor are somehow responsible for their own condition. At least from the time that Jefferson claimed that he had never seen a poor man in America, there has been a subtle feeling that it is faintly un-American to be poor. Thus, when contributory social insurance began in 1935, it was widely assumed that public assistance would just "wither away." Although the argument was less clearly articulated in 1965, there was an assumption among many that as Medicare and other programs developed, Medicaid would become less important and perhaps disappear.

This argument that a criterion of success would be that the program would diminish (i.e., that recipients and costs would steadily be reduced) might seem reasonable so long as medical services for the needy are regarded as one fringe benefit for those who already have a low income. Once income levels are raised by getting people back to work, it follows that the health programs too should diminish as recipients move above prevailing means-test levels. But the argument, while appealing to those anxious to reduce the welfare rolls, took no account of the two-way relationship between health and poverty. By 1965, health services had become an expensive, as well as essential, service to the whole population, and large medical bills could impoverish even the most hard-working and prudent members of the population. Sickness was both a cause of poverty and a barrier to getting off welfare, once there. The concept of medical indigency built into Medicaid was supposed to meet the needs of those impoverished because of large medical expenses. Because their number was growing, the concept conflicted with the aim of reducing the welfare population. As the number of welfare recipients rose rapidly after 1965, Medicaid promised to expand into a huge service program. The overwhelming ethic of Medicaid, however, soon became that of the old welfare programs. As costs rose, the cry was for retrenchment.

By building onto a welfare system that was itself under stress, the Medicaid program begged the question of what, indeed, were government goals in welfare or in medicine. Is welfare's justification primarily charity for the needy, getting persons back to work, preventing social unrest, or assuaging the middle-class conscience; or are there other reasons? Undoubtedly, each of these factors plays some part, but the litany of welfare is not yet clearly defined in America; without a generally accepted purpose, there can be no clear commitment through which policies can be transmitted. In Medicaid, the clearest commitments proved to be those of bodies most intimately involved in program operation: state welfare departments administering means tests and state legislatures concerned with cutting program costs. From these forces stemmed a series of practical goals not always the same as those of Congress.

It is easy to find fault from the arrogance of hindsight. It is important to stress, however, that apparently unanticipated consequences of Medicaid could in fact have been foreseen. The lack of specific goals for Medicaid is perhaps its most basic weakness. Similarly, Medicaid's potential impact on the health system was barely discussed in 1965. Yet the attempt to provide free private comprehensive health services to a limited sector of the population, defined either by their welfare category or by their income level, was bound to generate problems in both the health and the welfare systems. At least some of the fiscal and administrative problems were predictable.

The basic welfare decisions of eligibility for the program were also to provoke predictable dilemmas. By concentrating on a limited sector of the population, defined in terms of some concept of "indigence," Medicaid was automatically defined as a program revolving around a means test. This definition carried with it implications not only in terms of public attitudes toward the program (including the attitudes of potential recipients) but also in terms of social equity. If a system provides generous medical services without cost to someone with a given income, and no services to someone equally needy but with an income a dollar above the means-test level, what is the second person to do when he has heavy medical expenses? This so-called notch effect was to be continually vexing. The fact that recipients have normally been allowed to "spend down" to the means test level—i.e., to apply the amount of their medical bills against their income in determining eligibility, thus bringing their income below the means-test level—has meant in effect that Medicaid has encouraged pauperization.

The political problems continue, for even providing "adequate" medical care for the poor may mean that those meeting the means test will have better medical care than at least some of those outside it.[1] Yet this in turn is but the proverbial tip of the iceberg. If the state is to provide medical care for a certain segment of the medically indigent, are these persons to be provided with mainstream and middle-class medicine, or are they consciously to be provided with inferior medicine, or are barriers to be provided to discourage them from using such services? In other words, is the doctrine of "less eligibility," which underlay the provision of workhouses and poor farms in the nineteenth century, to underlie the provision of medical care in the twentieth?

Legislation rarely embodies a single doctrine. But in the health field there is a mass of conflicting policies. This situation raises peculiarly complex difficulties of translating rhetoric into reality. In terms of what the welfare state means in America, the rhetoric of "equality" and "democracy" may seem strangely at odds with the inadequate social services frequently provided. The fact that everyone has access to a high school education—even if the quality of that education may vary with the tax base of the school board—and the fact that at least a third of the nation's youth goes on to college are in strange contrast to some of the failings in other areas of the Welfare State—income security, housing, and health. Why should free education rarely be subjected to a means test, yet a means test lie at the root of programs of medical care? Why should it be the norm for government to provide educational services and innovative to suggest that recipients be given vouchers to purchase their own, while the norm for government assistance in medical care is to force recipients to seek their (reimbursed) care in the private sector, and the idea that government should provide the actual services is still regarded as dangerously radical? Such questions were skimmed over in Congressional debates in favor of a palatably vague notion of medical indigence that Medicaid brought into the welfare system. In contrast, Medicare was joined to a Social Security program which, while also a form of welfare, has avoided a welfare stigma. Meanwhile, the federal role in health remains largely undefined.

As we move through the progression of cost increases, cost controls, professional resistance, cost cutbacks, calls for federalization of the program and for the instituting of national health insurance, there are constant reminders of the disseminated power structure implicit in the initial legislation. At the federal level, Medicaid (together with Medicare) has highlighted the inevitable tensions between the legislature and the executive, especially between HEW on the one hand and the House Ways and Means Committee and the Senate Finance Committee on the other. Who makes decisions in these competing centers of power inevitably affects implementation.

At the state level, too, the pressures have been magnified. Economically, the states have been faced with rapidly rising budgets for social-welfare services and the headache of raising appropriate taxes. Politically, in the years covered by the book, both in the governors' mansions and in the state capitols, there has been a move to the political right, accompanied by fiscal retrenchment. At the same time, at the state level the administrative failings in Washington have been magnified fourfold by generally weak administrative departments in the states that attempt to resist pressures from the providers' organizations and from lobbying groups of welfare recipients and poor persons generally. Finally, the judiciary, at both the federal and the state levels, has also had to make basic decisions about eligibility and services, through a series of problems thrown to the courts for solution.

This piecemeal approach to a major social program is, at least in part, the result of a reluctance to admit in 1965 that Medicaid *was* a major social program. As long as Medicaid could be regarded as an extension of what was already in existence, the excuse could be given that administrative changes were unnecessary. The role of the providers is a case in point. So far, in this country, the discussion of the provision of medical care has been largely predicated on the assumption that any federal contribution can be neatly grafted onto the pre-existing private sector. That is the lesser of two evils as far as the providers are concerned. Yet one of the clearest lessons to be learned from Medicaid is that the larger the infusion of federal funds, the greater the demand for federal control; at a certain point this control may take the form of having to restructure the medical-care market.

From other points of view, however, it is amazing how much has been accomplished in Medicaid's few years, in terms of services provided, influences on the health care system, and changing political attitudes toward a stronger governmental role in health care provision. In most states, for those on Medicaid the provision of care is better than it was before 1965.

At least in established health facilities—OEO health centers and the like having a special status—there is now probably less of a gap between the services provided for the poor and the nonpoor than there was before. Even in the most conventional hospital, the notion of the "welfare patient" is less rampant. There has been an increasing realization that health care has to be approached as a "health service," which takes into account the organization of medical care for the whole population, rather than as an appendage of other social programs, including programs of income maintenance.

The history of Medicaid, then, offers a rich field for inquiring into the problems of medical care and the nature and limitations of public medical services. If a series of actions and consequences could have been foreseen in 1965 but were not, it is reasonable to ask whether we are poised in the 1970s to repeat the same, or at least similar, mistakes. Thus, even if the present program is transitional, the study of Medicaid is vital to current health and welfare debates. It is vital because, as has increasingly become clear, the program will not disappear overnight and national health insurance, in its various guises, still has many hurdles to clear. And it is vital, too, because while in so many ways Medicaid is a museum of the defects of a medical care program, it is a remarkably instructive museum for those who must plan for the future.

We have written this book as social historians. It thus begins with an examination of Medicaid's antecedents, moves through the initial legislation (the Social Security Amendments of 1965) to its implementation in the states and at the local level,[2] and concludes by analyzing the series of modifications that have marked the program in the last few years. While generous references are made to the activities in the various states—notably in New York and California, whose programs have dominated Medicaid—our intention was not to write case histories of selected states but to identify the generic themes underlying Medicaid at the federal, state, and local level from the perspectives of its various participants.

Medicaid might well be analyzed as an illustration of general principles or theories of political development.[3] Equally, quantitive studies of selected aspects of the program, and especially its costs and utilization, are sorely needed. These approaches remain for others; indeed, one of our hopes for this book is that it will stimulate further research on Medicaid from both the theoretical and quantitative points of view. We chose the historical method for ourselves in the hope of providing a comprehensive understanding of how and why Medicaid developed, its major characteristics, its strengths, its tensions, and its weaknesses. Although we make no claim to having developed some new value-free method of studying social issues, we have approached the study of social policy as scholars concerned with social problems, not as advocates for change or polemicists anxious to score debating points. Our aim has been to make it possible for our readers—whether they be scholars, civil servants, lawyers, social workers, welfare recipients, or politicians—to develop informed responses to the program's dilemmas and to be able to view other medical-care programs in perspective.

NOTES

1. The problem is not new. In England in 1850, the Poor Law Commissioners in London refused to approve the diet proposed by the Board of Guardians of the Bradfield Workhouse on the grounds that it was inadequate. The local Board replied that their scale gave the paupers more to eat than laborers outside could buy for their families out of their wages. Cited, E. L. Woodward, *The Age of Reform, 1815–1870* (Oxford, 1938), p. 435.

2. For an excellent study of another federal–state program and confirmation of the absence of a literature on implementation, see Jeffrey L. Pressman and Aaron Wildavsky, *Implementation: How great expectations in Washington are Dashed in Oakland; or, Why It's amazing that Federal Programs work at all: This Being a Saga of the Economic Development Administration as told by Two Sympathetic Observers who seek to build Morals on a Foundation of Ruined hopes* (Berkeley, 1973).

3. In many senses, for instance, our study reinforces the Lindblom thesis concerning the development of solutions to social policy problems. Historic comprehensive solutions are rarely available; means and ends are invariably interwoven; and solutions emerge rather than being created. In this sense Title XIX is an example of "disjointed incrementalism." See especially D. Braybrooke and C. E. Lindblom, *A Strategy of Decision* (New York, 1963).

For a useful attempt to analyze Medicaid in terms of different theories of administrative decision-making, see John T. Gentry and Morris Schaefer, "The Impact of State and Federal Policy Planning Decisions on the Implementation and Functional Adequacy of Title XIX Health Care Programs," *Medical Care*, vol. 7, 1969, p. 92.

List of Acronyms

AALL	American Association for Labor Legislation
AB	Aid to the Blind
ADC	Aid to Dependent Children
AFDC	Aid to Families with Dependent Children
AFDC–UP	Aid to Families with Dependent Children—Unemployed Parent
AFL–CIO	American Federation of Labor–Congress of Industrial Organizations
AMA	American Medical Association
APTD	Aid to the Permanently and Totally Disabled
CMA	California Medical Association
ECF	Extended Care Facility
EPSDT	Early and Periodic Screening, Diagnosis, and Treatment
FAP	Family Assistance Plan
FERA	Federal Emergency Relief Administration
FHIP	Family Health Insurance Program
GA	General Assistance
HASP	Hospital Admission and Surveillance Program [Illinois]
HEW	Department of Health, Education and Welfare
HIP	Health Insurance Plan [of Greater New York]
HMO	Health Maintenance Organization
ICF	Intermediate Care Facility
ILGWU	International Ladies' Garment Workers' Union
MAA	Medical Assistance to the Aged
MAAC	Medical Assistance Advisory Council
MSA	Medical Services Administration
OAA	Old-Age Assistance
OAI	Old-Age Insurance
OASDI	Old-Age, Survivors, and Disability Insurance
OASHDI	Old-Age, Survivors, Health, and Disability Insurance
OASI	Old Age and Survivors Insurance
OEO	Office of Economic Opportunity
OMB	Office of Management and Budget
PREP	Program Review and Evaluation Project
PSRO	Professional Standards Review Organization
SNF	Skilled Nursing Facility
SRS	Social and Rehabilitation Service
SSA	Social Security Administration
SSI	Supplementary Security Income

Welfare Medicine in America

A CASE STUDY OF MEDICAID

PART I

The Coming of Medicaid

INTRODUCTION

Like other social-welfare programs in America, which often represent a reluctant and veiled acceptance of past problems rather than any clean sweep of idealism, Medicaid can be fully understood only in its historical context. Its structure, administration, and in large part its degree of success and failure were predetermined by existing patterns of public assistance. Its role, particularly its growing political importance, has been emphasized by the failure of Congress to develop any systematic organization of health services outside the public-assistance system. Part I of this book begins the process of unraveling this structure and role.

The provision of medical care to the poor has long been a recognized part of the American system of public relief. Concern over the equitable provision of health services is, however, a twentieth-century phenomenon, born of the great strides in medical science made in the late nineteenth century and accelerating, as they have, to the present. The manifestations of this latter phenomenon have been on the one hand a series of proposals (as yet not enacted) for government-sponsored health insurance covering the whole working population, and on the other an accretion of special programs designed to attack particular deficiencies in the health-care system or in health-care provision.

The question of how and to whom government health services should be provided has woven through debate after debate. Out of the welfare system eventually came the system of federally subsidized vendor payments in 1950, which in turn generated the Kerr-Mills legislation, with its bold new concept of "medical indigence," and ultimately Medicaid. Meanwhile, out of a social insurance tradition dating back to nineteenth-century European income-protection schemes for the working population, have come a series of proposals for national health insurance, of which one—

Medicare—has been implemented, though effectively limited to the elderly. Whether the government should guarantee health care to the poor or to the whole population remains to this day an open question.

The long debates have, however, left important legacies. Both administratively and conceptually, the American welfare state remains in the shadow of Depression legislation. Indeed, the great Social Security Act of 1935 forms the basis of today's most important programs of cash assistance, social insurance, and health-care provision. The Social Security Act of 1935 provided a watershed for both the welfare and the health-care movements, in terms of not only what the Act included but also what it left out.[1] Out of this Act came the present structures of public assistance, modified and added to in subsequent years. The most notable legacy of the legislation, as far as welfare was concerned, was the so-called categorical structure of federally supported public assistance, divided into separate programs for the aged, the blind, dependent children, and, later, the disabled. These categories, which were seriously eroded for the first time by the Social Security Amendments of 1972, have left indelible marks on public assistance. Perhaps the most obvious has been the prevailing climate of restrictionism. To get on the federally supported public-assistance dole, one had to wear the appropriate label. To be just "poor" was not sufficient.

At the same time, in the failure to include a health insurance program for the whole population in the 1935 legislation, a major opportunity to institutionalize national health insurance as an essential part of the American welfare state was lost. Health benefits did not become a cherished right, as they have in most European countries or as educational benefits have in the United States. Although old-age social security, provided under the 1935 Social Security Act, was equally "socialistic," it took on a patina of eminent social respectability; indeed, the pension elements of social security have become part of the American way of life.[2] The dichotomy has continued, reflected in the contrasting attitudes toward Medicare (social insurance) and Medicaid (public assistance), although both were introduced by the Social Security Act of 1965.

With that introduction, we now look in more detail—but still in outline—at the rise of public assistance, the social insurance movement, and government interest in medical care (Chapter 1). We then examine, in more detail, the federal role in health between 1935 and the Kerr-Mills legislation in 1960 (Chapter 2). We follow this with a study of the passage of Medicare and Medicaid (Chapter 3). The final chapter in Part I (Chapter 4) provides a detailed analysis of Medicaid.[3]

NOTES

1. For general background on the development of the Social Security Act, see Roy Lubove, *The Struggle for Social Security 1900–1935* (Cambridge, Mass.,

1968); Edwin E. Witte, *The Development of the Social Security Act: A Memorandum on the history of the Committee on Economic Security and drafting and legislative history of the Social Security Act* (Madison, Wis., 1962); Arthur J. Altmeyer, *The Formative Years of Social Security* (Madison, Wis., 1966).

2. For an analysis of the misleading nature of the "insurance" aspects of Social Security, see Joseph A. Pechman, Murray J. Aaron, and Michael K. Taussig, *Social Security: Perspective for Reform* (Washington, 1968).

3. For those concerned primarily with the politics of Medicaid, this technical chapter may be read "lightly."

1

Competing Welfare Philosophies and the Provision of Medical Care

The Welfare Heritage

Before 1935, welfare provisions were entirely the responsibility of individual localities and states. Arrangements for medical care for those on assistance were made on an *ad hoc*, decentralized, and often erratic basis, following the existing patterns of cash relief. There were substantial variations in coverage and eligibility from place to place and from state to state. Two broad patterns of relief were, however, evident by the early 1930s, based on assumptions that the poor were parasites (to be deplored) or unfortunates (to be succored). On the one hand were the old arrangements for general assistance to paupers through indoor or outdoor relief dating to Colonial times and with roots in the Elizabethan Poor Law. Such assistance was typically given grudgingly by the towns and counties, and there continued to be more than vestiges of the attitude that pauperism was a form of social disease and degeneracy: the poor were "a population which floats between the alms houses, the jail and the slums."[1] In this context the proper role of assistance was seen to be to provide minimal help in unattractive circumstances, lest those on relief corrupt both themselves and ultimately other members of society.

The most obvious examples of the survival of the Elizabethan poor laws were in the indoor (i.e., workhouse) form of relief that remained an integral part of "income security" in America until the 1930s. In 1926, Harry Evans' book on the poor farms caused a minor stir: in virtually every state they were for the flotsam of society who could not be incarcerated in prison because they had committed no crime. They were also used as a residual depository for the aged, the sick, and the mentally retarded despite the fact that in most states institutions like asylums had been developed in the nineteenth century.[2] Only in the most progressive states were there public hospitals or adequate resources to cope with paupers in private or so-called charitable hospitals or homes.

Most communities also made some use of outdoor relief—cash handouts —but they attracted the same taint as indoor relief. Nevertheless, born of the recognition that there were identifiable groups of persons who could not be labeled social deviates or paupers by choice, a number of special assistance programs slowly grew up during the early twentieth century, geared to provide help to "deserving" individuals. Impoverished old people, underfed children, and the unemployable blind could scarcely be blamed for their condition nor envied for being the recipients of relief. For such groups there developed a more sophisticated form of outdoor relief. Thus, for the aged who had suddenly fallen on hard times, a number of states developed noncontributory old-age assistance "pension" programs. In 1915, Arizona passed the first state law designed to abolish almshouses and establish an old-age cash assistance program. While this legislation was ultimately declared unconstitutional by the courts, other states followed with their own old-age assistance provisions. By the end of 1934, 28 states and two territories had passed old-age assistance laws.[3]

Dependent children provided another special group. The early "mothers' pension" laws were designed—on a principle similar to that of the old-age assistance program—to keep children on relief in their own families rather than to send them to institutions. Geared to the needs of widows, rather than deserted wives or unmarried mothers, the idea spread across the country after 1911, the year statewide legislation appeared in Illinois. The Child-Saving Movement that had pressed for mothers' pensions was also instrumental in the establishment of the first federal office concerned with a specific age group: the Children's Bureau, created in 1912. The Bureau was to be a model for the later development of various welfare and Social Security programs, serving as one of the bases for the Federal Security Administration, which ultimately became the Department of Health, Education, and Welfare. As with old-age assistance, however, programs of direct financial aid to dependent children were undertaken until 1935 without federal assistance. By 1934 all states except Alabama, Georgia, and South Carolina provided some form of welfare aid to mothers of dependent children, but again the programs were rudimentary, while varying enormously even within the states. In most parts of the country, responsibility was vested at the county level; in New England it was vested in the towns and cities. Such programs thus added to the existing complexity of welfare programs and reinforced the idea of local responsibility for relief.

The third and final group of persons singled out for special assistance was the blind. Wisconsin enacted the first such program in 1907; by 1935, 27 states made some arrangements for providing cash payments to the blind. In some cases, counties were authorized to pay blind allowances from general county funds. In other cases specific state taxes were assigned for the purpose. In Arkansas, for example, aid to the blind was funded by a tax on billboard and pool rooms, in Wyoming by taxes on liquor. Such redistribution of wealth from a less moral to a more deserving cause was reflected in the conditions for receipt of aid. Recipients in ten states were not allowed to be professional beggars; in Missouri they had to accept training when offered; and in New York they were not allowed to retain their assistance if they married a blind or partially blind person.[4]

These early categorical programs are important because the divisions were carried over into the Social Security Act of 1935, to become—with the addition of a further category for the totally and permanently disabled in 1950—the framework on which Medicaid was drafted. But also carried over to the present were some of the older philosophies of public relief.

After 1929, it might have been expected that the widespread experience of poverty by the middle class during the worst of the Depression years would have caused a major shift in social attitudes toward the poor. In some states in 1933, 40 percent of the population was on relief. Existing programs of outdoor (or cash assistance) relief broke down under the onslaught. The Federal Emergency Relief Administration (FERA), established in 1933, virtually took over outdoor relief operations in the states and for the first time established a major federal responsibility for income maintenance. Yet FERA, with its potential for a direct continuing federal role in providing relief for all types of poverty, was not to survive the Depression. With the advent of World War II came full employment, and those employed were often only too happy to breathe a sigh of relief and shrug off poverty as a feature of the past and a matter of insignificance. The world was once again divided into "them" and "us."

The Social Security Act of 1935 was, however, extremely important in affecting these patterns in various respects. Indeed, it represents the major landmark to this date in American social-welfare legislation. From cradle to grave, deserving individuals would henceforth have some government protection against the ravages of time and the ills of misfortune. However limited the benefits, the vision was monumental. In his now famous Presidential message of June 8, 1934, underlining his own support of social security legislation, President Roosevelt claimed, as a purpose of his Administration, "the ultimate objective of making it possible for American families to live as Americans should."[5] Income protection was a major part of this goal.

The general tone of the social security debates, therefore, was one of providing for those made dependent through no fault of their own and, more generally, for eliminating destitution as a factor that in turn could lead to social unrest and to disturbances in the general economic system. Humanitarian, political, and economic principles were thus involved, with the last two at least as important as the first. Such principles continue to mark the American social-welfare system. Indeed, a major legacy of the Social Security Act was the acceptance of categories of "deserving" recipients: the elderly, dependent widow(er)s, children (and their caretakers), the blind, the disabled, and those unable to find work.

Two threads of social philosophy were, however, responsible for two very different emphases for the actual programs for the deserving poor included in the Social Security legislation. The first was a growing fascination with the principles of social insurance to protect the working population from unexpected calamities (notably, disablement at work and unemployment) and to provide a guaranteed pension. The second was a strong commitment, both in Congress and in the states, to states' rights in the provision of public assistance. Thus the FERA program was seen not as the beginning of a federal take-over of welfare, but as a necessary means of shoring up programs in the states.[6] Local responsibility for public assistance had become ingrained. In the meantime, however, a strong federal role in the provision of income maintenance programs through social insurance was becoming an integral part of the philosophy of the New Deal.[7] With the optimism that accompanies new "solutions" to major problems, there was an expectation that social security and unemployment insurance would ultimately monopolize income security and that public assistance would "wither away." Poverty would therefore be defeated.

The Social Insurance Tradition

While public assistance was born of a grudging paternalism, social insurance was in large part the product of enlightened capitalism. Emerging in Europe, the movement had four primary emphases: workmen's compensation, health insurance, contributory old-age pensions and unemployment insurance.

The first and most important was the provision of workmen's compensation. This meant, in effect, employer insurance to compensate workers in the event of industrial accidents. A second European program—not included in the Social Security Act—was health insurance for the working population. (Germany's program had begun as early as 1883.) This program, like workmen's compensation, had both a humanistic and an economic rationale; the sooner he was cured, the sooner the employee was back at work. The third type of program, again geared to the social dependency of workers, was old-age and disability insurance. The fourth type of program was unemployment insurance, providing some cash benefit to the worker who found himself unemployed through no fault of his own. The theory of these programs called for the provision of a trust fund into which contributions by the insured and his employer were paid and out of which specified benefits were paid as an "entitlement" to those eligible. Each was work-related: contributions and benefits depended on an individual's employment status.

As in Europe, workmen's compensation had the major initial appeal in America. The first effective compensation law was that established in 1908 for civil employees of the federal government. Montana was the first state to pass a compulsory act, limited to coal mining, in 1909; but it was held unconstitutional by the courts. In the same year, however, the American Federation of Labor began to support workmen's compensation laws. Manufacturers were also beginning to favor the concept. By 1910 the die was cast. Between 1910 and 1915, 30 states enacted workmen's compensation laws, and by 1920 all but six states had some such legislation.[8]

Workmen's compensation, however, was the only widespread insurance program in operation in this country before the 1930s. The combination of lobbying, publicity, and expertise represented in the American Association for Labor Legislation (AALL), whose membership of about 3000 included academics, lawyers, labor leaders, businessmen, social workers, and representatives from a host of occupations and interest groups, came just too late to catch the Progressive tide. The AALL can justly claim credit for its role in stimulating workmen's compensation laws. Its second plank, the stimulation of health insurance legislation in the states, was to prove less successful.

Health insurance, which became the focus of the AALL's Committee on Social Insurance from 1913 onward, called for the payment of regular sums of money by the working population in return for the provision of specified benefits when they were sick. In England, as the result of legislation passed in 1911, workers who earned less than a specified amount (although not their dependents) were entitled to the services of general medical practitioners and related care. There was little doubt that the underlying philosophy of the English program was to get the worker back on the job and (more generally) to reduce the cost to society of time lost through sickness.[9]

Under the leadership of AALL and with the support of the American Medical Association, official investigation of health insurance was organized in eight states between 1915 and 1918; and a standard health insurance bill was introduced in fifteen states in 1917.[10] The American Medical Association, which was later to prove a stalwart enemy of the compulsory health insurance concept, produced reports initially favorable in tone. For example, its Committee on Social Insurance noted in 1916 that the new British system had "unquestionably improved the condition of the working classes which have come under the law."[11]

But health insurance, being less directly related to the working situation, had less appeal to employers and employees alike than did workmen's compensation. Employers perhaps saw the thin end of a wedge of paternalistic legislation under which they would eventually be held responsible for contributing to large social-welfare programs for their employees. On the other hand, the employees were chary of compulsory reductions in their salaries for services they might not need or want. Meanwhile, private medical practitioners began to express opposition to a system that would inevitably lead to some controls over the way they practiced medicine, if only in the form of additional paperwork and some supervision of fees. World War I gave opponents of health insurance further opportunity to attack such proposals as "German" and thus "un-American"; after the war the American Medical Association was able to organize a powerful opposition lobby. An increasing number of articles against health insurance appeared in the medical press, and finally an AMA resolution of 1920 expressed a position of formal opposition—not yet abandoned—against such government intervention.[12] With respect to national health insurance, therefore, the United States did not follow the European experience.

The third plank of European social insurance, contributory old-age pensions, was also largely ignored in America until the 1930s. Indeed, *any* pension, public or private, was the exception rather than the rule. By 1932, for instance, only 15 percent of American workers were covered by private programs for their old age.[13] But the pension aspect of social insurance was to become the primary focus of the 1935 legislation and to remain by far the most obvious aspect of the social security system. The term *social security* has become virtually a synonym for contributory pensions.

One more aspect of social insurance was unemployment compensation, which had also developed in England and other European countries. Sparked by the rising unemployment rate in the early years of the Depression, the ranks of the unemployed became a major poverty category whose needs were rather different from the existing categories of public assistance. Desiring and able to be economically independent, they were unlike the elderly, the dependent children, or the blind. In need through no fault of their own, they were also largely free of the social taint still lingering over those traditionally regarded as "paupers." But unemployment compensation insurance appeared to make no sense in the bountiful America of the twenties, and it was not until 1932 that Wisconsin passed an unemployment insurance law. Unemployment compensation was to remain primarily a state responsibility, although given a federal framework and tax base under the 1935 Social Security Act. By 1937, federal tax incentives insured that all the states and territories had such a law.

1935: The Freezing of Theories

The various fragments of programs in operation or under discussion in the early 1920s formed a patchwork of programs and assumptions rather than a unified approach to social welfare. When the Social Security Act was passed in 1935, political attitudes to social welfare were evolving and incomplete.

The approaches to social-insurance schemes were motivated by the massive deprivations of the Depression, but this urgency could not obscure the fact that there was no comprehensive American model for a welfare state. Thus, although there was widespread agreement that some "cradle to grave" income protection was necessary, there was no unified social-welfare tradition on which this philosophy could be based.

Hence, as we have seen, in terms of both policy and administration, there were two important and interwoven questions, to which as yet there were only partial answers. The first was the relationship between social insurance and public assistance; but, when decisions had to be taken, a clear division was drawn between the "working poor" (including the unemployed) and the "poor" (those who needed direct relief). Social insurance was linked with the former. It was not to be confused with pauperism, although to develop political consensus it was argued that poverty (and thus the categorical programs) would just wither away and only social-insurance programs would survive. Benefits made available under social insurance were contributory, work-related, available to beneficiaries as a right, and determined by Congress. Public assistance, on the other hand, was a matter for administrative discretion at the lowest levels of government. Welfare caseworkers determined both eligibility and benefits; there was no direct contribution by individuals for their subsequent benefits (although they might have contributed indirectly through paying state and local taxes), and thus no similar right. In a holdover from earlier days, public assistance continued to carry the welfare stigma, while social insurance did not.

The Social Security Act of 1935 was to include programs encompassing both philosophies. Indeed, through its various titles, it provided an umbrella for divergent views. The Act provided both contributory old-age pensions (OAI) in Title II and federal grants to states for noncontributory old-age assistance (OAA) in Title I. Under Title II the federal government set up a national trust fund and arranged to collect contributions from employers and employees and to pay out benefits. Under Title I, however, the federal government was merely a paymaster. With remarkably few requirements imposed on state participation, it agreed to pay 60 percent of the cost of cash payments to the elderly, up to $50 a month, if the state chose to develop such a program.

This dichotomy was also reflected in other parts of the legislation. A federal-state program of unemployment compensation was approved in Title III. Federal grants were made available to states for public assistance programs for aid to dependent children (ADC) in Title IV and for the blind (AB) in Title X. There were also related programs of federal grants-in-aid for crippled children and maternal and child care. The whole Social Security Act was thus a hodgepodge of different income-maintenance programs. Over-all it set up a tripartite system of income security—social security, public assistance, and unemployment compensation—which has been the basis of American social-welfare programs from that day to this. And apart from the fragmentary children's services, the issue of health care was not faced.

Just as the program approach created one set of potential dichotomies, the level of administration of the programs provided another. The new system of compulsory old-age insurance, financed by contributions from employers and employees, was (and remains) a federal program. Local administration is undertaken through a network of district Social Security offices, responsible to regional offices which are themselves responsible to Washington—or, more strictly, to Baltimore, where the federal Social Security headquarters are now located. Not only federally administered, but increasingly receiving direct infusions of federal funds, social security has gone from strength to strength. Insurance for survivors (OASI) was added to the original OAI in 1939, and disability insurance (OASDI) in 1956. Finally, health insurance for those 65 years old and over was added, through Medicare, in 1965, creating the present OASDHI program. Moreover, by the 1970s virtually all the working population was covered by the program.

While OAI was wholly federally funded and the unemployment compensation program set up under the 1935 legislation relied on a system of federal-state cooperation, the categorical assistance programs were based on a system that today would be classified as federal revenue-sharing. Old-age assistance, aid to dependent children, aid to the blind, and, later, aid to the permanently and totally disabled, were federal-state programs only in the sense that federal grants-in-aid were available on some kind of matching basis; administration was left with the states. Each state was free to decide whether or not to include all or any of the new programs, and for all practical purposes, to set their own eligibility levels and entitlements as they saw fit.

Federal control over these programs was minimal. It was true that each state participating under the federally-assisted programs had to ensure some limited uniform operation statewide, supply some element of state supervision, and have state plans approved at the federal level. The threat of federal control of public assistance, seen by some in the hearings on the 1935 legislation as undermining state's rights, in practice proved hollow. The federal role in public assistance remained one of subsidizing programs in the states rather than providing federal income guarantees or administrative standards. Thus, while the OAI program had national rates for contributions and clearly defined benefits, assistance or welfare programs continued to vary dramatically from state to state, while recipients remained largely at the mercy of caseworkers' discretion.

To add to the confusion, there were, after 1935, two broad types of public-assistance programs in the states, those federally subsidized and those which were not. By the end of 1938 all states and territories had one or more of the federally assisted programs.[14] Not all the states chose, however, to adopt all the possible federal public-assistance programs. Even those that did, normally continued general relief payments for those not eligible for categorical assistance programs—for example, the unemployed who had no entitlement to unemployment benefits or whose benefits had run out. Thus general assistance (GA) continued to be administered by some 10,000 local units, financed entirely from state or local taxes.

Finally, in the Congressional debates over the 1935 legislation another major pattern, of a different variety, was established. In the House, the Ways and Means Committee and, in the Senate, the Finance Committee assumed committee responsibility for social insurance and public assistance. The Social Security provisions had sprung from concern over economic security: the security not only of individuals, but also of the nation. Economic aspects of income redistribution rather than strictly humanitarian aspects were—not surprisingly—to remain paramount in subsequent Congressional debates.

Income Security and Health Care

With the passage of the 1935 legislation, the provision of health services remained in limbo, both for the poor and for the working population. The public-assistance provisions of OAA, ADC, and AB provided that matching federal funds could be used for the medical care of recipients, but only as an allowance included in the monthly cash payment to the recipient, without restricting any part of the payment for this particular purpose. But there were readily apparent drawbacks to this mechanism. There was the probability that individuals on assistance would not earmark the allowance, when it was made, for health care on a month-to-month basis, amassing a reserve for health expenditures. And there were too the unpredictability of medical costs, the large amounts that could be incurred, and the often special medical needs of the poverty population. For instance, a report of the Social Security Board for 1943 noted that about one third of the children accepted for aid under ADC were in need because of the physical or mental incapicity of the parent and that an estimated one fourth of the blind could profit by medical care to improve or conserve vision.[15] These special needs, which were directly related to income security, were clearly not being met under existing assistance programs.

There were two approaches for providing medical care to needy groups. A wide-ranging compulsory health insurance program could encompass at least some of the population who would otherwise be on welfare. This approach demanded, however, a commitment to health insurance for the middle class. The second approach was the provision of tax-supported health services for the needy through a system of entitlements for care in the private health sector or through separate public hospitals and clinics. Such a system was already in operation in some places, including New York and California. Both approaches had been canvassed by the Committee on Economic Security as it worked on the Social Security Bill, but President Roosevelt took the view that the public (and the medical profession) was not yet ready for a major federal incursion into medical care.

The 1935 Act, it is true, did provide for federal grants to states for maternal and child health services and for crippled children, under Title V of the Act; but this program, too, emphasized the prevailing philosophy toward health-care provision. When health services were necessary as an essential part of income protection or national security, they were to be provided under government subsidy and supervision. Health protection thus continued to be subsidiary to income maintenance. Title V, for example, was an essential feature of assistance programs for the nine million children then on relief, designed both to ameliorate their condition and to fight the demoralizing and deteriorating effects of the Depression.[16]

In terms of the health services themselves, the new Title V programs added yet one more layer of publicly provided or subsidized health services to an already complex system of organization. The basic question of welfare medicine was already evident. Could health services for the poor continue to be left to the whims of local government through the direct provision of care or through purchase or charity in the private sector? Or should health services be organized in their own right, as a separate social goal, parallel to old-age insurance or education?

The philosophical differences we have described were having increasingly serious implications for, by the mid 1930s, the dilemmas of modern specialized medicine were posing acute financial and organizational questions. Hospital inpatient and outpatient departments were expanding, and drugs and diagnostic equipment were revolutionizing the potential of medicine to treat and to cure. On the other hand, these added services were accompanied by rising costs. The possibility of ill health became a characteristic American spectre:

> *Tens of millions of families live in dread of sickness. Millions of families that are independent and self-sustaining in respect to the ordinary, routine needs of life sacrifice other essentials of decent living in order to pay for medical service.*[17]

Competing social philosophies were coming face-to-face with the economics of modern medicine.

Three possibilities were available to the poor who were sick. They could avoid medical services, run into debt, or seek charity from public or private agencies. Unfortunately these last services were rarely adequate or available. By 1937 it was evident that the "policy of leaving to localities and states the entire responsibility for providing even nominal public health facilities and services had failed in large measure."[18]

Government and Medical Care

It was of course true that government was already involved in the provision of medical care, on an "essential service" basis. For members of the population whose services were considered socially necessary (in transportation, for example, or defense) government medical services were often provided at a relatively generous level. Similarly, for those considered socially dangerous (violent or contagious) services were also made available. There was thus a patchwork of government services revolving around different definitions of the public weal. Indeed the history of the governmental role in medicine in America—whether at the local, state, or federal level—has consistently emphasized the pluralism and incrementalism of policy-making, itself a function of differently perceived views at different times of the purposes of providing health services.

The United States Public Health Service, for example, now part of the Department of Health, Education, and Welfare, owes its formal birth to the protection of trade: an Act for the Relief of Sick and Disabled Seamen of 1798. This legislation imposed a compulsory tax on the employers of seamen working in the coastal trade along the United States and established a system of hospitals and medical care, of which the present Public Health Service hospitals are the lineal descendants. Even before this, the states had provided hospitals for sick seamen, and Congress had legislated to ensure that at least a minimum of medical supplies were carried aboard each American vessel.[19]

The provision of medical services to groups considered essential to the United States as well as the provision of places for isolation in cases of potentially dangerous epidemics had purposes similar to those of the present vast medical care system for the armed services. The goals were strategic and economic. Health services were secondary to more immediate social priorities—in the case of the merchant marine, that of keeping the shipping industry of the country vital. As the armed forces developed, the emergence of a medical branch maintaining a basic standard of readiness in both army and navy represented a policy very different from any modern concept of welfare.

Other publicly sponsored health services also rested on social expectations and goals in which the health of the individual was secondary, if not incidental. Isolation in special institutions of those with infectious diseases or with other potentially dangerous social traits, including mental illness, led, particularly during the nineteenth century, to the development of institutions whose purpose was as much for the protection of the healthy population as care for the unhealthy. Indeed, the containment of potentially dangerous persons was a natural outgrowth of the police power vesting in the states rather than the federal government. While attitudes toward mental health became more enlightened in the second half of the nineteenth century, the states have continued to play a major role in providing hospitalization for mental illness.[20]

The early programs for protecting the health of the middle-class population could be categorized as "welfare medicine" in the sense that they protected the common weal. But at the same time, they could not be seen as welfare medicine in the sense that the term is now used of the large poverty population. Lacking a system of national health insurance, there was no overriding philosophy of medical care which would encompass the poor with all other social groups. Services to those with contagious and mental diseases were related to other public health services. Medical care services to the armed services and merchant marine and those provided to veterans under a separate federal government system, beginning after World War I, provided free health services to the working population, but only to selected groups; beneficiaries considered these services as work-related entitlements. Those who were "just poor" fell into neither category.

The philosophy of containment of the poor that led to early attitudes toward welfare assistance had its effect, too, on health care for dependent groups. The creation of public hospitals and dispensaries is a notable case in point. By the early 1930s, hospitals for the care of the indigent were in existence in numerous counties and cities, in rural areas the poor farm and the workhouse were not quite dead. By 1935 New York City, for example, owned and operated 23 municipal hospitals, out of a total of 200 hospitals.[21] Such facilities were, however, typically limited to provisions of medical care to the poor.[22] Where they existed, there was thus a two-class system of medical care, a system of private hospitals and physicians for those able to afford them, and a public system—if system is the right word—for the indigent.

It is true that even in the early 1930s some cities and counties were paying for care of the indigent in nongovernmental hospitals on a daily reimbursement rate; but here too the patterns were discriminatory. As a general rule, welfare departments set their fees for paying private hospitals lower than the cost of services provided. Thus the private hospitals, too, were expected to regard welfare patients as charity cases. Charitable organizations were obviously heavily involved in the provision of medical services.

While the extent of care in public facilities increased rapidly in the early 1930s as a result of the Depression, basic integration of services was not achieved. No doubt many middle-class families benefited from the medical services provided by the Federal Emergency Relief Administration in the days of the New Deal, but this temporary merger of the poor and the middle class did not survive the 1935 Social Security Act. Indeed, the separatist pattern for health services paralleled the pattern of income protection which that Act emphasized. With respect to that, there was one system for the poor (public assistance) and another for the working population (Social

Security). Lacking a national health insurance system for both groups, government responsibility for the poor continued to be accepted, while government responsibility for the middle class was avoided or—as in the case of services for veterans—was not regarded as welfare medicine.[23]

NOTES

1. State of Wisconsin, State Board of Control of Charitable, Reformatory and Penal Institutions, *Annual State Conference of Charities and Corrections* (1893), p. 58, quoted by Joel F. Handler, Aaron E. Goodstein, "The Legislative Development of Public Assistance," *Wisconsin Law Review*, 1968, vol. 2, p. 416.

2. Harry C. Evans, *The American Poor Farm and Its Inmates* (Des Moines, 1926); Estelle M. Stewart, "The Cost of American Almshouses," *Bulletin of the U.S. Bureau of Labor Statistics*, No. 386 (U.S. Government Printing Office, 1925). See also David J. Rothman, *The Discovery of the Asylum* (Boston, 1971).

3. U.S. Commission on Economic Security, *Social Security in America: Factual background of the Social Security Act as summarized from staff reports to the Committee on Economic Security* (1937), p. 156 and *passim*.

4. *Ibid.*, pp. 302, 308–09.

5. U.S. Congress, House, *Presidential Message to the Congress Reviewing the Legislative Accomplishments of the Administration and Congress*, House Doc. 397, 73rd Cong., 2nd Sess., June 8, 1934, p. 2.

6. Edwin Witte, *The Development of the Social Security Act* (Madison, Wis., 1962); Gilbert Y. Steiner, *Social Insecurity: The Politics of Welfare* (Chicago, 1966).

7. Interest in social insurance in America was sparked as early as the 1880s by Bismarck's programs in Germany, which were rapidly emulated by other western European countries. But it was not until the establishment of the American Association for Labor Legislation (AALL), founded by a group of economists at the University of Wisconsin in 1906, that there was a serious platform for debate. Between 1906 and 1935 the ideas of social insurance were increasingly discussed and seemed the natural basis for reform during the economic crisis of the 1930s.

8. Herman M. Somers and Anne R. Somers, *Workmens Compensation: Prevention, Insurance and Rehabilitation of Occupational Disability* (New York, 1954), pp. 30–34.

9. For a contemporary analysis, see Haven Emerson, "The Social Cost of Sickness," *American Labor Legislation Review*, vol. 6 (1916), pp. 11–15.

10. See Odin W. Anderson, "Health Insurance in the United States 1910–1920," *Journal of History of Medicine and Allied Sciences*, vol. 5 (1950), pp. 363–96; Arthur J. Viseltear, "Compulsory Health Insurance in California 1915–1918," *ibid.*, vol. 24 (1969) pp. 151–82.

11. "Report of Committee on Social Insurance," *AMA Bulletin*, vol. 11 (1916), pp. 354 and *passim*.

12. See James G. Burrow, *AMA: Voice of American Medicine* (Baltimore, 1963), pp. 141–51 and *passim*.

13. Roy Lubove, *The Struggle for Social Security, 1900–1935* (Cambridge, Mass., 1968), p. 128.

14. Robert Stevens, *Statutory History of the United States: Income Security* (New York, 1970), p. 184.

15. U.S. Federal Security Administration, *Report of the Social Security Board for 1943, Social Security During and After the War,* quoted by Stevens; cf. *supra* note 14, p. 271.

16. U.S. Congress, House, Committee on Ways and Means, *Social Security Bill,* House Rept. No. 615, 74th Congress, 1st Sess., (April 5, 1935). While Title V is not limited by its wording to children on relief, it has been so interpreted.

17. *Social Security in America, supra,* note 3, p. 315.

18. *Ibid.*, p. 335.

19. See Ralph C. Williams, *The United States Public Health Service, 1798–1950* (Washington, 1951).

20. See Franz G. Alexander and Sheldon T. Selesnick, *The History of Psychiatry* (New York, 1966). Of the 494 psychiatric hospitals in the United States in 1970, 324 were government (primarily state) institutions. In addition, of the 108 tuberculosis hospitals, 101 were government-owned, again chiefly by the states; and of 126 hospitals for geriatric services and chronic diseases, many of which are converted infectious disease hospitals, 71 were under government sponsorship. U.S. Department of Health, Education, and Welfare, National Center for Health Statistics, *Health Resources Statistics,* 1971 edition (1972), p. 309.

21. United Hospital Fund of New York, *Report of the Hospital Survey of New York* (New York, 1937), p. 116.

22. Cincinnati and Buffalo were unusual in operating large public general hospitals that were open, under certain circumstances, to all residents. Committee on the Costs of Medical Care, *Medical Care for the American People* (Chicago, 1932; reprinted U.S. Public Health Service, 1970), p. 89.

23. Sar A. Levitan and Karen Cleary, *Old Wars Remain Unfinished: The Veterans Benefits System* (Baltimore, 1973).

2
Public and Political Concern with Medical Care

The Philosophies Congeal

While the Social Security Act of 1935 sidestepped the issue of medical care, the question of national health insurance by no means disappeared. For both the working population and the poor, some type of coverage of medical bills was becoming imperative. High medical bills were already a feature of modern specialized medicine. There was still no direct federal provision for medical care for those on welfare, a situation which continued until 1950. For the middle class, the alternative to a federal program was reliance on the private insurance sector. From 1935 to 1950, however, national health insurance continued to be actively debated.

Private health insurance schemes for the working population grew to fill the vacuum caused by the failure to implement public insurance or to offer a viable alternative. Both Blue Cross (for hospitals) and Blue Shield (for physician bills) were products of the late 1930s. The first fullfledged example of the latter was the California Physicians Service, started in 1939. By the end of 1946 this plan had over 419,000 subscribers.[1] These voluntary, nonprofit insurance plans filled a pressing need, by spreading the risk of large medical bills among the middle-class population. The programs were to expand rapidly in the 1940s, in large part through collective bargaining agreements negotiated after World War II.[2]

By 1940, however, only 9 percent of the civilian population were covered for any kind of hospital benefits through private health insurance. Only 4 percent were covered for surgical benefits and 2 percent for in-hospital medical benefits. Nevertheless the gap was closing. By 1950 these figures had grown dramatically to 51 percent, 36 percent, and 14 percent respectively.[3] So fast was the increase, indeed, that the private health insurance movement was used by some in the late 1940s as evidence that a government-supported health insurance scheme for the whole population was unnecessary.

During the 1940s innumerable bills proposing a government subsidy, organization, or provision of a socially inclusive health insurance system died in Congress.[4] President Truman's plea that every member of the population had a "right to adequate medical care and the opportunity to achieve and enjoy good health," as well as the "right to adequate protection from the economic fears of . . . sickness"[5] was apparently unpersuasive. The Congress was in favor of a new program to subsidize construction of hospitals and related facilities in rural areas, enacted as the Hill-Burton Act in 1946[6]—another government excursion along the same philosophical road of "gap-plugging" with respect to services for the socially deprived. But prepayment of medical costs for all was consistently defeated.

Compulsory government prepayment for health services for the working population fell once more under the stigma of political clichés. Whereas the earliest health insurance movement of 1915–20 had suffered the indignity of the times by being labelled "German," the health insurance movement of the 1940s found itself castigated as "socialized medicine" by the major lobbying groups against it (notably by the American Medical Association). Senator Wagner, one of the major proponents of compulsory national health insurance in the 1940s, insisted in vain that a system of insurance was not socialized medicine. No hospitals would be taken over, no physicians would be employed by the state; the scheme would primarily have guaranteed certain medical services to all those eligible when they needed it. Yet by 1949 the movement toward national health insurance for the whole population was moribund. It was to remain moribund until the 1970s.

If Congress or the states had enacted a comprehensive system of health insurance or service for the whole or a substantial sector of the population, health services and income-maintenance programs would have been long ago divorced in the United States, as they are in the United Kingdom and many other western European countries. Health services would have been made available to the poor and to other beneficiaries as an entitlement quite apart from programs of cash assistance and other supporting services. But the defeat of the Wagner-Murray-Dingell bills of the 1940s, like the earlier exclusion of health insurance from social security legislation, denied that there was a need for a separate system of health protection. Instead, government intervention in health services continued to focus on the health needs of specific groups and continued to be viewed as a subsidiary aspect of income protection.[7]

This philosophy of providing medical services only to those in approved financial need permeated a host of alternative proposals to the Wagner-Murray-Dingell bills. Although the provision of health services to essential personnel (and their dependents) in wartime clearly represented a different social goal from the provision of health services to those on public assistance, the same selective principle operated. There was tacit agreement that publicly organized health services were not necessary to the normal operation of a private enterprise system. Publicly supported medical care would be made available only to those who could not afford to purchase it privately. For those on public assistance (and for veterans in the expanding World War II veterans program, with respect to non-service-connected health conditions), this meant access to free health services only on passing a means test.

By 1950 the proponents of comprehensive national health insurance and those in favor of providing medical care only to those in proven need formed two distinct political camps. The two philosophies were once again in conflict. National health insurance, like other aspects of the contributory social security program, would provide specific benefits as a right for all beneficiaries. The public assistance approach, supported by Senator Robert Taft and others, regarded the need for government-sponsored health care as an aberrant necessity rather than being in any sense generally desirable and saw eligibility and benefits in terms of discretionary actions rather than clear-cut rights.

Senator Taft outlined this latter philosophy in a nutshell, in presenting his own proposed National Health Program of 1949:

> *It has always been assumed in this country that those able to pay for medical care would buy their own medical service, just as under any system, except a socialistic system, they buy their own food, their own housing, their own clothing, and their own automobiles. . . . Undoubtedly, in that system there are gaps, particularly in rural districts and poorer districts in the cities, and we have a very definite interest in trying to fill up those gaps.*[8]

It was in this context that "welfare medicine" was defined. Medical services to the poor were viewed as a reflection of unavoidable—but peripheral—breakdowns in the economic system, rather than as a pointer toward national health service benefits.

Vendor Payments Become the Order of the Day

The philosophical arguments could, however, have been made much more clearly if public assistance benefits had been both broader and more effective. But public assistance, too, was in a state of confusion and disarray. The structure of categorical federal grants to the states for public assistance was one drawback. Even with the inclusion of a new program of Aid to the Permanently and Totally Disabled (APTD) in 1950, under the same formula as OAA and AB, and even with the extension under the same legislation of ADC to cover a needy adult caring for a child, thus translating the program into the current Aid to Families with Dependent Children (AFDC), there were obvious gaps in the categorical system. The child of an unemployed father was not covered (a situation later somewhat alleviated by the development of the Aid to Families with Dependent Children-Unemployed Parent [AFDC-UP] program); the child of a father who had deserted his family was covered under AFDC.[9] The destitute person aged 64 was not covered; the person of 65 was eligible for OAA. Yet categorical assistance became the order of the day. Between 1940 and 1966 the number of individuals receiving cash payments under general assistance declined from four million to less than 600,000, while the number receiving categorical assistance rose from some three million to over seven million persons.[10]

Even within the categories the amounts of assistance were barely adequate. At the time the 1950 Amendments were being discussed the maximum possible federal contribution for OAA and AB was $30 of the first $50 a month spent by the state. For ADC the maximum was $16.50 of the first $27 a month spent by the state for the first child in a family, with a similar percentage of a lesser amount for other children. (States could, of course, choose to pay a sum lower than the federal maximum, thereby receiving less by way of matching funds). There was marked concern in some states over the inadequacy of these arrangements. A referendum in the California state elections of 1949 approved a constitutional amendment guaranteeing every old person a minimum of $75 a month. Similar pressures in Louisiana led to a doubling of old-age assistance grants and a definition of need so liberal that in 1949 as many as 79 percent of the elderly population were receiving relief.[11] But in many other states assistance provisions continued to be minimal. Thus, even where reasonably comprehensive health services were provided by the states and localities to those on assistance, in many states, including New York, there were large numbers of "deserving poor" who were not eligible.

The lack of separate provisions in the 1935 Act for federal cost-sharing of any health care provided to public assistance recipients proved another obvious deficiency in public assistance programs. Federal grants to the states applied only to payments made directly to welfare recipients. Although part of such payment could be earmarked by the state for medical care paid for out of the recipients' pocket, the existence of the relatively low federal ceilings on reimbursement made this possibility unlikely.

A survey of 20 states undertaken by the Bureau of Public Assistance in the late 1940s noted the absence of any provision for medical care as the major problem of public assistance. Even where there were programs, there were problems of administration. Especially where large amounts of money were involved, it was not surprising that the agencies preferred dealing directly with doctors, nurses or clinics rather than attempting to pay for services through the welfare recipient.[12] There was an implied possibility that the recipient might abscond with the funds, or at least use them for other purposes, and serious concern by welfare administrators about the provision of good medical care.

The debates over social security and public assistance roles, purposes, and levels in the 1940s (and after) formed an essential backdrop to concurrent discussions of health insurance. If the basic working population were to rely increasingly (as seemed likely) on private health insurance as a means of paying their medical bills, protection of the marginal worker and the nonworking population could be seen as a vital foundation for the remainder of the population. Indeed, if the poor were receiving adequate medical care from public sources and the main working population were covered by private insurance, there would be no obvious call for setting up compulsory state-run national health insurance. Providing better health services to the poor through available public assistance schemes thus offered a viable political alternative to national health insurance in the 1940s.

The Social Security Amendments of 1950 provided an important watershed in these debates, and a temporary victory for those opposing national health insurance. By expanding the federal public assistance categorical grants-in-aid to include federal cost-sharing with respect to charges for hospital and other medical care paid directly to providers by state welfare agencies, the amendments enlarged the potential scope of welfare medical care. State welfare administrators were mollified because states would henceforth be able to reimburse the providers of care directly—hence the coining of a new term, *vendor payments*. Opponents of national health insurance were also gratified in that—while funding continued to be low—the new arrangement opened the door for expanded health services for the poor and thus lessened the need for more draconian federal measures.

These hopes were not unfounded. With the availability of federal grants-in-aid for vendor payments, the states began providing medical services on a much larger scale. By 1960, medical vendor payments under all public-assistance programs had reached a total of $514 million, well over half of which was for hospital and nursing-home care.[13] These payments were, however, still limited to persons on the welfare rolls, for almost all of whom the states were also recovering part of their cash benefits from the federal government through one of the categorical assistance programs.

At the same time, the implementation of federally-subsidized vendor payments marked the end of serious discussions of comprehensive national health insurance by the Congress for 20 years. Yet it was clear from the beginning of the vendor payments scheme that the level of health care provided was likely to remain inadequate, at least for those receiving old-age pensions and old-age assistance, as well as for certain other groups.

Opinion polls late in the Depression had indicated widespread support for government disbursements to the aged needy; such concern continued in the 1940s.[14] Indeed, as already noted, some states were making assistance payments substantially above federally subsidized levels. Yet health needs and income needs could not be separated. The provision of medical care to the elderly was an essential part of their income protection; the aged, more than any other categorical group, were likely to fall sick, need hospitalization and nursing-home care, and incur major, long-term medical expenses without concomitant earning powers. But besides having increasingly evident medical needs—and medical bills—the elderly were becoming a potent force in American politics. In Massachusetts, for example, the demands of the old-age lobby affected health care services to the extent of a state policy amending the OAA state law as early as 1945, requiring old-age assistance to "provide for adequate medical care for every recipient of assistance. . . ." Under this, recipients were to have free choice of physician, subject to departmental rules and regulations.[15]

The availability of federal vendor payments after 1950, by providing state responsibility for reimbursement to providers, accelerated the movement toward the provision of standard medical benefits within each state. In Massachusetts, for instance, the movement led in 1954 to a state plan that set out liberal provisions for medical care for old-age assistance recipients, reimbursable under fee schedules negotiated with medical organizations. Yet the relatively low amounts provided by federal grants-in-aid (including vendor payments) meant that a state such as Massachusetts, with relatively liberal medical provisions, spent far more for the medical care of its OAA recipients than the sums received from the federal government under the vendor-payment formula. In many other states, however, medical care for the aged poor remained minimal or nonexistent, with considerable variations even within the states.

Medical Care and Geriatric Politics

During the 1950s there was a growing groundswell of concern from and about the increasing number of the aged who were not on public assistance but who, becoming sick through no fault of their own, frequently lacked adequate private insurance, with the result that their life's savings too often vanished in a spate of medical bills. In 1935 one of the major foci for welfare provision had been children. But while children remained an important sector of the welfare population, their assistance and health needs were (probably wrongly) assumed to be relatively well met in comparison with the conditions of the elderly. By the 1950s, moreover, the aged represented a special group of "deserving poor," with special needs with respect to medical bills. The very successes of modern medicine in preventing and controlling diseases meant that an increasing proportion of the population lived to reach the age of 65 and thus became susceptible to chronic and crippling conditions. Almost four out of five aged persons, it was reported, were afflicted with one or more chronic conditions. Few were able to buy private health insurance; as a result, almost three fourths of all health bills for the elderly had to be met by the aged themselves, from savings or by assuming debts or by their relatives—at the very moment that family structure was changing, and the social responsibility of children for their parents was being questioned. Moreover, the medical bills themselves were high. Because of their great need, the average health bill for those over 65 was twice that for the remainder of the population.[16]

Although the early years of the Eisenhower administration reflected a certain amount of complacency, a series of hearings in the late 1950s brought these demands into focus through poignant vignettes.[17] The political pressures were growing. In terms of policy, there were three ways in which the needs of such elderly persons, unable to pay their medical bills out of Social Security benefits (which had not kept pace with the cost of living) or from other funds, could be met. First, efforts could be made to remove the stigma of public assistance, making a minimum income a guaranteed right and with it providing basic health protection. The idea of a minimum income, while it had a period of popularity in the Townsend plan of the 1930s, was alien to the burgeoning prosperity of the 1950s; indeed, it has reappeared as a serious possibility only in the last few years. The second possibility was to provide health benefits as a part of the existing social security provisions for the elderly, regardless of their means. The third and most traditional approach was to create a new category of those to be recognized as deserving and poor, who would be clearly distinguished from others on public assistance. These last two possibilities, based on the very different insurance and assistance philosophies, formed the context of debate over welfare medicine in the 1950s.

The medical needs of the elderly had become a focus of attention for both Republicans and Democrats. In 1951, on the advice of Oscar Ewing, the Federal Security Administrator, President Truman's administration withdrew from its previous position as an advocate of national health insurance for the whole population. Instead, the administration focused its efforts on proposals for a subsidized hospital insurance scheme limited to the elderly.[18] This move defused the health insurance issue from the emotionalism caused by its apparent (if erroneous) kinship to "socialized medicine," in favor of building services on to the existing social security pension system. Between 1957 and 1965 (in which latter year the present Medicare program was passed) health insurance proposals instituted by both Republicans and Democrats were geared toward the special needs of the aged.[19]

There were both political as well as humanitarian reasons for taking this tack. Politically, the aged were becoming both more numerous and more articulate. By 1960, there were 16.5 million people 65 years of age and over, representing 15.4 percent of the population over 21. This sizable proportion of potential voters could not be ignored politically. While proposals for health insurance remained dormant during the first Eisenhower term,

Health Insurance for the Aged, the forerunner of hospital benefits under Medicare, appeared forcefully in 1957 under the sponsorship of Senator Aimé Forand.[20] His bill proposed that Social Security contributions should be raised to provide up to 120 combined days of hospital and skilled nursing home care, together with necessary surgery, for those receiving Social Security benefits. This proposal was thus much more limited in scope, as well as in coverage, than the earlier proposals for national health insurance. Nevertheless, the underlying principle was similar: Health benefits would be provided as a right to all eligible members of the population regardless of any means test. Such a health insurance system could, moreover, be extended in the future to other age groups and to other types of health care. As such the Forand bill and its successors were the thin end of a wedge of national health insurance. Meanwhile others were pressing for expanded medical care through the categorical forms of public assistance. From this latter pressure the Kerr-Mills compromise was to emerge.

Kerr-Mills

By 1960 health insurance for the aged had become a major political issue.[21] In part this was a reflection of inadequate levels of retirement benefits under Social Security; in part it was a reflection of the inadequate services made available under public assistance vendor payments to the two million persons on old-age assistance. In 1960 there were still 10 states and jurisdictions that made no vendor payments at all to provide medical care for those receiving public assistance. And in those states with a federal-state vendor-payments program, there were wide variations. Under OAA, the average monthly amount paid for medical care per recipient varied from 19 cents (Montana) to $43.93 (Wisconsin). Services covered under the programs also varied widely, some states covering hospitalization but not physician services, some excluding hospitalization, and so on; moreover there were often variations from county to county.[22]

The voluntary nature of the assistance grants programs encouraged such differences. States were not required to offer health programs or services under the vendor-payments scheme, although the federal government stood ready to provide matching funds when the states spent their share. Entitlements for care were rarely generous or open-ended. In Missouri recipients of old-age assistance were entitled to hospital care only for medical emergencies or acute serious illness, and care was limited to 14 days per admission. However, nursing-home care was also available, but only up to a maximum of $65 a month, or $100 a month if the patient was completely bedridden. Mississippi paid up to 15 days of acute hospital care for an OAA recipient in any one year at rates not to exceed $15 a day, at a time when the average daily cost of voluntary hospitals in the state was more than $25.

The state did, however, maintain three state charity hospitals for provision of care to the indigent (at a daily cost of well below $15). Louisiana had a unique state network of charity hospitals. Begun in 1814, and substantially developed by Huey Long, they comprised nine hospitals, two of which acted as specialist referral centers. Free ambulance and bus service was also provided.

Iowa made vendor payments for virtually all types of care except hospital care, but the latter was provided by the State University Hospital at Iowa City or locally, with the expense borne by the county poor fund. Delaware also left hospital care to the counties, which paid for ward care at the extremely low rates of between $2 and $4 a day; it was estimated that the hospitals themselves subsidized the poor to the extent of a quarter of a million dollars a year. Nationwide, the medical profession was expected to give free care: it was alleged, for instance, that physicians donated $658 million in services in 1960 alone.[23] Of course, relatives were expected to help finance their poor relations. In Texas it was estimated that in 1961 private charity contributed between $10 and $11 million to medical care of the indigent. Much of this was contributed (often under pressure from welfare departments) by the children of aged recipients. These patterns and their variations were duplicated from state to state and from place to place.

The combination of vendor-payment schemes and services provided by state, county, and city authorities created a web of enormous complexity. But it was clear that New York and California were providing substantial programs compared with most other states. New York, in particular, with its $80 million public health service expenditures (in 1959) and a total of $69 million in vendor medical payments, was providing a vast social service with respect to medical assistance. Yet even there, the payments made to providers of care were far lower than the standard prevailing fees. While there appeared to be general agreement in the states about the inevitability of low payments for the care of the poor, the expectation of charity by providers—hospitals, nursing homes, physicians and others—gave not only a continuing piquancy to the welfare stigma but also a direct incentive for the providers to welcome more generous public assistance reimbursement schemes.

The question of costs was to reverberate throughout all subsequent debates about welfare medicine. In 1960, however, it was largely as an aspect of consumer hardship rather than provider concern that costs were of vital political importance. The rising costs of medical care, especially as far as the elderly were concerned, were pricing vital health services out of reach. Hospital room rates more than tripled in cost between 1945 and 1958. While in retrospect the costs appear nostalgically low even in the latter year (an average of $28 a day), the price spiral of medical costs was already causing general concern.[24] For the elderly, rising costs were of special concern, or at least of special interest in view of the fact that they frequently had fixed incomes. The average annual medical bill per OAA recipient in New York in 1960 was $700.[25] This was not only higher than the average cash benefits provided to the elderly in that state, but it was appreciably more than many of those not on public assistance could afford for medical services.

That persons 65 and over were reportedly twice as likely as other members of the population to need medical care, and at the same time held significantly less private health insurance,[26] meant a continuing prominence for medical care costs in Congressional hearings and in the press. Concern with the problems of the aged was reinforced, in turn, by 1960 House and Senate hearings on the Forand bill, by then under the sponsorship of Senators Clinton Anderson and John Kennedy. Although the House Ways and Means Committee defeated the Forand proposals by a vote of 17–8, the mail continued so strongly in favor of the proposals that the Committee took up the proposals a second time. While its second vote, in June, was similar to the first, the proposals could not be lightly dismissed.

It was clear to the political realist that, if the movement for health insurance for the aged as part of the Social Security system were to be slowed down (if not stopped), there had to be a viable, or at least plausible, alternative. While the health insurance principle was vigorously opposed, there was thus a willingness to consider benefits for the elderly under an expanded form of welfare system. One form of expansion was already available. As a countermeasure to the proposals for hospital insurance for the aged, the Eisenhower Administration had proposed earlier in 1960 a new federal-state program to protect the low-income aged against the cost of long-term illness. This proposal would have established a national means-test eligibility level for medical assistance, with specified physician, hospital, and nursing benefits.[27] But a national means test was still unacceptable; this, too, was rejected by the House Ways and Means Committee.

This left as a third possibility the expansion of the existing system. Sponsored by Representative Wilbur Mills of Arkansas, and by Senator Robert Kerr of Oklahoma, the Kerr-Mills proposal was born. Added to the omnibus Social Security Bill of 1960 (H.R. 12580) the new proposals, representing the triumph of the welfare approach, were enacted into law as the Kerr-Mills Act of that year.[28]

The Kerr-Mills legislation rocked no boats. This, indeed, was the essence of its political success. Other proposals at the time for subsidizing health bills for the elderly would have required substantial administrative changes in the manner of paying medical bills as well as the acceptance of new concepts of entitlement to medical care. The Forand proposals, for example, would have demanded substantial expansion in the social security system, an expansion eventually achieved under Medicare in 1965. Proposals supported by the Administration in 1960 would have set an important precedent in providing federal subsidy of private insurance for the elderly. The Kerr-Mills legislation provided temporary relief to opponents of both philosophies, by accepting neither principle. Instead Kerr-Mills extended the existing system of vendor payments, turning an expedient blind eye to that system's deficiencies.

Social legislation is too often accompanied by hyperbole. As was later to be true of Medicaid, wide claims were made for the new legislation. According to Senator Kerr the plan was "to provide a program, in every State of the Union in which the individual State has or wants a medical-care program for its aged, whereby every aged person in each individual State can, under the provisions of a medical-care program approved by each state, have an adequate medical-care program." Two underlying themes were evident. The first was a strong commitment to continuing state responsibility for welfare medicine; the second, a kind of hopeful expectation that each state would indeed provide adequate care so that a national problem would be avoided. The legislation thus contained a built-in inconsistency. Senator Forand remarked:

> *It will not do any harm, but it will not do any good. Personally I think it is a shame, I think it is a mirage that we are holding up to the old folks to look at and think they are going to get something. I am sure all of you know enough about legislative bodies to realize that the list of items the States could provide under the plan just would never be realized.*[29]

The potential of Kerr-Mills was, however, substantial. The Act not only provided more generous federal matching grants for vendor medical payments for medical care provided to welfare recipients under old-age assistance;[30] it also—much more significantly—included a new category of vendor payments that would apply to elderly persons who were poor but not receiving cash assistance. To accomplish this, a separate program of federal grants to the states, Medical Assistance to the Aged (MAA), was established to pay for services with respect to the "medically needy" aged; after 1962 the blind and disabled were included under a similar category (Title XVI). These new beneficiaries were defined as elderly or blind persons or totally disabled persons over 21 who were not on public assistance and whose income might be above state eligibility levels for cash assistance but who nevertheless had incomes insufficient to meet their medical bills. Here, then, was a new assistance category, "medical indigence," for the deserving poor, primarily for those 65 years of age and over. The new program provided matching grants to participating states of 50 to 80 percent of the cost of vendor payments.

The structure, to be followed later by Medicaid, was one of open-ended federal cost-sharing, without limitations on individual payments or on total state expenditures; cost control was left to the states. The matching formula favored lower-income states, including incidentally those of Representative Mills and Senator Kerr, but state participation was optional, as with other public assistance categorical titles. Unlike the Eisenhower proposal, each state would set its own definition of the limits and scope of medical indigence. In other respects, too, most of the initiative was left to the states, although one important precedent was set with respect to future legislation. While the Act only suggested a broad range of hospital, nursing-home, physician, and other services that might be provided in the state plan, it required each plan to include both institutional and noninstitutional care as a condition of federal sharing.

Thus while the new program was left in the hands of state administrators, it included as an important precedent the concept of federal standard-setting: the provisions that a recipient could not receive medical care under both OAA and MAA,[31] that the states were not to set up enrollment fees for participation, and that (as with other categorical public assistance programs) the program had to be in effect in all administrative subdivisions of a state. Two innovations set the new MAA apart from other public assistance programs: States were not to impose residency requirements on participants except for current residence, nor were they to impose liens on the recipient's property during his lifetime or that of a surviving spouse.[32] The Department of Health, Education, and Welfare was made responsible for approving state plans, issuing guidelines, and receiving reports on their operation; the program was set to begin on October 1, 1960.[33]

In theory the new program could have provided extensive services to a substantial proportion of the elderly population and to the other two adult groups included in at least some of its provisions. It could have met a considerable share of the needs of those who fell into the gap between adequate coverage of their medical bills through private health insurance schemes and those receiving cash payments under public assistance.[34] But in fact the nature of Kerr-Mills was predetermined by its heritage as a political compromise in Congress, and by its formulation as a supplement to existing forms of public assistance.

Kerr-Mills was perhaps less a means of increasing aid to the elderly than it was a means for shifting the burden of that aid from others to the federal government. The many counties in the United States subsidizing medical relief could look upon Kerr-Mills as a golden egg of additional state support;[35] hospitals and doctors could view it as a means of reducing their own private charitable contributions to medical care to the indigent by its introduction of more realistic fees for welfare patients who were elderly; and the states had the pleasant prospect of expanded federal funding. The rhetoric of health was thus even more firmly wedded to the economic realities of the welfare system.

Insofar as it increased aid to the elderly, Kerr-Mills was predicated on a welfare, means-oriented, not a social security insurance oriented, theory. Thus the program was administered by the Bureau of Public Assistance, not by the Public Health Service. Here was a clear indication of its welfare image. Moreover, without exception, the states in implementing their programs designed means tests for the medically indigent under MAA, which, while more liberal than the means test for both cash and health programs under OAA, were similar in administration and intent.[36] Nor were the benefits much more generous than those available under the previous programs.[37] In terms of vendor payments, Kerr-Mills extended OAA at a somewhat higher income level. The atmosphere of welfare was all-pervasive.

No one seriously pretended that Kerr-Mills was the final answer to meeting the health needs of the elderly. Nevertheless the program was disappointing to conservatives and liberals alike. It did not vindicate those who saw the long-term answer to health care financing as a mix of private health insurance backed by public assistance, rather than comprehensive national health insurance; nor did it begin to meet the concern of those who looked for a full range of preventive as well as curative services for the elderly as a means to forestall possible indigence.

Indeed, perhaps the program's most serious flaw was this failure to act until sickness had struck and medical indigency was achieved. Under MAA, the elderly were forced to spend down to the relatively low income-eligibility limits of the program before receiving any benefits. As Secretary Celebrezze pointed out in the 1963 hearings on hospital insurance for the aged, Kerr-Mills did not prevent dependency but only dealt with it after it happened.[38] Like other welfare programs, moreover, its effect was often subtly punitive. A later report from the Subcommittee on Health of the Elderly of the Senate Special Committee on Aging was to catch this flavor of the program:

> *If the objective of a public program designed to assist with the expenses accompanying illness is the preservation of the financial independence of older persons, then any program employing means tests —such as MAA—cannot achieve that goal. For, such programs afford some help* only *after the older individual has depleted his irreplaceable assets to the point of semidependency or total dependency. . . . It is impossible to divorce consideration of how the aged person will manage after he is well from consideration of when and what benefits are available to him during illness.*[39]

Kerr-Mills Is Implemented

The implementation of Kerr-Mills in the states was similar in approach to the later implementation of Medicaid. The Secretary of Health, Education, and Welfare wrote to all the state governors recommending that each state take necessary action to implement the new law. The Bureau of Public Assistance of the Social Security Administration was renamed the Bureau of Family Services of the Welfare Administration, a name reflecting its increasing social role. The Bureau issued a series of State Letters summarizing the provisions of the legislation and reflecting the department's view that both the extended OAA vendor-payment provisions and the new MAA program would improve health care for the elderly. While the role of the Federal agency was limited, as in any other state-federal grant-in-aid program, the Bureau offered exhortation and advice. Its staff prepared information leaflets, met with state directors of public assistance, appointed a group of consultants on medical matters, prepared a guide and a handbook of regulations, published statistics, and assisted the states through technical medical consultation.[40] As a voluntary program of grants-in-aid, however, MAA imposed little responsibility on the Department of Health, Education, and Welfare. Success or failure rested with the states.

This degree of state responsibility could be regarded by proponents of states' rights as a natural development of state responsibility. On the other hand, it represented some buck-passing. Decisions made in Washington as a political alternative to expanded social security were thrown squarely into the laps of legislators in Sacramento and Albany. Each state could decide whether to join the program or not, with no penalty for not doing so. Each could set its own limits for defining the "medically needy," provided they were over 65; and aside from having to provide some institutional and some noninstitutional care, each state could choose the services to be covered and any limits on those services. Far from being taken over by the federal government, state medical services were given expanded responsibility. Indeed, the lack of guidance from Washington was soon to become a point of criticism, as it was even more strongly in respect to Medicaid. At the hearings on Kerr-Mills in 1963, Representatives Burns and Curtis in the House publicly asserted that HEW administrators were dragging their feet on approving programs and not giving even the guidance provided for in the Act.[41]

In fact, the states responded slowly to the new program. Twenty-eight states had Kerr-Mills programs by the end of 1962. Generally these were states which already had substantial vendor-payment programs, states such as Massachusetts, Michigan, Illinois, New York, California, Conecticut, and Pennsylvania. The federal cost-sharing provision was designed to encourage the poorer states to enter, but it was the richer states that saw the potential of the new programs as an extension of existing welfare programs and as a new source of federal budgetary assistance. Because of the higher federal sharing provisions under MAA there was an immediate incentive, particularly in the states with large vendor-payment programs, to shift part of their existing programs into the new category. This was also encouraged by the provision that a recipient could receive medical care through OAA or MAA, but not both.

Massachusetts, for example, began its Kerr-Mills program in October 1960 by transferring 14,000 persons—recipients needing and receiving long-term nursing home care—from other public assistance programs; these persons represented 89 percent of the initial recipients under MAA.[42] A study of MAA in Connecticut found that in its first month of operation (April 1962) 3887 of the total 3929 individuals on MAA were already receiving assistance through the OAA: and the transfers continued.[43] Altogether, it was estimated that nearly 100,000 persons then on other welfare programs in the states were moved to the new program.[44] There was nothing illegal about such transfers; indeed, from the state point of view, they were perfectly reasonable measures to protect their taxpayers against greater costs. But, at the same time, the transfers frustrated the alleged intention of the Kerr-Mills legislation to provide a major new source of services to the elderly and to serve an entirely new group of recipients. Indeed, one report in 1963 estimated that nationwide the combined percentage of old people who were covered for medical care under OAA and MAA had actually declined after the adoption of the new program, from 14 to 13 percent.[45]

Quite clearly, the rhetoric of federal policy did not jibe with the reality of state concerns. Since the states were given primary responsibility, their concerns predominated. An important by-product of the funding arrangement was that, instead of encouraging services where they were most needed through higher federal matching grants to the low-income states, Kerr-Mills provided substantial additional subsidies to states which already had large vendor programs. By 1965, the five states of New York, California, Massachusetts, Minnesota, and Pennsylvania, which together included 31 percent of the aged in the country, were receiving about 62 percent of federal MAA funds.[46] Forty-four of the 54 jurisdictions had some program in effect by 1965, but in many cases programs were minimal and there were wide and confusing variations. Only five jurisdictions were judged to provide comprehensive medical services.[47] Of the 29 jurisdictions with programs in effect in 1963, only 19 provided drugs (which on average accounted for one fourth of all per-capita health payments of the elderly); and, despite the importance of teeth to the elderly, only 17 states provided dental care.[48] Eligibility levels varied widely; indeed, in 14 states the MAA income levels were found in 1963 to be more rigidly interpreted and often lower than those for OAA.[49]

One major difficulty—which was to be transported lock, stock and barrel into Medicaid—was the financial inability and thus unwillingness of low-income states to afford a medical assistance program even when the federal matching grant was up to 80 percent of the total cost. Georgia, for example, authorized MAA in 1961 and Mississippi in 1964, but no state funds were ever appropriated. Even the richer states were already aware of state funding problems. Governor Brown of California stated in 1963 that the cost of making MAA a comprehensive medical care program in that state "would bankrupt the State and county governments."[50]

Another effect of federal funding, also noted by Governor Brown, was the incentive for states to subsidize costly institutional care (in hospitals and nursing homes) rather than other types of health services. In California, for example, institutional care was generous under MAA, while other services were parsimonious. Hospital coverage was provided during the first 30 days of care in county or county-connected hospitals or in nursing homes upon transfer from such facilities. The older person in a private institution could get help under MAA within the first 30 days only if he had already spent $2000 for care. There was thus an incentive to seek care in county institutions.[51]

The focus on institutional care was indeed widespread, for there were substantial advantages in transferring long-term hospital and nursing-home patients from the OAA to the MAA categories; OAA had upper limits on federal reimbursement for such care, MAA had no such limits. But by paying for long-term institutional care, the Kerr-Mills program also stimulated it, a factor to reappear with greater force in Medicaid. Medical vendor payments for nursing-home care had been rising rapidly even before Kerr-Mills. The new program encouraged the process. Vendor payments for nursing-home care (of all age groups) rose from $47 million in fiscal 1960 and then jumped to $449 million in fiscal 1965. Of the total vendor payments of $1.4 billion in fiscal 1965, $1.0 billion was for nursing-home or hospital care.[52]

Kerr-Mills was thus a program out of balance in several respects: in terms of state coverage, eligibility levels, and services. But perhaps more fundamental than these broad disparities was the failure of the program to develop any approach that might distinguish it from other welfare programs, at least one of the original claims made for Kerr-Mills. New York, despite its wide coverage of services, was a case in point. Although the income limits were below the $2500 (single) and $3800 (couple) suggested in the congressional debates, they were relatively generous in comparison with other jurisdictions.[53] Once eligible for the program the New York recipient was entitled to unlimited hospital and nursing-home care, the services of physicians, dentists, optometrists, and podiatrists, prescribed drugs, sickroom supplies, special nursing services, physical therapy and related rehabilitation services, laboratory and x-ray, outpatient hospital and clinic services, eyeglasses, dentures, and prosthetic appliances.

In theory this seemed a generous and comprehensive program. It was also by far the largest of all the MAA programs, providing services in 1962 to roughly one third of all Kerr-Mills recipients nationwide. Yet the means test provision soon became a rallying cry for opposition. Recipients who were "medically needy" were subject to the same rigorous scrutiny of their financial status as were other potential welfare recipients. The Congress might have believed it was enacting a new category of dignified assistance. To the states, MAA was just another welfare program. Recipients who were driven to MAA out of sheer need for assistance for medical bills faced what was to them often a humiliating situation of being a supplicant for relief. Indeed, the International Ladies' Garment Workers' Union (ILGWU) became so angry at the harshness of the means-test administration in New York City that it advised its members not to use Kerr-Mills.[54]

There were other administrative problems. One such was the continuation in the system in several states in 1962, including New York, of family responsibility for relatives such as existed in other forms of public assistance. If an individual applied for MAA in these states, he had to give the names and addresses of his children. Each of these was then sent a detailed, probing personal questionnaire. As the ILGWU testimony remarked: "this part of the investigation is devastating to many of our elderly patients."[55] The recipient thus also subjected his family to a means test.[56] In effect, too, the recipient had to make a public confession of his pauperization.

Kerr-Mills did indeed remove one distasteful aspect of public assistance: the lien on a recipient's property prior to his death. Nine states (again including New York) did, however, require applicants to give them the right to collect from his estate (or that of his surviving spouse) after death by use of post-mortem claims. This factor, too, undoubtedly inhibited applicants from approaching the MAA program, for it meant that the individual would not have anything to leave to his children, and in recognition of this fact 15 states (including Calfornia) did not make any lien requirements.[57] As a final disincentive to utilization, some states imposed deductibles before care was made available. Tennessee, for example, had a limited program, but it was made more limited by the requirement that an applicant first incur $25 of hospital expenses in a fiscal year. Oregon set a scale of deductibles, including $50 for physician services.[58]

Kerr-Mills thus had inherent drawbacks for potential recipients. With respect to providers, the system of below-cost fee schedules that generally prevailed in vendor payment programs was also beginning to cause difficulties. Some ominous cracks were appearing as the gap between welfare schedules and provider costs grew wider. Louisiana's Department of Public Welfare allowed hospitals to collect the difference between the hospital bill and the amount paid by the department from the MAA recipient or his relatives. Doctors in West Virginia fought with the welfare department for the right to charge MAA patients supplemental fees. The participation —or, rather nonparticipation—of both doctors and hospitals in Kerr-Mills began to cause consternation.[59] Several of the MAA programs also restricted the recipient's choice of hospital or physician. As has been noted,

California used incentives to see that care was provided in public hospitals. In the District of Columbia, hospital and clinic care was only provided in specified hospitals, and nursing-home care in one public institution. Here was no entitlement to care with dignity, which the elderly had asked for in the Congressional hearings.

In large part, however, the problems of Kerr-Mills reflected not so much the failings of welfare administration but the lack of alternative channels of medical care. Kerr-Mills was built on the dilemma that foreshadowed Medicaid. If benefits for the medically indigent were to be viewed as a program of health services, there was no particular virtue in attaching them administratively to a program of public assistance cash benefits, whose primary capability lay in determining individual eligibility through a means test. Educational services for the poor were not channelled through public welfare departments. The problem of health care was that no separately subsidized or organized alternative existed.

Public hospitals and clinics, where they existed, could be expanded as the basis for a separate program for health services to the medically indigent as well as those on cash assistance. This, indeed, was the logical approach if Kerr-Mills had been viewed primarily as a program of welfare assistance. Congress, however, had seen medical indigence as a concept to be differentiated from assistance. The report of the Senate Subcommittee on Aging in 1963 looked, indeed, with some alarm at California's MAA program built around its county hospitals and salaried staff physicians, as a "definite step toward 'socialized medicine.'"[60] While determination of medical indigence was universally interpreted in the states in terms of standard means-test provisions, the "medically indigent" were emphatically not "indigent" in the sense of being on cash relief; and public hospitals and clinics, with their stigma of welfare, were not necessarily appropriate places for treatment. Kerr-Mills thus fell between two stools. It was both a reflection of inadequate medical services to those with low and middle incomes and an extension of traditional notions of cash assistance under welfare programs.

NOTES

1. Joseph F. Follman, Jr., *Medical Care and Health Insurance* (Homewood, Ill., 1963), pp. 107–11.

2. See Raymond Munts, *Bargaining for Health: Labor Unions, Health Insurance, and Medical Care* (Madison, Wis., 1967), pp. 9–11 and *passim*.

3. Louis S. Reed, "Private Health Insurance: Coverage and Financial Experience, 1940–66," *Social Security Bulletin*, vol. 30 (November 1967), pp. 12–13.

4. Rosemary Stevens, *American Medicine and the Public Interest* (New Haven, 1971), pp. 272–77 and *passim*.

5. "Special Presidential Message to the Congress Recommending a Compre-

hensive Health Program," Nov. 19, 1945, *Public Papers of the Presidents of the United States: Harry S. Truman 1945* (Washington, 1961), p. 475.

6. Hospital Survey and Construction Act, P.L. 79–725, 60 Stat. 1040 (August 13, 1946).

7. Two programs which were phased out after World War II hammered home this point. The Farm Security Administration had begun a medical care program in California in 1938, as part of a program for the income security of farm workers. By 1944, when this program was transferred to the temporary War Food Administration, there were organizations for migratory farm workers in all states. The second notable group recognized as being the "deserving poor" at this period were the wives and children of servicemen in the four low-ranking grades of the armed forces and of aviation cadets. A large emergency maternity and infant care program (EMIC) was organized through the Children's Bureau in 1943. By 1945 this program, too, was in force in all the states. Indeed, it was estimated that the various services for physician and hospital care under the program had been used by 850,000 women and 110,000 infants. Nathan Sinai and Odin W. Anderson, *EMIC* (Univ. of Michigan, Ann Arbor, 1948), pp. 57–58.

8. Statement of Honorable Robert A. Taft, in U.S., Congress, Senate, Labor and Public Welfare Committee, *National Health Program of 1949, Hearings* on S. 1106, S. 1456, S. 1581 and S. 1679, before a Subcommittee of the Labor and Public Welfare Committee, 81st Cong., 1st Sess., 1949, p. 12.

9. Social Security Amendments of 1950, P.L. 81–734; 64 Stat. 477.

10. U.S. Department of Health, Education, and Welfare, Social Security Administration, *Social Security Programs in the United States* (1968), p. 14.

11. Testimony on Welfare Aspects of Social Security by Elizabeth Wickenden, Washington Representative, American Public Welfare Association, in U.S., Congress, House, Committee on Ways and Means, *Social Security Act Amendments of 1949, Hearings* on H.R. 2892 before the Committee on Ways and Means, House of Representatives, 81st Cong., 1st Sess., 1949, p. 226.

12. Statement of Arthur J. Altmeyer, *ibid.*, p. 17. For a useful study of the scope of the provision of medical care by selected local government units in 1951, see Oscar N. Serbein, Jr., *Paying for Medical Care in the United States* (New York, 1953), Ch. XXIV.

13. U.S., Department of Health, Education, and Welfare, *Medical Resources Available to Meet the Needs of Public Assistance Recipients* (Committee Print, House Ways and Means Committee), H.R. Rep. No. 1799, 87th Cong., 1st Sess., 1961, p. 31 and *passim.*

14. See Michael E. Schiltz, *Public Attitudes Toward Social Security 1935–1965*, U. S. Department of Health, Education, and Welfare, Social Security Administration, Office of Research and Statistics, Research Report #33, 1970, p. 49 and *passim.*

15. At the time, medical care for the poor was the responsibility of local agencies in the state. In response to the new policy, the state welfare department required agencies to submit medical plans for its approval, the first step toward eventual state standardization of health care. Martha Derthick, *The Influence of Federal Grants: Public Assistance in Massachusetts* (Cambridge, Mass., 1970), pp. 64–65.

16. U.S., Department of Health, Education, and Welfare, *The Health Care of the Aged: Background Facts Relating to the Financing Problem* (1962), pp. 17, 34, and *passim.*

17. See the hearings in Detroit in December 1959. U.S., Congress, Senate, Committee on Labor and Public Welfare, *The Aged and the Aging in the United States* (The Community Viewpoint), *Hearings* Before the Subcommittee on Problems of the Aged and Aging of the Committee of Labor and Public Welfare, Senate, 86th Cong., 1st Sess. (1959), pp. 2092–93.

> *I am one of your old retired teachers that has been forgotten. I am 80 years old and for 10 years I have been living on a bare nothing, two meals a day, one egg, a soup, because I want to be independent.*
> *I am of Scotch ancestry, my father fought in the Civil War to the end of the war, therefore, I have it in my blood to be independent and my dignity would not let me go down and be on welfare.*
> *And I worked so hard that I have pernicious anemia, $9.95 for a little bottle of liquid for shots, wholesale, I couldn't pay for it . . . .*

18. Richard Harris, *A Sacred Trust* (revised edition, New York, 1966), Ch. 10.

19. Robert Stevens, *Statutory History of the United States: Income Security* (New York, 1970), pp. 275–89, 401–36; Rosemary Stevens, *American Medicine and the Public Interest* (New Haven, 1971), Ch. 13 and *passim.*

20. H.R. 9467 (1957); and see H.R. 4700 (1959).

21. The development of the Forand bill and the subsequent bills and debates that led to Medicare in 1965 have been well documented. See Odin W. Anderson, *The Uneasy Equilibrium: Private and Public Financing of Health Services in the United States, 1875–1965* (New Haven, 1968); Peter A. Corning, *The Evolution of Medicare* (U.S. Department of Health, Education, and Welfare, Social Security Administration, Office of Research and Statistics, Research Report No. 29, 1969); Eugene Feingold (ed.), *Medicare Policy and Politics: A Case Study and Policy Analysis* (San Francisco, 1966); Richard Harris, *supra* note 18; Max J. Skidmore, *Medicare and the American Rhetoric of Reconciliation* (University of Alabama, 1970); Theodore Marmor, "The Congress: Medicare Politics and Policy," in *American Political Institutions and Public Policy; Five Contemporary Studies* 2–67 (Alvin Sindler [ed.], New York, 1969); James L. Sundquist, *Politics and Policy: The Eisenhower, Kennedy and Johnson Years* (Washington, 1968), pp. 287–321. On the development and implementation of the Kerr-Mills legislation we have also drawn on John C. Roberts, *Kerr-Mills and the States: An Evaluation of Medical Assistance for the Aged 1960–65* (1967) (paper presented at the Yale Law School, 1967).

22. U.S., Department of Health, Education, and Welfare, *Medical Resources Available to Meet the Needs of Public Assistance Recipients, supra* note 13.

23. Services given to the poor of all age levels by physicians were estimated in 1960 to be worth $658 million. Voluntary hospitals were estimated to be providing at least $180 million of care without charge from their own resources (income from endowments, fees from paying patients, gifts, and other income). Many of the providers of care, particularly physicians, were presumably subsidizing their welfare practice through higher charges to other patients; thus the net amount of charity was not as great as might be supposed. Nevertheless, hospitals were by 1960 beginning to feel crimped by rising prices and salary levels. *Ibid.*, pp. 69–70.

24. See for example Herman M. Somers and Anne R. Somers, *Doctors, Patients and Health Insurance* (Washington, 1961), p. 195 and *passim.*

25. W. Kaufman, *Analysis of Medical Care Expenditures by Local Public Welfare Districts for Public Assistance Recipients in New York State During 1960* (New York State Department of Public Welfare, Special Research Statistical Reports No. 17, Sept. 1961).

26. And because of their high medical risk were unable to buy health insurance at prices they could afford. U.S. Public Health Service, *Health Statistics from the U.S. National Health Survey: Older Persons, Selected Health Characteristics, July 1957–June 1959* (Public Health Service Pub. No. 584-C4, 1960).

27. The suggested income level was $2500 for an individual, $3800 for a couple. As an option, cash benefits would be provided for the purchase of private health insurance. The proposal was revealed in testimony before the House Ways and Means Committee on May 4, 1960. A strong supporter was Vice President Richard Nixon. See Congressional Quarterly Service, *Congress and the Nation 1945–1964* (Washington, 1965), pp. 1153–54; Sundquist, note 21, *supra,* pp. 287–305.

28. P.L. 86–778; 74 Stat. 987 (September 13, 1960).

29. *Congressional Record,* vol. 106, col. 16425 (1960).

30. Under the 1950 authorization for medical vendor payments for OAA, AB, and APTD, the federal government matched the state budget on the equivalent of $30 of the first $50 of a state's combined monthly payments for living expenses and vendor payments for welfare recipients. The formula was revised upwards in 1952, 1956, and 1958. Under the last change the federal share was between $41.50 and $46.75 of the first $65 a month of the state's combined outlay per client, with the greater share going to the poorer states. The Kerr-Mills Act added on to this a federal matching payment of 50 to 80 percent (depending on the per-capita income formula of the state) of the next $12 a month spent on medical care for OAA recipients (that is, over and above the $65 limit for all vendor-payment recipients of categorical assistance), *Congress and the Nation,* note 27, *supra,* p. 1154.

31. For the breakdown between OAA and MAA in these early years, see U.S. Department of Health, Education, and Welfare, *Medical Resources Available to Meet Needs of Public Assistance Recipients,* note 13, *supra,* p. 29.

32. Under other public assistance programs, it is open to the state to make a recipient liable in perpetuity should he ever earn enough to repay sums received by way of welfare payments. See James Graham, "Public Assistance: The Right to Receive; the Obligation to Repay," *New York University Law Review,* vol. 43, p. 451 (1968).

33. William L. Mitchell, "Social Security Legislation in the Eighty-Sixth Congress," *Social Security Bulletin,* vol. 23, No. 11 (Nov. 1960), pp. 12–15.

34. Secretary of Health, Education, and Welfare Arthur Flemming, speaking in favor of the original Eisenhower Administration proposal, estimated that 75 percent of all persons over 65 would be eligible to participate under the initial plan (thus providing a major system of free or "socialized" medicine to the elderly).

35. California defined its new MAA program quite clearly as being designed "to supplement the financial ability of counties to meet the health needs of aged persons." U.S., Congress, Senate, Special Committee on Aging, Subcommittee on Health of the Elderly, 88th Cong., 1st Sess., *Medical Assistance for the Aged, The Kerr-Mills Program 1960–63,* Committee Print (88th Cong., 1st Sess., Washington, 1963), p. 75.

36. E.g., New York's relatively comprehensive and liberal MAA program, begun in April 1961. The basic income levels were $1800 for a single applicant and $2600 for a married couple. Applicants might receive health insurance policy premiums of up to $150 for single applicants and $250 a year for a married couple. The home was exempt from means-test levels, as were clothes and house-

hold effects. Applicants could possess life insurance with a cash surrender of $500 and cash reserves of $900 for a single person and $1300 per married couple. "Nonessential" property (as defined by the public assistance caseworker in terms of regulations in the state manual and the plans of the local welfare district) and excess assets were applied against the costs of medical care. In addition there was provision for recovery from the estate of a deceased recipient (though not a live one), and the spouse, parents, and children of the recipient were liable for payment of medical bills when they were found able to assist. Patients in medical or nursing institutions for chronic care were allowed up to $10 a month for personal-care items. These provisions followed the provision of other state welfare programs. *Ibid.*, p. 80

37. E.g., Kentucky inaugurated a vendor payment plan under the federally aided programs (including MAA) in January 1961. Hospital care was included, but only in cases of acute, emergency, and life-endangering conditions, and only as of June 1, 1961, for 6 days per admission. *Medical Resources,* note 13 *supra,* p. 52. When asked what happened if the patient were still sick after 6 days, the Kentucky commissioner for economic security replied, "We pay only for 6 days. If the patient is in the hospital longer, the care may be paid for by a relative or a charity, or the hospital may discharge him. We do not know what happens after our responsibility is met." *Medical Assistance for the Aged,* note 35 *supra,* p. 5. For a survey of programs in effect in 1961, see U.S. Department of Health, Education, and Welfare, Social Security Administration, Division of Program Research, *The Health Care of the Aged: Background Facts Relating to the Financing Problems* (1962), pp. 122–23 and *passim.*

38. U.S., Congress, House, Committee on Ways and Means, *Medical Care for the Aged, Hearings* before the House Committee on Ways and Means, 88th Cong., 1st & 2nd Sess., 1963–64, p. 31.

39. *Medical Assistance for the Aged, supra,* note 35, pp. 30–31.

40. *Ibid.*, pp. 65–72.

41. *Medical Care for the Aged, Hearings, supra,* note 38, p. 258.

42. *Medical Assistance for the Aged, supra,* note 35, p. 86.

43. A ready device for such transfers was for states to drop the expensive services, notably nursing-home care, from OAA and transfer them to MAA: the person needing these services was thus transformed into an MAA recipient. Albert Snoke and Parnie Snoke, "How Kerr-Mills Works in Connecticut," *Modern Hospital,* vol. 101, Aug. 1963, p. 79.

44. *Medical Assistance for the Aged,* note 35, *supra,* p. 2.

45. New York State, Department of Social Welfare, Office of Medical Economics, *Medical Care Expenditures for the Aged in the United States under the Federally Aided Public Assistance Programs, January–March 1963* (1963).

46. Testimony of Wilbur Cohen, U.S., Congress, Senate, Committee on Finance, *Social Security, Hearings* before the Senate Committee on Finance on H.R. 6675, 89th Cong., 1st Sess., 1965, p. 166.

47. Indiana, Massachusetts, Minnesota, New York, and North Dakota. *Ibid.*, p. 163.

48. *Medical Assistance for the Aged, supra,* note 35, p. 49.

49. There was also the problem of the arbitrary cut-off if an applicant's income rose above the state eligibility level (nowadays referred to as the "notch" effect). In one Michigan case, a man was refused services under MAA because his annual income was $1542, while the MAA level was $1500. (In this case he was, how-

ever, still eligible for OAA under the more flexible eligibility provision.) *Ibid.*, pp. 35–36.

50. Testimony of Edmund Brown, *Medical Care for the Aged, Hearings, supra*, note 38, p. 920.

51. Such MAA however was made available for a range of inpatient services and outpatient services needed after the first 30 days. There were no upper limits on such services, provided a physician certified that they were necessary. Eligibility for MAA in 1963 was determined after the 30 days in a licensed medical institution. The level was set at the basic OAA level (then $171 a month) plus the estimated cost of medical care, and the individual was also allowed to retain real property up to $5000 value and personal property of $1200. *Medical Assistance for the Aged, supra* note 35, pp. 75–76.

52. Hospital care accounted for $582 million and nursing-home care for $448 million. Vendor payments as a whole were $212 million in fiscal 1955, $493 million in fiscal 1960, and $1,367 million in fiscal 1965. U.S., Department of Health, Education, and Welfare, Social Security Administration, Office of Research and Statistics, *Compendium of National Health Expenditures Data* (Washington, 1973), Tables 7, 8.

53. On a score card of the states in 1963, New York ranked fourth. The most generous jurisdiction was the District of Columbia with an individual income limit of $2100. *Medical Assistance for the Aged*, note 35, *supra*, p. 35.

54. *Medical Care for the Aged, Hearings*, pp. 552–53.

55. *Ibid.*, p. 553.

56. In Connecticut, for example, 75 percent of the MAA applications rejected were denied on the grounds that the family should provide. Testimony of Joseph C. Bober, *ibid.*, p. 1410.

57. *Medical Assistance for the Aged, supra*, note 35, p. 33 and *passim*.

58. *Ibid.*, p. 45.

59. *Ibid.*, pp. 50–51.

60. *Ibid.*, p. 45.

3
The Federal Role: An Aphilosophical Expansion

The lack of a strong federal role in the Kerr-Mills legislation was not merely a reaction against federal health insurance proposals. It was, rather, a reflection of a general groping for a federal role in programs that were federally subsidized but not federally organized or directed. Before 1960 the typical federal assistance program, whether it was for vendor payments, land grant colleges, highways, vocational education, or agricultural support, did not involve an expressly stated national purpose.[1] Federal programs were designated to support state and local efforts, financed through formula or other grants, and with federal advice but not control.

With the rapid and general rise in federal subsidies in the 1960s, such passivity began to be questioned. Nevertheless, the tendency for a federal role of support rather than direction continued in the wide variety of new health programs that blossomed in the early 1960s, for Kerr-Mills and the debates about health insurance were only one aspect—albeit the most important—of various health care debates. Indeed, in the Johnson administration alone, it has been estimated that Congress enacted 51 pieces of health legislation, administered through 400 different authorities.[2] Federal intervention in health services therefore remained indirect and diffuse rather than the product of a cohesive plan at the national level.

Other Federal Programs

Adding to the growing complexity of health services stimulated under federal largesse, the New Frontier and Great Society programs, together with those passed in earlier years, represented a series of distinct approaches to what the federal role in health should be. Some of the programs of the 1960s followed the earlier tendency of federal intervention: they provided health services as a secondary aspect of some other social goal. Such were the health services provided to Cuban refugees (1962), migrant farm workers (1962), participants in Head Start programs (1965), and residents of Appalachia (1965). Somewhat similar was the initial development of neighborhood health centers under the OEO "War on Poverty" legislation (1964), although the centers soon branched off into a separate program. The primary impetus for these programs was not to improve health but to ensure that health reforms and health costs did not obscure other functions—in the case of migrants, Appalachians, and other poor citizens, the function of general income maintenance, and for Head Start children, learning disabilities.

Other programs were primarily geared toward health but covered a series of specific and different purposes. They thus added to an increasing array of programs aided in some way through public subsidy. Early interest in the federal provision of health care for strategic groups has been noted. "Socialized" services for members of the merchant marine, for the armed forces, and for veterans, have long been accepted as "American." Indeed, after World War II veterans' benefits were vastly expanded and the now famous network of federal veterans' hospitals developed. Federal programs for 400,000 Indians and Alaska natives have also a long history and a ready acceptance. By fiscal year 1966, the Indian Health Program alone had an annual budget of over $80 million.[3]

Federal interest in the "deserving poor" has also been noted. Categorical grants-in-aid to states for maternal and child health services, including services for crippled children and grants for state and local health departments have continued since 1935 and have been interpreted to be primarily for the working poor; these were joined by the federal system of medical vendor payments in 1950. From about 1946 to 1963, however, the major thrust of federal involvement in health was not the provision or subsidy of services but the less direct function of long-term investment in hospital construction, biomedical research, and funding of health manpower programs.[4] The Hill-Burton Act of 1946 provided for a major impetus for hospital construction in the years following World War II, initially and particularly in rural areas. Federal subsidies for construction costs, limited to one third of such costs, were channeled through specially established state Hill-Burton agencies, typically the state health department. Between 1946 and 1968 nearly $3.2 billion in federal funds was channeled through the program, predominantly for building general hospitals in smaller towns and rural areas.[5] By 1965, moreover, the Hill-Burton program had been extended to construction of out-of-hospital community health facilities, to modernizing as well as constructing hospitals, and to subsidizing urban as well as rural facilities.

While Hill-Burton formed one aspect of federal investment in medical care, the phenomenal growth of grant support for medical research from the early 1950s to the late 1960s provided another focus for public beneficence. Under the benign gaze of an enthusiastic Congress the budget of the National Institutes of Health shot up from $2.5 million in 1945 to $285 million in 1960, to $1.6 billion in 1968.[6] Much of this research support was granted to investigators working in the nation's medical schools and was in turn having a profound effect on the schools, in terms of their size, structure, and major interests. For example, the average full-time faculty of American medical schools rose from 70 in 1949 to 250 in 1968, many of whom were predominantly engaged in medical research.[7] Indirectly, federal policies for biomedical research affected the direction of medical education. By 1965 the medical school was a highly scientific research institution. As with Hill-Burton and the much less significant manpower programs developed and brought together in manpower legislation of 1963, the federal role remained that of offering funds to those who sought them, rather than mandating changes in the system or consciously attempting to develop policies.

The period of rapid federal legislative activity between 1963 and 1966 provided, in some respects, a counter to the previous federal role in health, in other respects, some similarities. Mental health legislation of 1963 provided federal matching grants for the development of community mental health and mental retardation facilities. This was followed by an array of legislation of all kinds, some of which has already been mentioned. Indeed, by 1965 it had become necessary to issue a special guide to federal financial aid in the area of medical care.[8] There were programs for older people, for children, for particular diseases, for special ethnic and economic groups, for medical libraries, hospital housing, neighborhood facilities, and so on. Yet while there were programs for federal-local systems of Regional Medical Programs based on medical schools (1965) and federal-state systems of Comprehensive Health Planning agencies (1966) based on community-wide organizations, the federal role in health remained largely passive. The Uncle Sam of the mid-1960s was Sugar Daddy, not Stern Parent.

The idea of the federal government as a kind of friendly helper and innovator—some form of giant Ford Foundation—proved remarkably resilient. Yet at the same time federal grants were becoming a major source of health care funding in the 1960s, for mental health centers, health-planning agencies, regional educational networks, the building of hospitals and health centers, and a variety of training programs, "experiments," and "demonstrations." Implicit in this evolution was the notion that the proper role of government in a capitalistic society was to encourage innovation and monetary investment, reflecting a continuing faith in private enterprise. There was, perhaps, also a vague optimism that some new form of health organization would provide a magic solution to all of medicine's difficulties, without massive government direction. As long as a project was for demonstration purposes, the federal role was not—apparently—suspect. The curious result of the whole process was that, at the very time there was an explicit rejection of the need for a federally-organized welfare state, a welfare state was in fact developing. Rhetoric was once again at work, smoothing out the implications of the massive federal subsidy of the health sector that was the end result of literally hundreds of emerging programs.

Over-all, federal expenditures on health services and facilities increased from $2.9 billion in 1959–60 to $20.6 billion in 1970–71, a sevenfold increase within eleven years. By 1970 public spending as a whole (federal, state, and local) represented more than one third of all health expenditures.[9] Medicare and Medicaid, legislated into existence in 1965, were the most important influence in these changes, but they were part of a wider movement of increasing federal involvement in the health field, which was itself largely a product of the unsatisfactory implications of MAA.

The Fall of Kerr-Mills

If Kerr-Mills represented the triumph of the welfare approach to providing medical care to the aged, it was a triumph that was hollow indeed. Organized groups of senior citizens continued to support the principle of Social Security-based health insurance, providing specified benefits, even while Kerr-Mills was going into effect. To the elderly the question was simple: "Why should the aged citizens that have been forced into retirement have to accept welfare? They deserve independence, dignity, and respect that they have earned over the years."[10]

Indeed, on all sides Kerr-Mills appeared a temporary solution. The states, pressed by mounting costs and carrying the often considerable administrative costs for the program,[11] might welcome the additional aid but could scarcely count the program a success. At the federal level, Kerr-Mills was clearly no solution to the national problem of buying health care for the elderly. Health care costs, particularly hospital costs, were rising steadily—from an average per capita cost (for all age groups) of $142 in 1960 to $198 in 1965.[12] The increases fell particularly heavily on the aged.

In this context the movement for compulsory health insurance took on a new force. Even as the Kerr-Mills programs were being developed in the states side-by-side with the continuing vendor payments under the other categorical assistance programs, further pressures were building up in Congress for hospital insurance for the aged through Social Security for persons at all income levels; that is, the provision of specific services as a covered benefit under the Social Security program, free of variations by state and divorced from any means test. The two developments—the growing disappointment with Kerr-Mills and the pressures for health insurance for the aged—gathered momentum in the years after 1960, culminating in the Social Security Amendments of 1965, which established both Medicare and Medicaid.

President Kennedy strongly endorsed hospital insurance for the aged through Social Security in his health message to Congress in 1961.[13] This endorsement was followed by an Administration bill introduced by Senator Clinton Anderson and Representative Cecil King.[14] Opposed by the AMA and by the Health Insurance Institute representing the private insurance interests, and with little chance of support from Representative Mill's powerful Ways and Means Committee, the King-Anderson bill was initially unsuccessful; and a similar proposal offered by Senator Anderson as an amendment to the Public Welfare Amendments in 1962 suffered a resounding defeat.[15]

Nevertheless, a record was slowly being built up. Hearings by the Ways and Means Committee in 1961 had documented the continuing failure of the system to meet the medical bills of the elderly. Hospital expenses had risen from $9.39 a day in 1946 to $32.23 in 1960 and were rising increasingly rapidly.[16] Born of the continuing increase in medical costs and encouraged by the lack of effectiveness of the Kerr-Mills program, by the changed composition of the Senate after the 1962 elections, and perhaps even by the sheer familiarity of the emotive phrases and the lessening of credibility in the AMA's position, support for health insurance for the aged was rising. President Kennedy outlined his proposals for hospital insurance in a Special Message of February 1963; the King-Anderson bill was introduced again, and the House Ways and Means Committee again held hearings.[17] The following year, after bipartisan efforts to break the deadlock and reach agreement on some constructive health proposal, the Senate for the first time passed a proposal for hospital insurance for the aged as an amendment to the Social Security Bill; but it died in a House-Senate conference committee.[18]

With the Democratic landslide in the elections of November 1964, the composition of the House of Representatives (and of the Ways and Means Committee) was changed in favor of compulsory hospital insurance. President Johnson at once called for action on the King-Anderson proposals—Medicare—as a first priority of business. Hospital insurance for the aged through Social Security appeared as the first bill on the calendar for both Senate and House in 1965 (S. 1 and H.R. 1 of the 89th Congress), and the proposals were incorporated into the over-all aims of the new Administration's program for a "Great Society." Hearings were held by House Ways and Means Committee in January and February 1965. While the AMA continued to claim that "we physicians care for the elderly and know their health needs better than anyone else" and that health insurance controlled by Washington was incompatible with "good medicine,"[19] the tide was turning in favor of including compulsory hospital insurance as a benefit of Social Security.

Other proposals for financing health care were, however, by no means dead. Indeed, it was the eventual combination of several major proposals that was to give the 1965 legislation its peculiar and distinctive character. In 1961 Senator Jacob Javits had revived the Eisenhower proposal for federal support of extensive state programs for those over 65 whose individual incomes did not exceed $3000 or couples whose joint incomes did not exceed $4500. This again raised the question of national standards of eligibility and services, implemented under state administration. The AMA's "Eldercare" proposal, sponsored in the Congress by Representatives Curtis and Herlong and Senator Tower, also called for a federal-state program. This proposal would have subsidized private insurance policies for the elderly, with respect to hospital, doctor, and drug bills. A similar bill was sponsored by Representative John Byrnes and endorsed by the House Republican leadership. But the Byrnes bill, "Bettercare,"—there were as many catchy titles as ideas—suggested federal rather than state administration. The elderly would be encouraged to contribute part of the premiums of a voluntary health insurance program, nationally organized, with public subsidy of the remainder. There were also continuing proposals for tax credits and deductions for health insurance premiums and for expanding the struggling Kerr-Mills program.[20]

Representatives Mills, King, Herlong, Byrnes, and Curtis were all members of the House Ways and Means Committee. Thus, the full range of points of view was present in the crucial Congressional committee, and the outcome of the debate over Medicare was by no means predictable. In the end, the bill reported out of the Committee was not one bill but a compendium of three originally separate, and in some respects competing, proposals. The Administration's proposals for hospital insurance for the aged, financed through the Social Security system, would provide basic inpatient and nursing home coverage for all those eligible for Social Security retirement benefits. As a second layer, there would be a system of federal subsidies to enable old people to buy into a voluntary program of insurance for their doctors' bills (the Byrnes proposal), with the federal government setting premiums and benefits but the administration of the scheme being funneled through insurance companies and nonprofit agencies. These two proposals were to become, respectively, parts A and B of Title XVIII of the Social Security Amendments of 1965. They provided the two interlocking parts of Medicare.[21]

At the same time, a third proposal was made to liberalize and extend the program of federal grants to states for the indigent and medically needy. This last proposal became Title XIX of the Social Security Amendments, popularly known as Medicaid. The different points of view over medical care financing were thereby brought together. In one fell swoop the elderly were offered compulsory hospital insurance through Social Security, subsidized voluntary health insurance for their medical bills, and the expanded program of benefits under the rubric of "medical indigence," a program thereafter to be available on a more general basis. In terms of passage, this strange mixture, brewed by adept political alchemists, proved to be a brilliant political success. The revised proposals passed the House, survived hearings by the Senate Finance Committee, were voted with some modifications in the Senate, were further modified in conference committee, and Public Law 89–97 was signed by President Johnson, amid some flourish, on July 30, 1965.

Medicare

Part A of Title XVIII, largely unchanged to this day, is often termed "compulsory" health insurance, as individuals who pay Social Security contributions during their working lifetimes cannot opt out of the health insurance payments (although they can, of course, decline to accept its benefits). The second program, Title XVIII Part B, provides supplementary medical insurance, chiefly for physician bills. But contributions are based on quite different principles. Instead of being funded from regular Social Security payments, monthly contributions are made entirely at the election of the elderly. This part of the program is thus voluntary. The contributions are channeled into a separate trust fund, where they are matched by an equal contribution from federal general tax revenues.[22]

The Medicare legislation provided an extensive array of hospital services to the over 19 million persons enrolled in Part A. In addition, nearly 18 million of these persons also enrolled in Part B: a reflection in large part of a highly successful campaign launched by the Social Security Administration in 1965 to inform the elderly about the voluntary program. Well over a third (37%) of all eligible persons received some benefits under Medicare in its first year of operation;[23] and the program now accounts for about half of all the medical care payments of the elderly.

The new program was thus massive in proportions and intent. Under Part A of Medicare, beneficiaries became entitled to major subsidy of inpatient hospital services (now up to 90 days); to another 100 days of care, following hospitalization, in an extended care facility; to 100 home visits by health workers after hospitalization; and to services in a psychiatric hospital.[24] Outpatient diagnostic services were also initially made available under Part A, although these were later transferred to Part B, for general ease of administration.

Part A of Medicare thus followed quite closely the intention to provide hospital insurance for the elderly. Extended care in a nursing home and home health visits were subject to the patient having been in hospital for at least three days. Indeed, information presented at the 1965 hearings by the chief actuary of the Social Security Administration and by a representative of the private health insurance industry indicated that such care would act as an alternative to an otherwise longer period of hospitalization.[25] There were thus obvious cost incentives, rather than service alone, to providing out-of-hospital benefits. Generally, Part A resembled the Blue Cross benefits of the time. It was designed to deal with persons who were already sufficiently ill to have to enter a hospital and to protect them from heavy expenditures while there.[26]

Part B, in turn, in some respects resembled Blue Shield. After an initial fee the patient was to become eligible for an unlimited number of subsidized physician services in and out of hospital; for other medical services, including diagnostic tests, radiation therapy, medical supplies, ambulance services, and rental of medical equipment; for up to 100 home health services, without any requirement of prior hospitalization; and for a limited amount of out-of-hospital psychiatric treatment.[27] Ordinary preventive services were not, however, covered; nor were other services of particular concern to many of the elderly, notably eyeglasses, hearing aids, and dental care. Like Part A, therefore, Part B of Medicare provided income protection, of particular value for large expenditures, rather than full service care.

Both parts of Medicare inherited from private health insurance two major features—"deductibles" and "co-insurance"—which required at least some direct patient contribution for the costs of sickness. For inpatient hospital care under Part A, for example, the patient was made responsible for the first $40 of the bill; this was termed the "deductible." In addition, he had to pay a flat sum of $10 a day as "co-insurance" after the first 60 days of hospitalization.[28] Part B was established with an annual deductible of $50. The plan then paid 80 percent of subsequent bills that fell under the program, thus leaving the patient to pick up 20 percent of the bill as co-insurance. While these provisions were generous in terms of the annual amount of funding available—Part B paid out $1.2 billion in benefit payments in its first full year of operation—they were still not comprehensive. For example, persons with medical bills of $1000 in a given year would have to contribute $240 toward this amount (the $50 deductible plus 20 percent of the remainder). If they did not have this amount, they would be forced to seek help through Medicaid.

The limitations of co-insurance and deductibles were also compounded in Part B by two other factors. The first was the necessity for old people to keep proper records, i.e., to submit their bills to Medicare so that they could establish their payment record with respect to the deductible and to subsequent benefits. The second was the opportunity for physicians who so chose to set charges above recognized Medicare levels. Thus the patient might find himself responsible for more than 20 percent of the bill.[29] In addition, at the commencement of Medicare, the patient might have to pay the total bill before he could claim reimbursement.[30] These factors, too, militated against the Medicare program as a means of divorcing health costs from income considerations.

Besides the incorporation of deductibles and co-insurance, Medicare also mimicked the private health insurance industry in terms of organization and administration. As the rhetoric demanded, it was insisted that this was no scheme of "socialized medicine." The law was specific in its statement that there would be no supervision or control by any federal office or employer over the practice of medicine or the way in which medical services would be provided.[31] As with most other federal health programs of the time, Medicare was designed as a program of entitlement rather than control. This was nowhere more clearly seen than in the structure through which federal money was to be channeled to the providers of health services. Hospitals, nursing homes, and home health agencies remained private institutions, mostly (with the notable exception of nursing homes) operating on a technically nonprofit basis. Doctors and other professionals were also to remain strictly independent of government supervision, except in certain specified (minimal) respects. The broad assumption was that a multibillion-dollar program would be quietly absorbed into the private "mainstream" system.

The absorption itself was facilitated by the use of private insurance carriers, including both commercial carriers and nonprofit Blue Cross and Blue Shield agencies, to administer Medicare on the government's behalf. Under the hospital insurance of Part A, groups of hospitals and other facilities were able to nominate private organizations to act as so-called fiscal intermediaries. The intermediaries were to handle all Medicare claims arising under Part A and to bill the Social Security Administration for these sums together with their estimated administrative costs. Most hospitals nominated Blue Cross plans for this role.[32] These intermediaries became, in effect, agents of the federal government. In Medicare's early years, moreover, they operated remarkably free of government regulation.

Part B of Medicare (medical insurance) followed a similar pattern, although in this case the choice of insurance agent (called a "carrier" in a Part B program) was made by the Secretary of Health, Education, and Welfare. Most (33 of 49) of the Part B carriers turned out to be Blue Shield plans. Again, federal direction of the program was minimal.

The use of fiscal intermediaries and carriers for Medicare was important in one respect, in that a smooth implementation of the program was assured. These agencies were already used to the mechanics of health insurance payments. But the system had advantages in the political as well as the administrative arena. Blue Cross had close ties with the hospital establishment; Blue Shield with physicians. There was at least the appearance of—once again—not rocking any boat. Medicare thus began with an apparent paradox. Private enterprise had failed, markedly, to provide adequate health insurance for the elderly: hence the passage of Medicare.

Yet private insurance was chosen to administer the new governmental system.

In other respects, too, the rhetoric of the private sector prevailed, more strongly at the beginning of Medicare than in its later manifestations. Hospitals were to be reimbursed under Part A on the basis of "reasonable costs," physicians according to a system of "reasonable charges." (The quotation marks indicate that these phrases rapidly became charged with administrative complexity.) All licensed physicians became eligible to participate in Medicare. Generally, judgment of the propriety and costs of medical care was left to individual physicians with controls coming into operation after the event. Under Medicare, hospitals had to establish utilization review committees, to oversee the reasons for patient admission and stay: these were, of course, staffed by hospital physicians. Fee review outside hospitals was left to the traditional peer-review structure of medical committee appraisal on behalf of the insurance agencies.

For the individual elderly patient these mechanisms were to be welcomed at the beginning of Medicare, for they stated quite unequivocally that the Medicare beneficiary was not to be seen as an object of charity, a second-class citizen. He was a full-fledged private patient, paid-up through an insurance scheme. The fact that the insurance scheme was government-run was to be regarded as incidental. Medicare was a "right." Its contributions and benefits were clearly specified entitlements. Nor was there any reason why hospitals or doctors should reject Medicare patients or patients feel apologetic in applying to them. At least in theory, their bills were to have the same character as those of everyone else.

Medicaid and Federal Health Care

Compared with Medicare, which had cut-and-dried provisions for eligibility and benefits, Medicaid (Title XIX of the Social Security Act) was relatively ill-designed, its future vague. Medicaid was, in fact, Kerr-Mills applied to a wider constituency: an extension of medical payments under state welfare provisions rather than a new health service program. Indeed, the section of the Senate report dealing with Title XIX was entitled, "Improvement and Extension of Kerr-Mills Medical Assistance Program."[33] But, at the same time, Medicaid's potential for providing medical care to dependent groups was at least as wide as that of Medicare.

By providing more generous federal matching funds to the states and by extending the principle of "medical indigency" to all welfare categories, Medicaid offered to the states the opportunity not only for vast expansion in public assistance medical services but also for a rethinking of their goals and philosophy. Some observers of the time saw Title XIX as the "sleeper" of the 1965 legislation. Social welfare analysts noted the relatively limited scope of Title XVIII (Medicare) in terms of persons covered (the elderly only), the types of health care covered (chiefly hospital and related care), and the presence of deductibles and co-insurance. In this respect Title XIX (Medicaid) was intended as a catch-all program to "pick up the pieces," most notably with respect to covering needy groups other than the aged, to paying for out-of-hospital and nursing-home care, and to paying the remaining charges imposed on impoverished Medicare patients.[34] Both liberal and conservative commentators, in the climate of social justice and poverty eradication of the mid-1960s, wondered whether the Medicaid legislation would not go further. For in theory Medicaid could establish schemes of "socialized medicine" for large sectors of the population in the states, or at least point the way to the state provision of medicine. Was Medicaid to become the exemplar of a national health program of the future?[35]

The appearance of Medicare and Medicaid in the same legislative package appeared to make a test of philosophies inevitable. In providing compulsory (Part A) and voluntary (Part B) health insurance Title XVIII offered a proving-ground for the effectiveness of national health insurance in America. Title XIX (Medicaid) was based not on the insurance principles of specified benefits for specified contributions but on the time-worn structure of federal grants-in-aid to states for medical assistance. Its origins and underlying assumptions were quite different. It thus provided a natural basis for comparison: Which would prove more successful, a federally organized insurance scheme run as part of the social security contributory system but administered through private insurance agencies, or state-organized plans for providing care only to those judged to need it?

President Johnson, in signing the 1965 legislation, remarked, "We marvel not simply at the passage of this bill but what we marvel at is that it took so many years to pass it."[36] These comments were directed specifically at Title XVIII (Medicare), but they were also applicable to the potentially vast system of federal-state medical care programs, whose bare outlines were sketched in Title XIX (Medicaid). Whatever the rhetoric of change, provision of medical care to the poor appeared at last to be accepted as a national problem, requiring at least some federal responsibility.

To see the passage of Medicare and Medicaid solely in terms of ideas "whose time has come"—a phrase which appears continually in health services debates—takes, however, an unnecessarily simplistic view of the events surrounding the passage and implementation of Public Law 89-97. Legislation is seldom the product solely of ideas. And quite clearly there were important economic and political factors underlying the passage of Medicare that were phenomena of the 1960s: the rising costs of health services, the articulation of the special needs of the elderly, and the rise of poverty groups and the equal-rights movement focussing attention on the needs of impoverished minorities.

The rhetoric of Medicare and Medicaid was an important ingredient in their legislative provision and in their subsequent implementation. Yet there was relatively little commitment to any social philosophy that health care should be provided to those who need it. As is perhaps inevitable in the political process, the Congressional debates seemed to be on a different plane altogether. Medicare appeared in virtually opposing guises, in which the provision of health care seemed of relatively minor importance. Its opponents labeled the proposed increased government role in medicine as "not only socialism—it is brazen socialism."[37] On the other hand, Medicare's proponents saw it as an important means of forestalling socialism, by enabling the population to buy insurance to protect their health costs in old age and allowing the elderly to preserve their economic independence. On the one side Medicare was thoroughly "un-American"; on the other, thoroughly "American."[38]

The legacy of these debates was a relative blindness to the scope and purposes of the new health programs. The myopia was both philosophical and structural. The absence of any clear commitment, on the part of either Medicare or Medicaid, to the goal ensuring a basic right to health services meant that both programs were open to future cutbacks in entitlements, funding, and eligibility. If anything, the basic concerns of both programs appeared to be fiscal. Medicare was to maintain the incomes of the deserving elderly when faced by large health bills. Medicaid was to help get people off the welfare rolls and generally to ease welfare budgets in the states. These goals were quite different from the social goals of health services in Western European welfare states. In Britain, for example, health services are regarded as necessary social services: questions of costs and income protection have been treated as secondary. In the United States, the reverse philosophy obtained. Medicare and Medicaid would rise and fall according to fiscal rather than humanitarian objectives.

It was both logical and unfortunate that the second major aspect of having the new legislation appear as "American" as possible was to impose ground rules on the new programs that militated against their very success. Far from being presented as the triumph of a long movement for compulsory health insurance or as a needed social service provided under governmental guarantee, Medicare appeared in the guise of an insurance company, and Medicaid as an extension of welfare programs in the states. Indeed the dilemmas of Medicare and Medicaid were the more general dilemmas of the proper role of government. It was to become increasingly difficult to view them as philosophical entities, representing different aspects of "Americanism"—insurance principles on the one hand, states' rights on the other—when the combined impact of these programs, compared with others developing concurrently, was to raise costs and encourage inefficiency in the whole health care system.

NOTES

1. James L. Sundquist, *Making Federalism Work* (Washington, 1969), p. 3 and *passim.*

2. U.S., Congress, Senate, Committee on Government Operations, Subcommittee on Executive Reorganization and Government Research, *Federal Role in Health,* S. Report 809, 91st Cong., 2nd Sess., 1970, p. 18.

3. U.S., Department of Health, Education, and Welfare, *To Improve Medical Care: A Guide to Federal Financial Aid for the Development of Medical Care Services, Facilities, Personnel,* revised edition, 1966, p. 32.

4. For an interesting review of the changing federal role see William L. Kissick, "Health Policy Directions for the 1970's," *New England Journal of Medicine,* vol. 282, 1970, pp. 1343–54.

5. Rosemary Stevens, *American Medicine and the Public Interest* (New Haven, 1971), pp. 509–10.

6. *Ibid.,* p. 360 and *passim.*

7. *Ibid.,* p. 359

8. *To Improve Medical Care, supra,* note 3.

9. Rosemary Stevens, *supra,* note 5, p. 501.

10. Letter from John F. Kinder, Rhode Island State Council of Senior Citizens, in U.S., Congress, House, Committee on Ways and Means, *Medical Care for the Aged, Hearings* before the Committee on Ways and Means, House of Representatives, 88th Cong., 1st and 2nd Sess., 1963–64, p. 2210.

11. New York, for example, had an annual administrative cost of $4.1 million, a significant portion of it reportedly resulting from the process of collecting contributions from relatives toward paying for the care given to MAA recipients. U.S., Congress, Senate, Special Committee on Aging, Subcommittee on Health of the Elderly, 88th Cong., 1st Sess., *Medical Assistance for the Aged, The Kerr-Mills Program 1960–63,* Committee Print (88th Cong., 1st Sess., Washington, 1963), p. 32.

12. U.S., Department of Health, Education, and Welfare, Social Security Administration, Office of Research and Statistics, *Compendium of National Health Expenditures Data* (Washington, 1973), Table 1.

13. Congressional Quarterly Service, *Congressional Quarterly Almanac 1961* (Washington, 1972), p. 870.

14. Congressional Quarterly Service, *Congress and the Nation, 1945–1964* (Washington, 1965), p. 1154.

15. *Ibid.,* pp. 1154–55.

16. U.S., Congress, House, Committee on Ways and Means, *Health Services for the Aged Under the Social Security Insurance System, Hearings* before the Committee on Ways and Means, House of Representatives, on H.R. 4222, 87th Cong., 1st Sess., 1961, p. 40.

17. President Kennedy's proposals were submitted to Congress on February 21, 1963, as part of the message "Aiding Our Senior Citizens." He called for Social Security payment of all costs of inpatient hospital care for the elderly up to 45 days, support for up to 90 days with some contribution from the patient, and support for up to 180 days with the patient making a greater contribution. The proposals also included up to 180 days of nursing-home care and 240 home health care visits. The Administration bill was introduced by Representative

King (H.R. 3920) and Senator Anderson (S. 880) in February 1963, and initial hearings were held in November. *Congress and the Nation, supra,* note 14, p. 1155.

18. *Ibid.*

19. Testimony of Dr. Donovan Ward, President, AMA, in U.S., Congress, House, Committee on Ways and Means, *Medical Care for the Aged, Executive Hearings* before the Committee on Ways and Means, House of Representatives, on H.R. 1, 89th Cong., 1st Sess., 1965, pp. 745–46.

20. For a report of the congressional history of the different bills, see Congressional Quarterly Service, *Congressional Quarterly Almanac 1965* (Washington, 1966), pp. 248–69.

21. Social Security Amendments of 1965 Public Law No. 89–97, July 30, 1965 79 Stat. 343. For a discussion of the impact of Medicare, see Herman A. Somers and Anne R. Somers, *Medicare and the Hospitals* (Washington, 1967).

22. Both Part A and Part B went into effect in July 1966. An exception was benefits for post-hospital care in skilled nursing homes. This part of the program took effect in January 1967.

23. U.S., Department of Health, Education, and Welfare, Social Security Administration, *Social Security Programs in the United States* (Washington, 1968), p. 20.

24. Subject to a limit of 190 days during a lifetime.

25. *Medical Care for the Aged, supra,* note 19, pp. 436–41.

26. In its first year of operation, fiscal 1967, hospital costs accounted for $2.4 billion of the combined expenditure of $3.4 billion for Medicare, Parts A and B. Total expenditures for hospitalization of the elderly in that year were $5.6 billion. *Compendium of National Health Expenditures Data, supra,* note 12, pp. 53, 83.

27. Initially this was linked to payment in a calendar year of up to (a) $312.50, or (b) 62.5% of the expense, whichever was smaller.

28. Calendar year 1967. Robert J. Myers, *Medicare* (Bryn Mawr, 1970), p. 250.

29. Physicians could submit bills directly to Medicare for payment on behalf of the patient, but in this case they had to accept Medicare reimbursements levels. In the first eighteen months of operation, only 38 percent of Part B bills were paid this way. See Rosemary Stevens, *supra,* note 5, p. 448.

30. This billing method was modified in the Social Security Amendments of 1967 (P.L. 90–248; 8 Stat. 821) to enable patients to present an itemized (unpaid) bill to the carriers for reimbursement. But the two methods—direct payment to the physician ("assignment") and payment via the patient—remain.

31. Public Law 89–97, Title XVIII, Sec. 1801.

32. 6876 of 7906 hospitals nominated the Blue Cross Association and its associated plans. See Rosemary Stevens, *supra,* note 5, p. 447.

33. U.S., Congress, Senate, Committee on Finance, *Social Security Amendments of 1965,* S. Report 404 to Accompany H.R. 6675, 89th Cong., 1st Sess., 1965, p. 73.

34. See Eveline M. Burns, "Some Major Policy Decisions Facing the United States in the Financing and Organization of Health Care," *Bulletin of the New York Academy of Medicine,* vol. 42, 1966, pp. 1072–1080.

35. See Benjamin Werne, "Medicaid: Has National Health Insurance Entered by the Back Door?" *Syracuse Law Review,* vol. 18, 1966, p. 49.

36. Quoted by Richard Harris, *A Sacred Trust* (revised edition, New York, 1966), p. 4.

37. Senator Carl Curtis (Republican, Nebraska), *Congressional Record,* vol. CXL, col. 15870 (1965).

38. For an interesting analysis of this definition process, see Max J. Skidmore, *Medicare and the American Rhetoric of Reconciliation* (University, Alabama, 1970). Skidmore argues that the passage of Medicare represents a general feature of American society, namely, that the need to reconcile philosophical opposites, e.g., the ideology of free enterprise versus the desirability of social welfare programs, is met by rhetoric. We are indebted to this approach in the development of our own analysis.

4

Basic Provisions of Medicaid

The basic purpose of Title XIX (Medicaid), as outlined in the 1965 legislation, was comprehensive and far-reaching. Each state was to be encouraged "as far as practicable under the conditions in such state," to provide medical assistance to families with dependent children and to aged, blind, or permanently and totally disabled individuals "whose income and resources are insufficient to meet the costs of necessary medical services."[1] In addition, the law called upon states to offer rehabilitation and other services that would help such persons attain (or retain) their independence.

The interpretation of this general purpose was a matter for discussion and implementation in each state, within broad guidelines set up under the legislation. Perhaps of most importance in the ensuing debates was, however, not so much what was in the legislation but what was left out. Three major characteristics of the new legislation should be stressed. First, this was not a sweeping program of assistance to all those who were poor, even within a state. Like its welfare predecessors, the Medicaid program was "categorical": the federal subsidy followed (and expanded) the existing welfare classifications of AFDC, OAA, AB, and APTD. Second, the definition of medical services and the amount of each type to be provided to those eligible was not standardized from state to state. As will be seen, the law contained important provisions for minimal coverage of specified types of care, which put Medicaid far beyond the Kerr-Mills program and were designed to lead to comprehensive care. Nevertheless there was considerable room for maneuvering as to what should be covered in each state. And, finally, the decision as to what "income and resources" ought to be included in determining eligibility for services within the various categories was left up to each state. Here was no nationwide program to provide a standard of care to all those whose incomes fell below a certain level. Rather, the actions of each state were critical. The program would stand or fall by the combined activities of fifty different legislatures. In this respect, the implementation of Medicaid was a rerun of Kerr-Mills.

The Structure of State Programs as Outlined in Public Law 89-97

Since Title XIX, as enacted, extended and revised Kerr-Mills, it set requirements for state plans in some aspects comparable to existing provisions in the law. As with other welfare programs, including Kerr-Mills, the federal budget was open-ended. The law called for a sum to be appropriated "sufficient to carry out [its] purposes." Because Medicaid was a program of federal matching grants, the size of the sum would depend on the number of states participating and the size of approved programs in those states. Congress thus could not control the costs of the program through limiting appropriations but only by cutting back on the program itself.

Each state had to submit its state plan for medical assistance to the Department of Health, Education, and Welfare (technically to the Secretary of HEW) for approval. Theoretically, this approval could be used as a formidable weapon of federal influence over the states. In fact, however, it was a weapon that with respect to welfare programs generally had not been used. The federal government had traditionally relied on the states to exercise fiscal restraint in assistance programs. The review was used primarily to ensure that certain basic conditions in the law were fulfilled.

Several conditions were built into Medicaid. The first of these was that to become eligible for federal matching funds, a state plan had to be in effect in all political subdivisions of the state.[2] This same provision had been part of Kerr-Mills, as well as other public assistance programs, and was important in ensuring that the program was indeed a state program, not subject to county variations. Each state was also required to provide for such methods of administration as the Secretary of HEW might deem "necessary for the proper and efficient operation of the plan,"[3] a statement that might have heralded (but did not) a strong federal role in this part of state welfare administration. Similarly, the state had to provide for the making of such reports as the Secretary might require, as well as to comply with provisions for federal auditing procedures, as and where called for, to assure that the reports were correct.[4]

With respect to the services themselves, the state was required to provide the opportunity for all potential recipients to apply for assistance under the plan and to act "with reasonable promptness" on such applications.[5] Any individual whose claim for medical assistance was denied or was not acted upon with reasonable promptness was to be entitled to a fair hearing.[6] Recipients were also to be protected through safeguards designed to protect the confidentiality of information concerning applicants and recipients.[7] In addition, the states were required to establish or designate state authorities responsible for establishing and maintaining standards for private or public institutions in which the recipients of Medicaid would receive care.[8]

True to the general (if limited) emphasis on standardization of the vendor-payment program within a state, each state was to establish or designate a "single state agency" to administer the plan. Which agency this was to be was left unspecified by the vague and outline form of Title XIX. The additional requirement, however, that the determination of eligibility for medical assistance under the plan should be made by the state or local agency administering Titles I or XVI of the Social Security Act (almost invariably the welfare departments)[9] in large part preordained this choice. To have eligibility determined by the state welfare department but the program run by the state health department would have added, rather than reduced, confusion. Thus while the requirement that welfare departments be used to determine eligibility was due to Congressional confidence in the welfare department's "long experience and skill in determination of eligibility,"[10] it also helped set the underlying approach of the Medicaid program. In practice most of the states designated their welfare departments as the "single state agency" for all other aspects of Medicaid as well.[11]

Having met all these requirements, together with those for eligibility and services, and produced a document describing the program in detail, the state could look for a substantial subsidy for its Medicaid program from the federal government. The minimum federal contribution for medical assistance expenditures to the states' approved Medicaid programs was 50 percent with a maximum of 83 percent, based on a variable-grant, federal-state matching formula, which paid most to the state with the lowest per capita income.[12] Additionally, the federal government would pay 75 percent of the administrative costs attributable to skilled professional medical personnel and 50 percent of other administrative costs in the states. As a further wrinkle, Title XIX provided that if the matching federal medical assistance percentage for any state, as computed by this formula, was less than 105 percent of the federal share of the medical expenditures made by the state during fiscal year 1965, then 105 percent of the 1965 federal share would be the state's federal medical assistance percentage for fiscal years 1966 through 1969. Federal payments were to be made by HEW based upon quarterly estimates supplied by the states, with corrections in each quarter for previous overpayments and underpayments.[13]

As far as the state's own share of funding was concerned, each state was initially required to pay at least 40 percent of the nonfederal share out of state monies, with the remainder being allowed to come from local funds. By July 1, 1970, however, all of the nonfederal share had to be provided by the state government or through an approved tax-equalization formula with the same effect.[14] Once again, therefore, these provisions encouraged the notion of state rather than local responsibility. Responsibility for welfare medicine was moving upward, from the county to the state.

A complementary shift in responsibility from state to federal government was, as we have noted, barely visible in the initial legislation. But beside the concept of state (rather than local) standards for Medicaid, the legislation attempted to influence state spending in another important administrative respect. Since the program was intended to provide additional services, the law sought to prevent the states from using the new federal medical care dollars to replace their existing medical assistance expenditures, as had happened extensively in the Kerr-Mills program.[15] In other words, Medicaid programs had to be incremental. This principle of using additional federal money for additional programs rather than for funding programs previously paid for by the state was known, rather quaintly, as the concept of "state effort." Medicaid was not to be regarded (at least, not according to the legislation) as a welcome windfall that would release dollars for other purposes in the states.

Such were the bare bones of the administrative arrangements between the participating state and HEW. In theory, the Department could be quite tough on program management and dollar use in the states. But the sanctions available to the Secretary of HEW in cases of noncompliance were not wholly clear, nor does the legislative history provide any significant clarification. Title XIX provides that if, after reasonable notice and an opportunity for hearing, the Secretary finds that a state plan has been so altered that it no longer complies with the statutory requirements or if the administration of the plan is substantially out of compliance, then he is entitled to cut off funds until the failure is corrected. However, in a rather cryptic parenthetical expression, he is also given discretion to determine "that payments will be limited to categories under or parts of the State plan not affected by such failure."[16] The meaning is clearly that total cut-off of federal funds is not to be the only sanction available to HEW, but it is not at all clear what facets of any state program are separable from the remainder of the program for purposes of this part of the statute. While the possibility of selective federal cut-off of funds was an advance on the all-or-nothing approach of earlier legislation establishing federal grants-in-aid for public assistance categorical programs, the lack of precision in this section may well have encouraged HEW's reluctance to make use of it. On the one hand HEW has been unwilling to use a sledgehammer for a task that would more appropriately demand use of a scalpel, yet on the other, the new Medicaid section gave no instructions in the use of the scalpel.

The act did not require the states to establish a Medicaid program, but it put considerable pressure on them to do so: a reaction to, and a considerable advance on, the Kerr-Mills legislation. In particular, the Medicaid legislation provided that after December 31, 1969, there would be no further federal matching funds for state medical vendor expenditures under the categorical titles for OAA, AFDC, AB, APTD, and Kerr-Mills. Thus each state had to opt for Medicaid or forego federal help for vendor payments. Perhaps even more important as an inducement, especially to the larger states, was the provision in Title XI (section 1118) allowing states establishing Medicaid programs to use the more favorable Title XIX reimbursement formula for their other categorical assistance programs, since this offered a significant windfall. Together, these pressures were effective. Although some states barely made the deadline—for example, Alabama, Arkansas, and Mississippi commenced their programs on January 1, 1970 —only two, Alaska and Arizona, failed to implement Medicaid by the deadline. (They explained that, since virtually all Eskimos and Indians would be eligible, the potential costs would be "unbearable," although Alaska finally undertook a Medicaid program in 1972.) The combination of carrot and stick inherent in the 1965 legislation was thus highly successful in encouraging the states to participate. In this respect, if not in others, Medicaid far surpassed Kerr-Mills.

Who Is Eligible under Title XIX?

Perhaps the murkiest language of Title XIX as enacted was that which specified eligibility standards. Indeed, even the welfare and health departments concerned had difficulty in comprehending all the implications of the legislation. The key to—and the problem of—understanding exactly who was eligible for the new program was the categorical nature of the existing welfare programs. Medicaid eligibility, too, generated other categories. In the legislation as originally written, the exact nature of these categories was by no means clear. Nevertheless, it is now generally agreed that potential recipients fall into four basic classes. It says something for the bureaucratic flavor of Medicaid that these are technically known as the "categorically needy," the "categorically related needy," "the categorically related medically needy," and the "noncategorically related medically needy."[17]

First, the state Medicaid plan had to include those receiving aid under the four categorical assistance programs (OAA, AB, AFDC, APTD) or the expanded Kerr-Mills program (Title XVI),[18] the group known as the "categorically needy." Second, the state had to include certain groups from the "categorically related needy" category: those who would be included in these five programs were it not for a specific state provision overridden by Title XIX [for example, section 1902(b) (3) prohibited durational residence requirements, which many states still had in 1965 for their public assistance programs]; where there were age requirements for cash benefits in excess of 65 years; or, effective July 1, 1967, where a state imposed age requirements that excluded persons between ages 18 and 21 who would otherwise be eligible for AFDC.[19]

In short, everyone deemed eligible for cash assistance or the earlier Kerr-Mills program, or who would be eligible if it were not for specified state provisions invalidated by Title XIX, was automatically to be covered in a state's Medicaid plan. For convenience, we sometimes refer somewhat inaccurately to the persons in these mandatory classes simply as the "needy" or "indigent" or "welfare recipients" or most commonly, as the "categorically needy." We use this in contrast to those in other categories that a state might or might not cover for medical assistance, for whom federal matching funds were available if the state so chose. All these other potential nonmandatory recipients of Medicaid we generally describe as "medically needy," a generic term which in turn includes at least two other categories of potential recipients.

Besides, then, the groups who must be covered in a state Medicaid plan, there are specified groups who may be included in the Medicaid program at the option of the state, but for whom federal cost-sharing is available. (States may, of course, also include whomever else they please, but no federal matching money is available.) In discussing the optional groups, there are terminological problems springing from the unfortunate wording of the Act. In fact, the first two groups properly belong in the category of "categorically related needy," whose other groups it is mandatory to cover.

The first of these optional "categorically related needy" groups comprised persons who would be eligible for federal-state categorical programs if the state had adopted the broadest coverage possible for those programs: for example, a person who would be eligible for AFDC-UP except for the fact that his state had no such program. The second group included persons who would be eligible for assistance if they were not in a medical facility, including those over 65 who are in mental or tuberculosis institutions. Eligibility for this last group was derived from the so-called Long Amendment, which marked the first time federal participation in medical vendor payments had been authorized for this institutionalized population. Federal payments, however, on behalf of anyone under age 65 in mental and tuberculosis institutions (which are usually state-financed) were explicitly forbidden.[20] For other persons who were chronically sick and, significantly, for all the elderly in medical institutions, this provision of Medicaid provided an extraordinarily important innovation.

The second optional category, the "categorically related medically needy," allowed the states to include "all individuals who would, if needy, be eligible for aid or assistance under any such State plan and who have insufficient (as determined in accordance with comparable standards) income and resources to meet the costs of necessary medical or remedial care and services." This meant, in brief, persons who were children (and their families), elderly, blind, or disabled but with income above prevailing means-test levels for cash assistance.

The Kerr-Mills legislation had set the precedent of providing vendor medical payments for the medically indigent: persons whose incomes and assets were above the eligibility levels for welfare payments but were still insufficient (according to states' criteria) to meet medical bills. In practice, eligibility was determined by the establishment of a second (somewhat higher) means test. Those who fell within this means-test criterion became eligible for medical benefits but not for cash assistance. Kerr-Mills, sparked by Congressional demands for care for the elderly, had originally focussed on one category of recipients, those aged 65 years and above, although it was later expanded to the blind and disabled. Medicaid provided a further major extension by offering a federal subsidy of state programs for those who were medically needy and whose status corresponded with all categorical assistance groups. These were the "categorically related medically needy"—persons who would have qualified as "categorically needy" by virtue of being elderly, blind, disabled, or a member of a family with dependent child or children, except that their income fell above the cut-off level imposed in their state for cash assistance.[21] It was the extension of the concept of "medically needy" to the family as a whole that was to prove the most significant development in Title XIX.

As with Kerr-Mills, each state could set up programs for the "medically needy" at its own option. A state could thus develop a Medicaid program limited to those as poor as persons receiving state welfare payments, or it could go well beyond this by adding the "medically needy," using eligibility levels developed in that state up to any given level. One important specification, however, was made with respect to these eligibility levels. While each state choosing to cover this class of "categorically related medically needy" was allowed to set its own income-level standard for this group, that standard had to be the same for all individuals regardless of the category to which they were related. In other words, the blind recipient, the disabled, the elderly, and the mother in the family categorically related to AFDC were all to be judged eligible or ineligible with respect to "medical indigence" according to a common set of criteria. This provision may sound straightforward, but it differed from the income eligibility standards for categorical recipients—where the states were allowed to, and frequently did, set different income maxim for the different categories.

In addition, the states were required to provide equal medical or remedial care and services to all persons classed—to revert to our terminology for the mandatory and voluntary categories—as "medically needy," just as they were required to provide equal treatment for all those in the "categorically needy" category as well.[22] There were to be no special concessions to advanced age or childhood. Rather, the legislation sought deliberately to rationalize the patchwork of programs in the states. Medicaid, where offered, was to apply equally across county lines and across welfare categories, requiring one standard of eligibility for one group of beneficiaries.

Besides this relatively clear-cut underlying assumption there were, however, obscurely drafted provisions as to how the categories were to be achieved. Probably the most opaque provision in the whole of Title XIX related to how the "medically needy" were to be defined. States were required under the legislation to take into account the costs incurred for medical care (including health insurance premiums) when determining whether an individual was eligible for Medicaid.[23] Exactly how this was to be done was not specified in the law, which merely noted that state standards should "provide for flexibility"; but subsequent interpretation produced the so-called spend-down provision, which requires the states in determining eligibility to take into account the amount spent by the recipient on medical care. For example, if the state's income eligibility level for a "medically needy" individual is $3000 annually and his income is $3200, then he becomes eligible for Medicaid payments for all but $200 in medical expenses.

It says much of the general lack of clarity in the legislation that it does not specifically state to which group(s) of recipients this provision refers. Indeed, it is only after analysis of the standards for the "categorically needy" (i.e., those on cash assistance and the mandatory groups of the "categorically related needy") that one realizes that the "spend-down" provision cannot apply to them as well, an interpretation of the statute that has been upheld by the courts.[24] Whether Congress genuinely "intended" this result is open to question, for a serious anomaly is created by it.[25] What it means is that a person in a state whose plan is minimal, providing services only for the "categorically needy," loses all his Medicaid entitlements merely by earning a few dollars above the categorical (cash) assistance level. On the other hand, a person in a state that also provides for the "medically needy" will never lose eligibility so long as he "spends down" to the appropriate medical assistance level. He could, for example, be earning $6000 but have medical bills of $3000, which would bring him down to our hypothetical $3000 for the state's "medically needy" Medicaid level. Other bills would then be paid. Yet if the state covered only the categorically needy, that is, those receiving or eligible for cash assistance, he would not be eligible for Medicaid help. Such an individual is said to be a victim of the "Medicaid notch," of which much was to be made in later years. For some of the victims themselves the legislation caused tragic and probably incomprehensible results.

The final category of persons who could be covered—but need not be—under Medicaid, and for whom matching funds were available, is mercifully less obscure syntactically, a quality more than compensated for by the obscurity surrounding its implementation. This might be called the "children's clause," but its technical term is the "noncategorically related medically needy." We have already seen that children were covered by virtue of being eligible for AFDC or otherwise eligible but with income above the AFDC limits. In addition, however, the Ribicoff Amendment[26] offered states the option of extending coverage to all persons under the age of 21 who were either "medically needy" or "categorically related needy." In plain words, these were children who for technical reasons did not qualify for AFDC but who were equally needy with respect to medical assistance. In fact, details of this aspect of the program have been hard to come by, and coverage is thought to have been sparse.

As noted, only the first class of persons, the categorically needy and two groups of the categorically related needy, had to be included in a state's Medicaid plan. Inclusion of the medically needy was entirely voluntary. States that elected to do so might add the appropriate groups to their plan and collect federal subsidies for services subsequently provided. A state which included all of the eligible classes was, however, still tied to the definition of the population by the former welfare categories, with the notable exception of the category of children under 21. This meant potentially that substantial federal-state programs could be made available to the young, the blind, the disabled, and the old (65 years and over), together with relatives living with eligible children.

But, except for families with eligible children and blind and disabled persons, the large group of persons between the ages of 21 and 65 was not covered, however needy they were, however large their bills or desperate their medical condition. Each state was certainly free to include a program of medical services for those in this age group or indeed in any age group and at any financial level they chose, but it had to do so out of state and local taxes. Federal funds were made available to help cover the administrative costs of such programs, but no federal funds were available to support the programs themselves. Again, not surprisingly, the availability (more accurately, the nonavailability) of services to those who were just "poor" but not categorically eligible or related was to provide a further source of confusion in the interpretation of Medicaid in the states.

What Was Provided under Title XIX?

The statute was considerably clearer in describing what the recipients might receive than in identifying who they might be. Effective July 1, 1967, all persons covered by a state plan, whether "categorically needy" or "medically needy," had to be provided, through vendor payments, with five basic services: inpatient hospital services (other than in an institution for tuberculosis or mental diseases); outpatient hospital services; other laboratory and x-ray services; skilled nursing-home services for persons aged 21 and older (again, with the exception of care in a tuberculosis or mental institution); and physicians' services when given in hospital, nursing home, private office or elsewhere.[27] The amounts of these services were not specified; the statute left it open for states to provide unlimited coverage within the mandatory categories or to impose limits on coverage (for example, on the number of days in a nursing home). However, all five services had to be included.

As these were vendor payments, the reimbursement would go directly from the state to the providers. The legislation specified that payment to hospitals for inpatient care was to be on the basis of a "reasonable cost,"[28] a phrase to be interpreted according to standards approved by the Secretary of HEW. Methods of reimbursing other providers of care were left unspecified. The hospitals thus had a potential head start over other providers, since presumably "reasonable cost," as defined in subsequent regulations, would bear a direct relationship to the actual cost of the services provided: as costs went up, so would reimbursement levels. In this, Title XIX followed the reimbursement pattern for Title XVIII (Medicare).[29] For other services provided under Medicaid states could, however, choose their own formulae and set their own payment schedules. These alternatives could include the continuation of the long welfare tradition of reimbursing at less than cost, in other words, expecting providers to donate out of charity. The inclusion of skilled nursing-home services in both Medicare and Medicaid suggested, however, that another acceptable method of reimbursement would be for Medicaid to follow the Medicare formula of "reasonable cost," with respect to nursing homes. In any event it was predictable that some states would find themselves under pressure from professional groups to follow the Medicare formulae, including paying physicians and other eligible professionals their "reasonable charges." By leaving such questions open, Title XIX was to open a Pandora's box for medical costs.

The essential service features of Medicaid were, in short, relatively straightforward. Five services had to be provided, with federal standards awaited for reimbursement of inpatient hospital care. But in addition to these mandatory services, the states could also receive federal matching funds for any of ten other types of services. These included: medical or remedial care furnished by other practitioners licensed under state law (e.g., chiropractors); home health care services; private-duty nursing care; clinic services; dental services; physical therapy and related services; prescribed drugs, dentures, prosthetic devices, and eyeglasses; other diagnostic, screening, preventive, and rehabilitative services; inpatient hospital and skilled nursing-home services for persons aged 65 or older in a TB or mental institution (the Long Amendment referred to earlier); and any other type of medical or remedial care approved by the Secretary of

HEW.[30] Here was a large array of services from which the richer states could build the outlines of their new Medicaid programs. States that were more parsimonious could remain with the basic five.[31] Each state had to decide where it would place its priorities. Given a limited amount of money for the program, was it more desirable to give relatively few services to a large number of recipients or to give a wide array of services to relatively few?

The thrust of the Medicaid legislation was quite clearly expansionist in both directions. Indeed, the Secretary was empowered to withhold funds from any state not "making efforts in the direction of broadening the scope of the care and services made available under the plan and in the direction of liberalizing the eligibility requirements for medical assistance," the ultimate goal being "comprehensive care" for substantially all eligible individuals by 1975.[32] But while this might sound as if all states would be required to provide all 15 services (mandatory and voluntary) by 1975 to both "categorically needy" and "medically needy" individuals, no further definition or limits on implementation were included in the legislation. "Comprehensive care" was to remain a phrase of high hope and incrementalism, rather than a requirement of specified services in each state by the target date.[33] Its appearance in the legislation did, however, point toward an eventual goal for Medicaid that subsequent regulations might develop.

In other respects, too, the legislation pressed for a more organized program of medical care. The sections relating to mental institutions are of particular note, as they represent the most explicit recognition to be found in the 1965 legislation of Medicaid's potential function as a lever for raising health care standards generally.[34] States which chose to include such services for those age 65 and older were required to show that they were "making satisfactory progress toward developing and implementing a comprehensive mental health program" and to arrange with institutions involved for "joint planning and for developing alternate methods of care," i.e., care outside the mental hospital. Additionally, each patient in such institutions was to be provided with "an individual plan" to be developed "in his best interest," including guarantees of initial and periodic review of his condition, appropriate medical treatment, and a periodic determination as to whether he should continue his stay in the institution. Standards for no other type of health care were prescribed so explicitly in Title XIX; arguably, some of the later problems facing Medicaid would have been less serious if there had been a greater willingness to spell out standards and purposes.

For other services the 1965 legislation merely provided that the state enter into "cooperative arrangements" with appropriate state agencies (e.g., the State Health Department) in aiming toward "maximum utilization" of health and rehabilitation services under the plan.[35] Although hospitals and nursing homes were required under Title XVIII (Medicare) to set up committees to review the appropriate use of inpatient services for Medicare beneficiaries,[36] no similar provisions were made for Medicaid. Nor, in the 1965 legislation, were there any similar review groups at the national level to advise on matters of utilization or general policy such as were built into Medicare in the (now defunct) National Medical Review Committee[37] and Health Insurance Benefits Advisory Council.[38] Apart from the inclusion of the Medicare formula for hospital reimbursement, Medicaid's initial shape took little recognition of Medicare's parallel development.

General Considerations

In part, of course, the differences between Medicare and Medicaid provisions reflect the distinction between a national and a federal-state program. But the lack of specificity in Medicaid must also be ascribed to the apparent haste with which it was written and the lack of detailed Congressional review in comparison to the interest generated by Medicare. Much of the confusion in the Title XIX legislation could have been cleared up in regulations—and, indeed, the pattern of eligibility determination outlined above gradually became clearer through administrative interpretation—but regulations were slow in appearing.

Some important additional parts of the legislation were quite specific. State Medicaid programs might "buy in" to Medicare for eligible recipients over the age of 65, with the states paying all or part of the monthly premium for Medicare Part B, as well as paying the deductibles and coinsurance payments required under that title.[39] With respect to Title XIX itself, states were prohibited in the 1965 law from imposing on any Medicaid recipient any "deduction, cost sharing or similar charge . . . with respect to inpatient hospital services furnished him under the plan." Any such charge, including enrollment fee or premiums, with respect to other services had to be reasonably related to the recipient's income and resources.[40] Additionally, certain impediments on eligible recipients found in some state assistance programs were prohibited under Medicaid. As under Kerr-Mills, no lien might be imposed against a deceased recipient's property prior to the death of his surviving spouse.[41] Special arrangements had to be made for furnishing medical assistance for persons temporarily out of the state.[42] Finally, the financial responsibility of relatives was to be limited to a married recipient's spouse or a minor recipient's parent.[43] This latter prohibition finally removed from adults the burden of being billed for the medical care of elderly, impoverished parents. Taken together with other sections of the Act, it was to have an important effect on the expanded utilization of nursing homes.

These and other specific provisions of the legislation caused relatively little difficulty in interpretation. The more general provisions pointed to a potentially ambitious scheme of medical services for the poor in terms of previous welfare medicine, even where the program was limited to providing the five basic services to the "categorically needy." Under the legislation a state could provide virtually all medical services to those in the appropriate categories and open such categories to those with relatively high income levels. In theory the Secretary of HEW could issue a series of tough interpretative regulations, which would give the general provisions the teeth of specificity.

Within the legislation were, however, the seeds of Medicaid's future difficulties: a lack of clarity as to who was covered and for what, factors which were to make the Medicaid program a target for action in behalf of the poor by legal services programs; a gap between the rhetoric of expansion and equality on the one hand and the flexibility allowed to individual states on the other; the dilemma of grafting a health program on to a still partly voluntary system of state welfare assistance; the failure to give to HEW the authority to administer the program in specific respects; and, finally, the lack of any time frame in which HEW might develop regulations before state programs might be submitted. As it was, the states began to develop their interpretation of the law before the new Medical Services Administration of the Social and Rehabilitation Services in HEW was fully activated.

Yet the prevailing mood of Title XIX was cautiously optimistic. Instead of a series of vendor payment programs there was to be one (Medicaid) program in each state, with each state moving toward providing comprehensive health care. The federal Welfare Administration (renamed the Social and Rehabilitation Service) stated, "A basic concept of Title XIX is that of equality of medical and remedial care and services."[44] At least some states took the encouragement seriously, more seriously perhaps than Congress had expected, for the Congress had projected the additional cost of the new program at only $238 million annually.[45] The period of reality was about to set in.

NOTES

1. Public Law 89–97, Sec. 1901.
2. *Ibid.*, Sec. 1902 (a) (1).
3. *Ibid.*, Sec. 1902 (a) (4).
4. *Ibid.*, Sec. 1902 (a) (6).
5. *Ibid.*, Sec. 1902 (a) (8).
6. *Ibid.*, Sec. 1902 (a) (3).
7. *Ibid.*, Sec. 1902 (a) (7).
8. *Ibid.*, Sec. 1902 (a) (9).

9. *Ibid.*, Sec. 1902 (a) (5).

10. U.S., Senate, Committee on Finance, *Social Security Amendments of 1965*, Senate Report 89–404, 89th Cong., 1st Sess., 1965, p. 76.

11. The one exception allowed by law to the "single state agency" approach was that states which previously had a separate Title X (AB) agency could continue to use that agency in administering the portion of its Medicaid program related to blind persons. P.L. 89–97, Sec. 1902 (a) (22).

12. Specifically, the nonfederal percentage is determined by the following formula:

$$\text{nonfederal percentage} = \frac{45\% \times (\text{Per capita state income})^2}{(\text{Per capita national income})^2}$$

For example, if the national per capita income is $5000 a year, while that of the individual state is $4000, then the state would be required to provide 28.8 percent of the Medicaid assistance bill, while the federal government would supply the remaining 71.2 percent.

13. P.L. 89–97, Sec. 1903 (a), (c), (1), (d).

14. *Ibid.*, Sec. 1902 (a) (2). In 1967 the deadline was changed to July 1, 1969.

15. *Ibid.*, Sec. 1903 (a); Sec. 1903 (c) (1); Sec. 1903 (d).

16. *Ibid.*, Sec. 1904.

17. The generally accepted categories of covered persons were clarified in U.S. Advisory Commission on Intergovernmental Relations, *Intergovernmental Problems in Medicaid* (Washington, 1968), pp. 10–12. See also CCH, *Medicare & Medicaid Guide*, par. 14,211–71; U.S. Department of Health, Education, and Welfare, Welfare Administration, Bureau of Family Services, *Medical Assistance Programs Under Title XIX of the Social Security Act*, Handbook of Public Assistance Administration: Supplement D, pars. D-4010-50 (1966). We use the terminology of *Intergovernmental Problems*, rather than *Supplement D*. Their relationship is described in CCH, *Medicare & Medicaid Guide*, par. 14,251. Also useful is Sydney Bernard and Eugene Feingold, "The Impact of Medicaid," *Wisconsin Law Review*, 1970, No. 3, pp. 726–732.

18. P.L. 89–97, Sec. 1902 (a) (10).

19. *Ibid.*, Sec. 1902 (b).

20. *Ibid.*, Sec. 1905 (a) (15) (A) and (B).

21. *Ibid.*, Sec. 1902 (a) (10) (B) (i).

22. *Ibid.*, Sec. 1902 (a) (10) (B) (ii); Sec. 1902 (a) (10) (A) (i).

23. *Ibid.*, Sec. 1902 (a) (17).

24. *Fullington v. Shea*, 320 F. Supp. 500 (D. Colo., 1970).

25. The legislative history would indicate a divergence between what Congress intended and what it enacted. See S. Report 89–404, *supra*, note 10, p. 78, which seems to assume that Title XIX would correct this anomaly.

26. P.L. 89–97, Sec. 1905 (a) (i).

27. *Ibid.*, Sec. 1902 (a) (13) (A). Up to July 1, 1967, states might provide merely "some institutional and some noninstitutional care and services" (the Kerr-Mills formula).

28. *Ibid.*, Sec. 1902 (a) (13) (B).

29. *Ibid.*, Sec. 1814 (b).

30. *Ibid.*, Sec. 1905 (a) (6)–(15).

31. In the event, at least in the early years of Medicaid, the existence of the voluntary services did provoke a wider array of services. Of the 27 programs in existence in early 1968, only 2 (Idaho and Maine) were limited to the basic five; these programs were also limited to the categorically needy. Tax Foundation Inc., *Medicaid: State Programs After Two Years* (New York, 1968), pp. 13, 63.

32. P.L. 89–97, Sec. 1903 (e).

33. The interpretation offered by the federal Welfare Administration in June 1966 was that a state should show "progressive steps in the direction of a comprehensive scope of medical care and services." *Supplement D, supra,* note 17, d-1100.

34. P.L. 89–97, Sec. 1902 (a) (20)–(21).

35. *Ibid.*, Sec. 1902 (a) (11).

36. *Ibid.*, Sec. 1861 (k).

37. *Ibid.*, Sec. 1868.

38. *Ibid.*, Sec. 1867.

39. *Ibid.*, Sec. 1902 (a) (15). See also Sec. 1843.

40. *Ibid.*, Sec. 1902 (a) (14).

41. *Ibid.*, Sec. 1902 (a) (18).

42. *Ibid.*, Sec. 1902 (a) (16).

43. *Ibid.*, Sec. 1902 (a) (17) (D).

44. *Supplement D, supra,* note 17, d-5143.

45. S. Report 89–404, *supra,* note 10, p. 85.

PART II
The Euphoric Demise

JULY 1965 – JANUARY 1968

INTRODUCTION

The passage of Medicaid provided the states with legislation, giving them a green light to reorganize and expand their vendor payment schemes. Action thus moved to the states and to the various groups and individuals with particular interest in Medicaid's implementation: the state legislatures, welfare rights organizations, medical societies, and nursing-home representatives. Idealists may frame laws; realists have to administer them. Although optimists saw in Medicaid something much grander than its public assistance heritage justified, Medicaid was, after all, the logical culmination of the development of welfare medicine. Not surprisingly, there were to be almost immediate tensions between the practical realities of welfare administration and the expansionist rhetoric of mainstream medicine.

Title XIX was signed into law on July 30, 1965, with a blaze of publicity. Two-and-a-half years later, on January 2, 1968, its author and supporter, President Lyndon Johnson, was constrained to sign a bill which signalled the beginning of the demise of Medicaid. In Medicaid's brief youth it was estimated that if all states developed broad and extensive plans, as many as 35 million people could be covered, close to 20 percent of the population.[1] Yet less than three years after its passage, when Medicaid was covering some eight million recipients,[2] the major cries were for cutbacks, both in program and in eligibility. By 1968, much of the present pattern of concern over Medicaid was set. An era of optimistic expansion was to be replaced by one of questioning, retraction, and criticism.

What happened? As might be expected, Medicaid was differently interpreted in different states; but equality was to be a relatively minor issue. Rather, Medicaid began almost at once to exhibit the inherent stress built into it. As with Kerr-Mills, state and federal goals were not aligned. It was the experience in the states which was to ricochet to Washington to form the rationale of the 1967 Amendments. But even this does not totally explain the shift in attitudes, which must be seen in the Great Society's larger context. For many of the programs launched in the mid-1960s, the spirit of prodigality—services at any cost—was to be replaced by the spirit of managerial efficiency. For Medicaid the process was accelerated for two reasons: first, because, as part of the welfare galaxy, it attracted relatively low political priority; second, because of the demand created by Medicaid and other programs, Medicaid was caught in the rapidly rising price spiral of medical care.

Whatever the reasons for Medicaid's lack of a constituency, the first 50 months of the program were critical. During this time the basic interpretations of the 1965 legislation were established, not always, it would seem, entirely in accordance with the original intention of either the legislators or the legislation, as far as these could be ascertained. Throughout this period, too, the equivocal role of the federal government in health was constantly being underlined. In Medicaid Congress had passed a program of massive proportions and minimal federal accountability.

NOTES

1. Robert J. Myers, *Medicare* (Bryn Mawr, 1970), p. 266.

2. U.S., Department of Health, Education, and Welfare, *Report of the State-Federal Task Force on Costs of Medical Assistance and Public Assistance*, October, 1968, p. 113.

5
Implementation

In terms of implementing the often vague and confusing provisions of Title XIX (Medicaid), an important basic point should be made. Once Medicaid had been signed into law, in July 1965, states could proceed to develop their plans instantly. While federal payments to states were not begun until January 1966, there was no specified period of gestation for appropriate interpretations to be made and federal regulations written before the law took effect within the states. States with a well-organized planning staff, experience with Kerr-Mills, and an eye to early federal subsidies quickly moved into action. From the beginning, therefore, there was little chance for federal initiative. In this as well as in other respects, Medicaid's implementation, through independent state readings of the federal legislation, was different from the relatively orderly and straightforward development of federal standards and procedures for Medicare, which came into effect on July 1, 1966.

The contrasting style of implementation of Medicare deserves emphasis. In the year between the signing of the law and the implementation of that program, the Social Security Administration, the federal agency responsible for Medicare, building on pre-1965 planning, recruited staff, issued basic regulations, including standards for provider participation, surveyed thousands of hospitals and other health facilities to determine eligibility to participate, worked with state health agencies, which were made responsible for standards of health-care providers under Medicare, negotiated contracts with the nonprofit agencies (Blue Cross and Blue Shield) and the commercial insurance carriers that were to act as fiscal intermediaries for Medicare Part A and carriers for Part B, and conducted a massive public relations campaign to inform the 19 million people aged 65 years and over of the benefits of Part A and of the necessity for signing up for Part B of Medicare.[1] In all these respects Medicare had the administrative advantages of being both a completely new program and one administered solely from the federal level, by a well-established, well-ordered and well-accepted entity within HEW. Regulations could be made and channeled down through SSA's existing network of regional and district offices, through which the basic Social Security insurance benefits are organized. By July 1966, sufficient groundwork had been laid for Medicare to take effect with minimal confusion and disorganization.[2]

The implementation of Medicaid was quite different. In some respects Medicaid was a new program; but in others, it was merely an extension of what was going on before. States were quick to grasp the potential expansionist element in Medicaid, in the same way that they had grasped the potential of Kerr-Mills five years earlier. For some states, already engaged in expanding programs of medical assistance, Medicaid provided enabling legislation to allow for a rather faster progress than would otherwise be possible. New York was one example; California and Connecticut were others. As a result, the development of state plans for Medicaid was underway before the basic provisions of the law were fully clarified and interpreted in the series of letters and documents that began emerging from HEW in the fall of 1965. Thus, in the Medicaid program, implementation proceeded simultaneously at the state and federal levels.[3]

The Federal Response

At the federal level, the distance between the euphoria over the potential of Medicaid and the realities of federal welfare administration could not have been greater. The New Society programs of President Lyndon Johnson were in full flood. The year 1965 was the *annus mirabilis.* Federal aid to education was expanded at all levels, expenditures in the War on Poverty were moving into high gear, special social programs were initiated for older Americans, and legislation for Regional Medical Programs authorized regional cooperative arrangements with respect to heart disease, cancer, and stroke. Federal aid for domestic social programs, in this short period before the wave of ghetto riots and the disillusion of Vietnam, appeared to be an unending and beneficent stream in which the problems of inequity would finally be tackled. The President and his Secretary of HEW, John Gardner, could not contain their excitement:

> *The Nation is going through an intensely creative period. . . . We are not just giving out money. We are trying to strengthen all the Nation's social institutions so that they can continue to play a creative and independent role. That may be the most revolutionary single thing that we are doing today. It means that the Federal Government, far from trying to dominate, is trying increasingly to preserve the pluralism of our society. We are heading toward a new kind of creative federalism, toward*

the establishment of new relationships that will see us through not only the complexity of today but the increasing complexity of the decades to come.[4]

Strengthening the institutions concerned with medical vendor payments was not, however, quite so simple. Medicaid, a state program made possible through federal funds, provided a prime example of the potential of "creative federalism." But there was a long weight of tradition in federal-state relationships with respect to welfare payments. Title XIX was, inevitably, to be administered by the Department of Health, Education, and Welfare. The legislation itself did not consign the program to any particular branch of HEW. In theory, a new division could have been established for Medicaid, outside the existing structure of the Welfare Administration. But HEW itself, struggling to implement a plethora of new and expanding social welfare programs, was scarcely in a position to establish a strong new division prepared, if necessary, to hassle and to confront the states and the providers of medical care.

Nor, indeed, was HEW in a position to provide a unified base for the various health programs developing in 1965. With each new piece of legislation came another layer of bureaucracy at the federal level. One set of persons was working on Hill-Burton grants to hospitals, another on grants for community mental health and retardation centers, another on community centers for older Americans (and individual centers might include health services), another on regional medical programs, and others on programs for special population groups—Indians or Cubans, as well as those who lived in Appalachia, or in the urban ghettos. As different bureaus and divisions were involved, there was no structure on which to attach Medicaid as a basic new program designed to give health care to the poor. In particular, ever since the Department had been created early in the Eisenhower administration, HEW had defied even the most aggressive Secretary in his efforts to make it operate as a coherent effective whole. Although this is a subject to which we shall have to return from time to time, at the moment we merely adopt President Johnson's frustrated reaction: the HEW of the mid-1960s, he said, was "a programmatic and bureaucratic nightmare."[5]

Whether Medicaid was to be regarded as a "health" or as a "welfare" program was to become increasingly important in ensuing debates. Many in 1965 assumed that Medicaid would provide the basis for widespread health care for the poor, yet its historical evolution pointed clearly to the narrower welfare mold. President Johnson might well announce that "Today we expect what yesterday we could not have envisioned—adequate medical care for every citizen."[6] But, by assigning responsibility for Title XIX to the Welfare Administration rather than to the Health arm of HEW, its creators ensured that Medicaid would inevitably be regarded as an intrinsic part of the administrative system of federal welfare grants to the states.

While this assignment may have been the only realistic alternative at the time, the effect was to recognize Medicaid—federally as well as in the states—as an extension of Kerr-Mills and other vendor payment programs rather than as a new philosophy or new approach. At the same time, some important limitations on the federal role in Medicaid were implicitly assumed. Traditionally, as we have noted, the states have had enormous freedom in determining the size and scope of categorical assistance—or indeed whether to have such a program at all. Federal regulations have tended to establish minimal criteria to be met in the states' welfare plans—for example, criteria for age, residence, and citizenship qualifications—but once approved programs are in operation, the states have had wide flexibility in developing welfare programs as they think fit. Effective federal control has been kept to a minimum.[7]

This tradition was important with respect to Medicaid. While federal control was being exercised firmly in other new programs of the 1960s, which also involved federal-state cooperation, Medicaid was attached to a relatively permissive ongoing system. Urban renewal grants, for example, made federal aid contingent on federal approval of such questions as the participation of local communities, and the legislation for Comprehensive Health Planning in 1966 was to take a similar line. But public assistance grants-in-aid were channeled to the states with very little standard-setting. As Gilbert Steiner has noted, "funds that may not be provided to support the cost of a highway that is too narrow or a building that is inadequately wired may be provided to support relief benefits below minimum standards of health and decency."[8] Whether desirable or not, this was the political reality within which Medicaid was to be administered.

The administering agent for Kerr-Mills, and then for Medicaid, was the Division of Medical Services of the Bureau of Family Services, which was in turn a part of the Welfare Administration. On July 1, 1965, the Medical Services Division had only 23 employees, including clerical staff. Many of the professional staff had spent all or most of their professional life in social work or in fields related to social work, and they were attuned to the traditional view of the vested power of the states in welfare administration, including the administration of medical vendor payments. Although, with passage of Title XIX, a further 35 positions were created, the 58 persons in the Division were expected to implement poorly drafted legislation, negotiate with powerful states, and administer a budget that was soon consuming a fifth of all federal expenses in medical care—a sum running into billions of dollars.[9] To add to their woes, leadership in the Division was not strong, and senior positions often remained unfilled for significant periods. There is also some evidence that the Welfare Administration establishment deliberately kept the Medical Services Division weak. Thus no changes were made until August 1967, when the renamed Medical Services Administration (MSA) was given bureau status; and even then the increase in staff was minuscule.[10]

If Congress and the federal bureaucracy failed to provide appropriate manpower to cope with Title XIX, the states, smelling easy federal money under the new Title, began putting on the pressure for implementation. Even as Title XIX was going through Congress, Pennsylvania had a bill in its legislature designed to obtain maximum funds for that state. Within a month of the passage of P.L. 89–97, the Pennsylvania bill was law.[11] California, too, would have been waiting on the doorstep with some version of its so-called Casey Bill but for the fact that at the last moment the County Supervisors Association of California managed to have the measures defeated, arguing that the new program would increase county costs.[12] Other states, too, saw Medicaid as a vehicle for accelerating already accepted welfare developments.[13] Nor were these states by any means alone; in a number of states action was being taken to develop the shape of Medicaid programs appreciably before HEW had clarified its own mind about the direction Medicaid should take.

In the absence of regulations, the meager staff of the Medical Services Division worked hard in 1965 and 1966 to develop guidelines and interpretations for the states. The process was perhaps more akin to the development of the Common Law than to the writing of a Napoleonic Code. The guidelines for Medicaid, published as Supplement D of the earlier and much-used Handbook of Public Assistance, sought to rationalize rather than dictate. Supplement D, a document of several hundred pages, provided states with the basic information on Title XIX. It was not, however, issued until June 1966, by which time the pattern of Medicaid was set in several influential states, most notably California and New York.

Supplement D itself (now superceded) had an odd status. For each provision of Title XIX it offered four sections: the provision as stated in the act; the requirements flowing from this which had to be included in the state plan; the criteria to be used in the administration of the plan; and, finally, the more free-form "interpretation" of what was intended. Except for the first (the provisions themselves), none of the sections had the force of law. They were signed by the Welfare Commissioner (then Dr. Ellen Winston), but their legal status was, to put it mildly, somewhat vague. Yet, for several years, Supplement D remained the primary vehicle for the federal view of the states' responsibilities.

Nowhere was the dichotomy between the "health" (expansionist) and "welfare" (restrictionist) aspects of Medicaid more apparent than in the sections of Supplement D labeled "interpretation." From the arid provisions of the legislation relating to the amount, direction, and scope of assistance emerged an impassioned optimism on the part of some HEW bureaucrats as to what these provisions meant:

> *The passage of Title XIX marks the beginning of a new era in medical care for low income families. The potential of this new title can hardly be over-estimated, as its ultimate goal is the assurance of complete, continuous, family-centered medical care of high quality to persons who are unable to pay for it themselves. The law aims much higher than the mere paying of medical bills, and States, in order to achieve its high purpose, will need to assume responsibility for planning and establishing systems of high quality medical care, comprehensive in scope and wide in coverage.*[14]

As we have seen, however, in terms of what was to be required in the state plan, the actual specifications were minimal.[15]

On the one hand, then, the states were looking at Medicaid as a new source for increasing vendor payments largely according to the states' own criteria. On the other hand, there was the desire on the part of at least some in the federal agency concerned to encourage and to exhort, in the hope that states would indeed seek comprehensive coverage and benefits. Throughout Supplement D the mood was bullish:

> *In seeking to put Title XIX into effect, States are expected to approach the provision of such health services with the aim of making them readily available to all eligible persons. The States are expected, furthermore, to set standards that will be appropriate to insure that the services will be of high quality and to adopt methods of administration designed to assure that the services are furnished in a sympathetic and dignified manner. The emphasis will be focused on medical care as part of a comprehensive plan for services, not just on payment of the medical bill.*[16]

There should have been no surprise when some states took these statements as more than rhetoric and requested federal funding to carry them out.

The State Legislatures Act

The states that already had burgeoning vendor payment programs had a head start in gearing up for Medicaid. Massachusetts, for example, which had been quick to recognize the potential of Kerr-Mills and which had a generous vendor payment program, hoped to realize an additional $15.6 million in federal funds from Medicaid merely by continuing at its current (1965) levels of medical assistance.[17] In general, the order in which the states moved in establishing Medicaid programs was dictated by concerns about maximizing the federal share of vendor programs. As the large states normally already had some provision for medical care in addition to minimal vendor payments, they had the staff to enable them to gear up for larger programs and to make whatever state effort was called for in a new program, and they were well aware of the political and economic advantages of moving quickly. It was these states, therefore, which rudely jostled their way towards the Title XIX trough, to the increasing consternation of legislators and administrators in Washington.

Certainly those with fairly generous medical vendor programs could hardly afford to stay out. Yet only six states met the earliest initiation date for Title XIX, with programs beginning in January 1966—Hawaii, Illinois, Minnesota, North Dakota, Oklahoma, and Pennsylvania;[18] and despite exhortations from the federal level that Medicaid meant comprehensive care to all those eligible, the first states moving to implement Medicaid did so at fairly modest levels. All the earliest programs offered services at about the same level as their Kerr-Mills predecessor or with only a moderate expansion. Eligibility levels for the new program were certainly not overgenerous. Pennsylvania, for example, set a limit of $4000 as the means test for "medical dependency" for a family of four ("Pennsycare") while Illinois set it at $3600.

It was left to the large states of California (whose program began in March 1966) and New York (April 1966), in both of which serious extensions of welfare medicine were in process or proposed, to leave their permanent mark on Medicaid. As with other states implementing or considering Medicaid at the time, their actions were predicated on pre-existing developments in welfare policy and vendor payment programs in those states. While both states saw the fiscal potential of Medicaid's higher matching percentages, their reactions were quite different. California and New York provide massive case studies of the implementation of different elements of federal rhetoric: the one in terms of "comprehensive care" and equality of services; the other in terms of defining the potential scope of "medical indigency."

Sacramento

In 1965 California had a costly,[19] fragmented, uneven, and largely disorganized system of public medical care. Services varied for each category of medical assistance.[20] The variety of programs was made more complex by the existence of an extensive county hospital system.[21] (State aid was also administered at the county level.) Although the public-assistance medical care and Kerr-Mills programs had eliminated many of the variations in county requirements, the county system for the medically indigent continued to vary widely in the provision of services such as dentistry, drugs, home health services, eye care, and appliances. Generally, those who were poor were expected to utilize the county facilities, and, as has been seen, Kerr-Mills recipients were financially penalized for entering a private hospital or nursing home.[22] Finally, there remained considerable hidden subsidies for welfare medicine from the private medical sector.[23]

Taken together, California medical assistance programs provided a patchwork of services, parts of which were generous and comprehensive, but parts of which were relatively minimal. Standardization of programs across assistance categories and across county lines, two notable provisions of Medicaid, automatically implied program expansion. But at the same time there were lobbies in the state anxious to reform the existing programs. Physicians were reported to be expressing "widespread and vocal dissatisfaction with the fees they received, as well as with other program restrictions or impositions."[24] County administrators, represented by the County Supervisors Association of California, were adamant that they should not be forced to provide expanded mandatory programs from local taxes. More generally, too, there was a powerful groundswell to move away from the concept of indigence implied in the county hospital system. From both lobbies came recommendations to give persons eligible for medical assistance the right to seek services from any part of the health care sector and at the same time to develop the county hospitals into community hospitals that would accept private patients.

These movements and recommendations predated Medicaid. They surfaced in the original Casey Bill, A.B. 760, introduced in February 1965. Under this, medically indigent recipients of Kerr-Mills would be given a form of state-organized health insurance,[25] which would remove the stigma of welfare assistance from them. While the Casey Bill was not passed, a bill for implementing Title XIX was introduced into a special session of the legislature in Sacramento in September 1965. Some of its chief items were lineal descendants of the earlier Casey Bill, but the chief selling point of its proponents was cost-saving. In 1964–65, public assistance medical care (including Kerr-Mills) had cost state and county funds 12 million dollars a month, with the federal government adding 8 million; if Title XIX had been in effect, legislators were told, the state and county effort would have been matched by 12 million dollars in federal funds.[26] The new Casey Bill was passed in November 1965.[27] Henceforth, at least in theory, the poor of California were to be brought into the mainstream of middle-class medicine, eligible to seek their medical care equally in both the public and the private sectors.

The two most pressing battles fought during the short, but intense, debates on the legislation were about the relationships of such programs to county governments and the issue of where, in the state administrative hierarchy, responsibility for the new program (Medi-Cal) was to lodge. The county boards of supervisors saw the extension of medical care, thereafter to be recognized as equivalent to that in the private hospitals, as having the potential for putting disastrous strains on their budgets. The fears were by no means unfounded, but the counties were eventually "bought off" with a formula that made the state responsible for all medical costs over each county's traditional share.[28]

The administrative dispute revolved around which of the divisions within the Health and Welfare Agency (HWA) should be given responsibility for administering Medi-Cal. Once again the old question arose: Was this a health or a welfare program? The two candidates for administration were the Department of Public Health (DPH) and the Department of Social Welfare (DSW).[29] The split and social gulf between these two sides of the bureaucracy was as evident in state administrations as it was at the federal level. The Secretary of HEW, John Gardner, was thought to favor Medicaid's being administered by health departments to spare it the welfare image and, in California at least, some members of the DPH were eager to have responsibility for Title XIX within that department. The health department was not, however, trusted by the medical establishment whose support had been crucial for the passage of the Casey Bill. Yet when Governor Brown opted for welfare department administration there was another outcry: The DSW was not acceptable to the counties. The ultimate solution was to give administration of Title XIX to the umbrella department, the Health and Welfare Agency. California's program thus became more health-oriented and less welfare-oriented than programs in most other states. It could be argued that, of all the states, it most fully approached the ideals set forth in HEW's "interpretations": a program of comprehensive care.[30]

The health emphasis was by no means accidental. Assemblyman Casey declared that the bill:

> *. . . gives us the tools with which to break down the barrier between the poor people of this state and high quality comprehensive medical care. We are now able to achieve one high standard of medical and health service for all Californians. By passing this bill, the legislature has recognised an important principle of our society: the right of every human being to good medical care, which is the foundation of productivity and self-support.*[31]

The same day, Senator John Schmitz (Republican, Orange County) characterized the bill as "the most massive step toward socialized medicine that the state has taken."[32]

By entering Medicaid, California was automatically committed to a program of adjusting services upwards to the standards available in its more comprehensive programs. Medi-Cal provided a wide range of fourteen different services, and it set about making these as comprehensive as possible. Continuity of health care was to be encouraged, and prevention and rehabilitation stressed. For those previously covered by Kerr-Mills the 30-day waiting period for hospital and nursing-home care was removed. Care was henceforth available for inpatients and outpatients in both private and public institutions.

At the same time, to comply with the federal legislation, services were to be made available to all groups for whom federal matching was available. Prior to Medi-Cal, services for the medically needy had been restricted to the aged. They were thereafter to be extended (effective 1967) to the other categorically related groups. Care available for parents in AFDC families, for example, was greatly increased. Altogether, an additional 1.2 million persons were eventually to become eligible.[33]

The Medi-Cal legislation was also sophisticated in various administrative aspects: It called for administration either through fiscal agents or through prepaid health care insurance. Blue Cross and Blue Shield were thus designated as state fiscal agents of Medi-Cal for processing and reviewing claims. There were incentives for county hospitals to reorganize as community hospitals. Medi-Cal introduced a system of payment to physicians according to their usual and customary fees, instead of through the fixed-fee schedules of earlier assistance programs. Taken together these moves represented a significant shift in emphasis, away from a minimal direct-service welfare system to a system more like private health insurance.

With these various changes the California program for welfare medicine was virtually transformed, from an erratic program administered through county social welfare departments to a state-run program with a strong service commitment. But in terms of eligibility, the legislation was restrained. Until 1967, Medi-Cal was to be open only to those who had been qualified for medical assistance programs in 1965. Even with expansion of the program scheduled in September 1967, the income limit for a family of four was $4092,[34] a limit similar to those set by the other industrialized and wealthy states. California's generosity lay not in its eligibility levels but in its vision of comprehensive medical care throughout the state and its willingness to consider the restructuring of the institutional provision of health care. It says much for this vision, as well as for the condition of federal-state relations under Medicaid, that Medi-Cal took effect in the state in March 1966, although the state plan was not approved by HEW until May.

Albany

New York,[35] it is true, did not move as fast as California. But when it did, its program was equally significant. New York already had a relatively comprehensive although sometimes erratic array of health benefits available through state programs to welfare recipients and the elderly "medically indigent." In New York City the services themselves were provided through a bewildering variety of sources although efforts were being made to coordinate the public medical sector and to extend services generally. The affiliation of municipal hospitals with voluntary hospitals—in the hope of attracting better staff and upgrading their quality—was already in progress. (The merger would ride forward on the wave of Medicaid funds.) Some hospitals had established home-care programs for poverty groups and comprehensive services for the poor.[36] On an experimental basis, several thousand indigent patients were having their premiums for health services paid through the privately-organized Health Insurance Plan of Greater New York (HIP). Although medical services were often hopelessly disorganized—the kinder critics would call them "pluralistic"—and although an individual might receive care at several clinics or institutions, each ignorant of the care provided by the others, New York City had already accepted a measure of integration of the public and the private sectors.

New York State had always had a relatively generous medical care program of services for those on public assistance or medically indigent within the meaning of Kerr-Mills, and generous eligibility levels.[37] By 1963, for instance, under the expanded Kerr-Mills program, the state welfare department allowed a family of four up to $4700 per annum, while meeting its general medical care expenses. If hospitalization was involved the maximum figure for eligibility might go as high as $5200.[38] This relatively high figure can be explained on economic and political grounds. Politically, in an effort to prevent discrimination against blacks, the Federal Social Security Act of 1935 had required of all categorical assistance programs that they be applied equally in all the political subdivisions of the state. This requirement was carried over into Kerr-Mills and ultimately into Medicaid. The economic fact with which New York had to grapple, however, was highlighted in the Bureau of Labor Statistics data for the cost of living; it was (and is) just much more expensive to live in New York City than upstate. This fact was already beginning to distort MAA (Kerr-Mills).[39] The same distortion passed into Medicaid. New York's reaction to Medicaid was thus quite different from California's. Whereas California's main impetus was to rationalize benefits, New York's major headache was to provide a sufficiently high eligibility level to cover the ever-increasing indigent population of New York City, whether services were given in the public or the private sector, without bankrupting the state or city treasury.

The New York legislature was not in session in the latter part of 1965. But, in any event, the understanding had been that if a state plan were submitted to HEW by March 31, 1966 (some were later to say April 30), it would qualify for reïmbursement backdated to January 1, the commencement day for Title XIX. Thus, on March 9th, Governor Rockefeller sent a Medicaid Bill to the State Legislature with the instruction that time was of the essence.[40]

The bill suggested avoiding the thorny issue of income levels by putting in no maximum limits for Medicaid. Ten days later, however, the Governor came forward with income standards, which, for instance, had a limit of $5700 for a family of four.[41] In response, the Democratic leader, Speaker Travia, produced a more generous set of standards, with the limit for a family of four at $6700.[42] The Republican leaders promptly labelled Travia as the "tool" of Senator Robert Kennedy, and his proposal as "designed to steal Republican thunder." The Governor and Speaker Travia also disagreed on the form of administration of the new program. The Governor's bill called for administration by the State Board of Social Welfare.[43] Speaker Travia wanted administration in the hands of the health department to avoid the "stigma of relief."[44]

There was remarkably little discussion of either bill. Travia's bill passed the Democratically controlled Assembly on March 28, without even appearing on the day's calendar. There had been no hearings on the bill, unless one counts four days of legislative hearings in 1965 before any specific measure had been submitted to the legislature. The Rockefeller bill, after a brief one-day public hearing, had been passed by the Republican-controlled Senate on March 23. With this the two factions sat back.

On April 27, the Governor attempted to force the issue. He sent a message to the legislature warning that it should take immediate steps to implement Medicaid. Indeed he warned that if the bill were not passed by April 30, the state stood in danger of losing $17 million in federal aid for the quarter. Moreover, "the longer the legislation is delayed, the more the chances of complication."[45] This was language everyone understood. Rockefeller and Travia met and hammered out a compromise. The income limits for a family of four were set at $6000; overall administration was to be in the hands of the Department of Social Welfare, but it was obliged to contract with the Health Department with respect to the medical aspects of the program. The compromise bill then passed the Assembly 136–15 and the Senate 64–1. It was all surprisingly unquestioned and harmonious. Noting that few legislators appreciated the scope of the program, one Senator later commented: "And it's a damn good thing . . . because they would never have voted for it if they had."[46] But such thoughts seemed far from the mind of Governor Rockefeller when he signed the bill on April 30, 1966. It was, he claimed, "the most significant social legislation in three decades."[47]

With the passage of New York's legislation, the form of the two major state Medicaid programs was set. The New York program went into effect immediately—again, and significantly, before federal approval of the state plan had been gained. Thus, before Supplement D had even been issued, California and New York were off and running, together with programs in six other states.

Being expansionist in nature, the new programs were naturally expansionist in cost. Indeed, a number of different actors were set to gain financially from Medicaid. Recipients stood to gain from expansion in

service and eligibility and were increasingly willing to express their demands; states looked for additional federal revenue; hospitals had the guarantee of higher reimbursement levels through Medicaid's adoption of "reasonable costs"; and physicians and other providers, interpreting Medicaid's rhetoric of equality literally, were pushing for reimbursement at their private fee levels. Each of these factors alone might have generated a relatively modest and steady increase in Medicaid funding. It was the combined impact of expansion in coverage (in services and eligibility) with an extension of the meaning of vendor payments to purchase in the private sector at private reimbursement levels, that was to create Medicaid's initial headaches. The provisions of the law, reinforced by federal exhortations, were inherently inflationary.

In terms of federal-state relationships there was an apparent assumption that Medicaid costs would be regulated by state constraints. The early enthusiasm of New York and California for considerable expansion in services offered and persons served made it quite evident that state policies would be geared toward program extension. If the costs of medical care had remained stationary, the states would, indeed, have had much to gain. In the event, costs rose rapidly; and, as they did, the early euphoria emanating from HEW came to appear both naive and irresponsible.

NOTES

1. U.S., Congress, House, *First Annual Report on Medicare,* House Doc. No. 331, 90th Cong., 2nd Sess., 1968, p. 3.

2. In retrospect the achievement was extraordinary. In its first full year of operation (July 1966–June 1967), Medicare paid 34 percent of all medical bills of those aged 65 or over, chiefly for hospital and posthospital care. Dorothy P. Rice and Barbara S. Cooper, *Outlays for Medical Care of Aged and Nonaged Persons, Fiscal Years 1966–68* (U.S., Department of Health, Education, and Welfare, Social Security Administration, Office of Research and Statistics, Research and Statistics Note, #12), p. 4.

3. Technically Medicaid became operative on Jan. 1, 1966, the earliest date on which federal payments could be made to states for the new program, under Sec. 1903 (a). However, as no money would be paid until a state plan had been approved, states had to move to develop these plans immediately the legislation was passed, if they wanted early funding of Medicaid.

4. John W. Gardner, Secretary of HEW, "Foreword," *1965: Year of Legislative Achievements* (U.S., Department of Health, Education, and Welfare, Office of the Assistant Secretary, 1965), pp. iii–iv.

5. *Public Papers of the Presidents of the United States: Lyndon B. Johnson 1967* (Washington, 1968), Book II, p. 1099.

6. Quoted in U.S., Department of Health, Education, and Welfare, Office of the Assistant Secretary, *Human Investment Programs, Delivery of Health Services for the Poor* (Washington, 1967), p. i.

7. Gilbert Steiner, writing in 1965, noted that no federal funds had been withheld for noncompliance since a dispute over confidentiality in Indiana in 1951, even though the federal government had by no means won all other disputes concerning federal standards since that case. Gilbert Y. Steiner, *Social Insecurity: the Politics of Welfare* (Chicago, 1966), p. 243.

8. *Ibid.*, p. 247.

9. U.S., Congress, Senate, Committee on Finance, *Medicare and Medicaid, Hearings,* before the Committee on Finance, Senate, 91st Cong., 1st Sess., 1969, p. 112.

10. At this time Social and Rehabilitation Service (SRS) was created, replacing the old Welfare Administration. MSA became a bureau of SRS.

11. Sydney E. Barnard and Eugene Feingold, "The Impact of Medicaid," *Wisconsin Law Review,* 1970, pp. 726–743.

12. For details see U.S., Department of Health, Education, and Welfare, Public Health Service, Margaret Greenfield, *Medi-Cal, The California Medicaid Program* (*Title XIX*) (Washington, 1969), Ch. 2.

13. New York City, for example, was in the process of affiliating its municipal hospitals, a process begun in 1961 but reinforced by the introduction of Medicaid. Connecticut, under the leadership of a progressive welfare administrator, was already in the process of liberalizing eligibility for medical services. Gerald E. Bisbee, *The Growth of the Connecticut State Department of Welfare 1953–72,* paper presented at the Yale Medical School, 1973; Eli Ginsberg *et al., Urban Health Services: The Case of New York* (New York, 1971), p. 115.

14. U.S., Department of Health, Education, and Welfare, Welfare Administration, Bureau of Family Services, *Medical Assistance Programs Under Title XIX of the Social Security Act,* Handbook of Public Assistance Administration, Supplement D (Washington, December 1, 1966), Sec. D–5140.

15. *Ibid.*, Sec. D–5120. States were, for example, to specify the items of medical care and the amounts to be provided to the categorical needy and medically needy; and they were to meet the basic requirements for five services effective July 1967. The plan was to guarantee equivalent entitlements to all beneficiaries and groups of recipients; it was also to describe the methods to be used "to assure that the medical and remedial care and services are of high quality," to provide for "broadening the scope" of services to meet the provision of comprehensive care (a term which remained undefined) to substantially all eligible individuals by July 1975.

16. *Ibid.*, Sec. D–1000.

17. Martha Derthick, *The Influence of Federal Grants: Public Assistance in Massachusetts* (Cambridge, Mass., 1970), pp. 66–67. But this time, perhaps as a result of the understaffed and ill-prepared haste with which Massachusetts had rushed to embrace Kerr-Mills, and the resulting friction between the state and the federal agency, Massachusetts was more wary; its program did not begin until September 1966. *Ibid.*, p. 65 and *passim.*

18. Tax Foundation Inc., *Medicaid: State Programs After Two Years* (New York, 1968), p. 11 and *passim.*

19. In the period July 1, 1965–June 30, 1966, $230 million was spent on medical care through California's various assistance programs. State of California, *Public Welfare in California, 1965–66,* Statistical Series AR 1–8.

20. For example, the services available to those eligible for AB were quite comprehensive, including both inpatient and outpatient benefits, while those

available to parents in the AFDC program were quite restricted. Besides the large programs of Public Assistance Medical Care and Medical Assistance to the Aged (Kerr-Mills), the state operated other medical care programs (including mental health, vocational rehabilitation, crippled children, and tuberculosis) for which public assistance recipients were eligible. Additionally, the state operated a special program for the prevention of blindness. Over and above these medical programs, a number of medical aids and dentures were provided through supplements to the cash grants of recipients, as were supplemental grants for the salaries of aides required at home for medical reasons. On California's programs, see Acton W. Barnes, *A Description of the Organization and Administration of the California Medical Assistance Programs: Title XIX*, mimeograph, School of Public Health, Univ. of North Carolina, 1968; and Greenfield, *supra*, note 12.

21. See Barnes, *supra*, note 20, pp. 18–20 and *passim*. In 1965, California provided 59 county hospitals, in 47 out of the 50 counties. Financial eligibility for county care was a matter of local interpretation.

22. See *supra*, Chs. 2 and 3.

23. Barnes, *supra*, note 20, pp. 21, 23. Five medical schools, for instance, provided care for individuals suitable as "teaching material." More significant was the amount of time donated by private physicians in the county and voluntary hospitals and the low charges and free care provided to welfare patients in their private offices.

24. California Medical Association, *Professional Services to Welfare Recipients in California* (January 1965), quoted by Greenfield, *supra*, note 12, p. 4.

25. See Greenfield, *supra*, note 12, p. 4.

26. In another claim, the mathematics of which are not at once apparent, it was said that failure to pass the new Casey bill (AB 5) would cost the state $6.5 million in federal funds each month.

27. Greenfield, *supra*, note 12, ch. 3.

28. Barnes, *supra*, note 20, pp. 38–39.

29. For the genesis of the HWA, see Greenfield, *supra*, note 12, ch. 4.

30. As required in the federal statute, eligibility determination was the responsibility of the Department of Social Welfare, but services were administered at the "umbrella" level. Greenfield, *supra*, note 12, ch. 3.

31. *Sacramento Bee*, November 4, 1965.

32. *San Francisco Chronicle*, November 4, 1965. In 1972, Sen. Schmitz ran as Presidential candidate on the American Independence Party ticket.

33. *Medicaid*, *supra*, note 18, p. 21.

34. Greenfield, *supra*, note 12, p. 31.

35. On New York's experience, see Benjamin Werne, "Medicaid: Has National Health Insurance Entered by the Back Door?" 18 *Syracuse Law Review* 49 (1966); Comment, "Furor Over Medicaid," 3 *Columbia Journal of Law & Social Problems* 158 (1967); R. B. Titus, *New York's Medicaid: A Study of the Development of a State Title XIX Program—Its Problems and Prospects*, 1968 (paper presented at Yale Law School). The authors acknowledge their debt, especially to the last of these, in their description of the early stages of Medicaid in New York.

36. See George A. Silver, Charles H. Goodrich, Margaret C. Olendzki, and George G. Reader, *Family Medical Care: A Report on the Family Health*

Maintenance Demonstration (Cambridge, Mass., 1963); Charles H. Goodrich *et al., Welfare Care: An Experiment* (Cambridge, Mass., 1970).

37. Indeed, as early as 1929, provision was made for some kinds of medical care to be provided under home relief. Schneider and Deutsch, *The History of Public Welfare in New York State: 1867–1940* (New York, 1969, reprint of 1941 edition), p. 287. The program was extended at the time New York established its old-age assistance program in 1930. *Ibid.*, p. 347.

38. *New York Times,* May 23, 1966, p. 1, reporting a television appearance by Governor Rockefeller later in the year.

39. The State Department of Social Welfare had reported that, during the first three years of Kerr-Mills, 13,281 out of the 28,747 average monthly recipients had been New York City residents, who had accounted for $187,291,499 out of a total expenditure of $289,416,309. In other words, the 46 percent of recipients in New York City had absorbed 64 percent of the costs. *New York Times,* July 30, 1964, p. 28.

40. The Governor's Message appears in *1966 Session Laws of New York* 2989 (McKinney, 1966).

41. *New York Times,* March 21, 1966, p. 26.

42. *Ibid.*, March 21, 1966, p. 26, col. 2; *Ibid.*, March 29, 1966, p. 27, col. 1.

43. *Ibid.*, March 30, 1966, p. 48, col. 1.

44. *Ibid.*, March 29, 1966, p. 27.

45. 1966 *Session Laws of New York* 2990 (McKinney, 1966).

46. *New York Times,* May 21, 1966, p. 14, col. 6. For what legislators had thought they were voting for, see "New Worry for Medicare," *U.S. News & World Report,* June 20, 1966, p. 54.

47. *New York Times,* May 1, 1966, p. 1, col. 2.

6
The Beginning of Disillusion

Even in the spring of 1966, when the majority of states were still only contemplating a Medicaid program, it was clear that the total costs of Medicaid would be far greater than expected. But the moment for general disillusion with Medicaid and other federal health programs, on the grounds of costs, had not yet arrived. An idealistic mood of expansion prevailed. President Johnson, in his Special Message to Congress on Domestic Health and Education on March 1, 1966, recommended further "advances" (and, implicitly, expenditures) to provide "good health for every citizen to the limits of our country's capacity to provide it."[1] Among the recommendations still pouring forth from HEW was that for grants to states for comprehensive health services, legislation which was to be passed in 1966 with a further fanfare of statements on health benefits and rights.[2] But the euphoria of the War on Poverty, especially in Congress, was waning; restrictionist attitudes toward welfare were gaining strength.

In terms of Congressional affection, as well as in terms of prestige within the executive, health has always outstripped welfare. Senators and Representatives sometimes seem to be vying for the position as spokesman for the health side of HEW, and this was especially true in the middle sixties. The Welfare lobby attracts Congressional attention for a totally different reason; a number of influential Congressmen have made their reputation flailing the profligacy of welfare programs and the immorality of welfare recipients.[3] To a varying extent, such phenomena have been paralleled in the states. While the language of Medicaid mouthed "comprehensive care," the ears of the legislators were attuned to the sterner issues of welfare spending. Thus, almost as soon as the first program began, a backlash set in. At first isolated voices in New York and California began a process of disparagement and dissent, but the sentiments voiced were soon reflected by critics on Congressional committees. Medicaid was a welfare program that appeared, to an increasing number of observers, to be an irresponsible junket in which vast public sums were being dissipated.

The First Crisis: The Backlash in New York

New York provided the first series of alarms. However, it was only after the state legislation had passed that the fireworks began. Almost at once the eligibility standards[4] came under vigorous attack. It was appreciated, by many for the first time, that some 8,000,000 people, or 45 percent of the population of the state, would technically be eligible for Medicaid, and nobody seriously contested this. Indeed the Department of Social Welfare conceded this figure as the basis of their calculations.[5] Governor Rockefeller, however, defended himself in a way which tells much about the American approach to medical care. The Governor claimed that experience showed that only 25 percent of persons actually eligible in fact signed up for public-assistance medical care programs. For instance, while 5.5 million persons had been eligible for medical care programs before 1965, the Governor pointed out that only 1.5 million had actually signed up.[6]

The Governor's estimate, moreover, was borne out by the facts. Only 11 percent of the population of the state (roughly 2,000,000 persons) signed up in the first year, not an appreciably higher percentage than in many other states with more limited programs. What distinguished New York was the potential percentage of the population who could be covered. Forty-five percent seemed very large when contrasted with 20 percent in Utah, 16 percent in Oklahoma, 13 percent in California, 10 percent in Connecticut, 9.7 percent in Maryland, 8 percent in Rhode Island and Washington, and 7 percent in Massachusetts.[7] Such a high percentage posed, moreover, a direct threat to the working population earning above the eligibility levels. If the "medically indigent" were to be given equivalent care in the private sector, they were not to be regarded as social failures but rather as competitors for that scarce resource—medical care. From the point of view of those somewhat above the means-test levels, condescension toward assistance recipients was replaced by spirited indignation.

The Governor tried to remedy the situation. In addition to the low utilization argument, he claimed that while the cost of medical assistance would rise sharply, the new formula meant that the brunt of the cost would be carried by the federal government. He expected the state burden to stay about the same, and the local authorities (who covered a quarter of the cost) to find that their contributions would drop appreciably.[8] The Governor appeared on television in a vain effort to quell the rising hostility,[9] most of it from upper New York State, where average incomes were lower than in and around New York City. It was claimed that in some upstate counties 70 percent of the population would be eligible for Medicaid, and the statistics certainly lent credence to this assertion. Moreover, the Governor was ultimately forced to admit that while New York City might be expected to save $54 million and large upstate communities might be helped, many upstate communities would have to pay out far more in medical care costs. Local welfare commissioners, employers' lobbies, even the State Farm Bureau set up a clamor, all saying that far too many persons were covered by Medicaid. The problem was that there was no generally accepted notion of what proportion of the population ought to be covered. It was the inevitable reaction to be expected when means-test medicine was expanded. Those a little or somewhat above the level of "medical indigency" were not likely to be enamored.

The medical profession was in a somewhat odd position. The AMA, it will be remembered, had favored "welfare medicine" and vigorously opposed anything savoring of health insurance. As one president of the AMA had put it: "Medicaid is the expression of a philosophy the American Medical Association has expounded since 1960."[10] Indeed the State Medical Society had earlier called for raising the level of eligibility for MAA assistance. While the New York bill was still being discussed, the President of the State Medical Society (Dr. James Blake) had sent telegrams to legislators urging its passage—provided that the State Medical Advisory Board include at least seven doctors, that only doctors approved by local medical societies be appointed as local medical directors, and that freedom of choice of physician be written into the legislation.[11]

As the bill was passed without these "safeguards," the State Medical Society convened a special meeting of its House of Delegates. Held on May 26, the meeting represented a wide spectrum of views. Several upstate medical societies (e.g., Niagara, Montgomery, Genesee) called for outright repeal of the new state program. The Erie County Medical Society urged the Secretary of HEW not to approve the state plan as it was currently drafted. But the leaders of the Society managed to hold to a more moderate position. The resolution which finally emerged called for implementation of the three demands made during the passage of the legislation, together with a demand that reimbursement be "on a usual, customary and prevailing basis," that is, that the prevailing fee schedules for welfare patients (which were generally low) be replaced by the equivalent of private fees. It also demanded that no "prior authorization" for medical services be required, that only Blue Cross and Blue Shield be used as fiscal agents, and that "continued consideration be given to the feasibility of deductible and coinsurance features."[12]

While the State Medical Society managed to maintain a remarkably balanced "face," some of the local medical societies were making more hawkish noises. The Suffolk County Medical Society, for instance, resolved that Medicaid was "socialized medicine" and that it operated "to deprive physicians of their constitutional rights to practice medicine in a free society."[13] By July a new lobbying organization had been formed, representing some 2900 doctors and dentists, the Association of New York State Physicians and Dentists, Inc. The Association filed a brief with HEW asking that approval not be given to the New York plan, arguing that the New York plan violated congressional intent with respect to the definition of "needy persons" and, among other things, claiming that the proposals would lead to declining standards of medical care.[14]

It was not only the medical profession which was disturbed about the Medicaid proposals; diverse interests, including industry, appeared to protest the legislation.[15] As the post-passage outcry grew, the Governor and the key Republican leadership decided that "a massive publicity campaign was needed to overcome widespread 'misimpressions' of the program's scope and cost."[16] Among other moves, it was decided to hold the hearings that had not been held before passage of the bill, and a Joint Legislative Committee was designated for this purpose. At first Speaker Travia refused to appoint any Assembly members to such a committee. But he ultimately agreed, and the three days of hearings began on May 24. These gave the medical groups and the employers' groups an opportunity to have their say.[17]

Nevertheless, few suggested amendments emerged from these hearings. At the end of June, the Republican-controlled Senate passed five amendments, including the right of choice of physician as demanded by the State Medical Society and three amendments relating to changes in the financial status of recipients. The most serious amendment was a "deductible" clause, designed to curb excessive use and small claims,[18] even though the use of deductibles, at least for the "categorically needy," was prohibited by the wording of Title XIX. Travia remained opposed to this last amendment, and it looked as if the measure would remain bottled up in the Rules Committee. At that point the Republicans threatened not to vote the New York City budget package.[19] A compromise deductible arrangement then mysteriously emerged, whereby families with $4500 or more would have to pay out 1 percent of their income before being eligible for Medicaid.[20] As thus compromised, the amendment passed.

But even then there were still hurdles to be cleared. In June, in what was to be the first judicial test of Medicaid, the Citizens Committee for Responsible Government began a soon-aborted action against the Department of Social Welfare alleging abuse of administrative authority as the Department set about to implement the Act.[21] When the movement failed to have the Medicaid legislation annulled either by the state legislature or the courts, it shifted its assault to Washington, where the state plan still had to be approved by HEW. Even before the Governor had signed the bill on April 30, the Department of Social Welfare had been at work consolidating all existing programs into a massive new Medicaid program, and early in

May a plan was submitted to HEW. Already the "doctors and dentists" brief was on the desk of the General Counsel and further attempts to pressure the Secretary of HEW were soon under way. On May 18 eight upstate New York legislators called on the federal government to withhold approval; while Representative Stratton, representing eight mid-upstate counties in the House, led a major attack to discourage the Secretary of HEW from approving the state plan.

While HEW vacillated, the lobbying continued. The situation was extraordinary. The federal welfare agency was being asked by the opponents to overrule a state on a welfare program without having any legislative authority to do so, for, if nothing else, P.L. 89-97 had given states clear responsibility to establish their own eligibility levels. The state interest was obviously being pressed: Governor Rockefeller, Commissioner of Welfare Wyman, Commissioner of Health Ingraham, Senator Javits, 18 of New York's 43 Congressmen, and four state legislators met with HEW Under-Secretary Wilbur Cohen early in June.

By law[22] HEW had 90 days from the submission of the plan on May 1 to approve or disapprove it. In a way that was to characterize much of the administration of Medicaid, such legal requirements were ignored, for fiscal and political reality had caught up with the administration. In the hallowed tradition of welfare, costs were becoming more important than services. In short, the problem was that the revised figures under the New York plan would call for a federal sharing of $145 million more than the state had been receiving under Kerr-Mills and the other public assistance medical programs. Unfortunately HEW had predicted that, nationwide, Title XIX would only cost $155 million more than Kerr-Mills; thus New York's plan alone would eat up most of the budget. Yet HEW had just approved California's plan (in May) which was also to be extremely expensive. And a number of other states were lining up for the federal largesse. Meanwhile, in June, Representative Stratton introduced a bill to cut back on Title XIX; and by August the House Ways and Means Committee was holding closed hearings on Medicaid. In fact Congress did not act that session, adjourning in October; but it threatened to return to the matter of Medicaid the following session.

HEW, after six and a half months, at last felt free to act. On November 15, the New York plan was approved, the final estimated federal share for the first year being $217 million.[23] But HEW did make some economies. It refused to reimburse New York for the first quarter of 1966, on the ground that the plan had not been submitted before March 31. The state protested vigorously, alleging that Senator Kennedy's office had been assured by HEW Welfare Commissioner Ellen Winston that there was "no magic in the March date." The Governor estimated that some $30 million had been lost by this maneuver.[24] But by this time New York had other problems.

Problems in State Administration: New York and California Contrasted

Against the furor in New York, California's Medicaid extensions moved relatively smoothly. Indeed, in the first part of 1966, the political opposition to Medi-Cal was chiefly on the ground that it was too restrictive.[25] New York jumped in at the deep end with inadequate administrative machinery. With better administration, California still moved slowly.

California, had, of course, six months lead on New York. The California plan was ready for submission in Washington in January 1966; state regulations were adopted in February.[26] Although there were some bureaucratic rivalries, both DSW and DPH were within the umbrella of the Health and Welfare Agency, and a series of formal agreements between the different departments were drawn up.[27] An Office of Health Care Services (OHCS), reporting directly to the Administrator of the Health and Welfare Agency, was also established to run Medi-Cal. Moreover, as has been seen, for the purposes of payment of providers, California opted for the fiscal agent system.[28]

On paper California looked eminently well prepared for implementing Title XIX, but even there problems soon began to arise. The OHCS turned out to be a thorn in the flesh of more established parts of the bureaucracy and to be lacking in at least some administrative skills. Differences in interpretation of the agreements between the various departments gave rise to increasing friction. By the fall of 1966, there was open hostility between OHCS and DPH about responsibility for medical consultants. It was never clear whether OHCS was a staff service or a line agency. OHCS increasingly complained about the attitude of DPH and DSW. There were specific fights about which prescription drugs would be paid for and about payment to hospital-based physicians.[29] But the blow-up in California, as in New York, was to be fiscal and political. The "county formula" proved to be very complex to operate, and there were political charges and countercharges. After November 1966 the Republicans were in control of the executive, and Governor Ronald Reagan espoused fiscal control. It was already evident that Medi-Cal was a true "sleeper" in terms of the costs of the program, although the exact amounts involved were not readily available.

While the California program was liberalizing available services and upgrading the county hospital system, during 1966 New York was struggling to implement its as yet unapproved program.[30] The operation was somewhat less elegant than California's. There was far more devolution, with New York City *de facto* running its own program. There was a great urge to get everyone who might be eligible off existing welfare programs and onto Title XIX where the reimbursement formula was more generous. But California's planning and phasing were noticeably absent. It was not easy to persuade persons to sign up for Medicaid.[31] In at least one sense the state predictions had been right. The over-all state costs under Medicaid were no higher than the costs under the earlier vendor payment programs,[32] and utilization—as Governor Rockefeller had predicted—was likely to be no more than 25 percent of those eligible.

While those on welfare were automatically eligible for Medicaid, few of the "medically indigent" signed up, although New York City planned a major sign-up drive.[33] Even though it was assumed that some four million persons in New York City were eligible for Medicaid, only 18,500 registered during the first six weeks,[34] and by the end of 1966, only 600,000 had signed up. The *New York Times* suggested the complex application form was the chief barrier ("at least as difficult as the long-form tax return").[35] Nine out of twelve processing centers in New York City had to close because of the light turnout. Early in 1967, a new drive was launched in the City—"Medicaid Alert"—with a house-to-house canvass undertaken by welfare recipients earning $1.50 an hour for enrolling persons.[36] Such problems illustrated that if Sacramento had the burden of dealing with the counties, Albany had the problem of dealing with "Fun City."

To serve this population effectively, the cooperation of private physicians was essential. Every effort had been made to placate the doctors, but New York, unlike California, had no fiscal agent to shelter behind. The law had been amended to ensure medical representation on state and local committees,[37] and free choice of physician had eventually been assured by regulation.[38] But the State Medical Society was still disturbed about the fee schedule. In May 1966 a Task Force headed by the Director of the State Budget Bureau came up with a suggested fee scale, which differed markedly from the medical society's demands. (For example, the Task Force suggested $6.50 for an initial office visit; the medical society wanted $10.)[39] When Governor Rockefeller pointed out that many of the proposed fees exceeded those paid by private insurers,[40] the society took the position that the private schedules were out of date.[41] Ultimately, in August 1966, the Governor, in an effort to placate the medical profession, created an Interdepartmental Committee on Health Economics,[42] and a five-man Advisory Committee from the medical society was established to assist the Interdepartmental Committee.[43]

The physicians, however, had still other gripes. They would have preferred to deal with an "agent," such as Blue Shield, over fees.[44] The State Medical Society, instead, urged Congress to pass legislation requiring states to pay recipients, who would then pay providers.[45] The Suffolk County Medical Society still refused to cooperate at all in Medicaid. Moreover, state-wide, physicians showed no enthusiasm for signing up for the program. The Department of Social Welfare required doctors wishing to participate in Medicaid to sign up by January 1, 1967. By that date, only 4500 of New York City's 15,000 physicians had signed up. "I wouldn't call it a boycott—

this is merely an expression of the way doctors feel about the program," said Dr. Himler, Chairman of the Coordinating Council of the Five County Medical Societies of the City of New York.[46] And, as he made clear a few days later, enthusiasm for the program would not return until doctors were paid their "usual and customary fees."[47] But it was also clear that the physicians feared utilization control. When the City promulgated a utilization regulation for providers beginning "Penalties for inappropriate utilization or practice shall be determined by the (New York City) Health Services Administration" and providing removal from the registry for non-cooperating practitioners, the State Health Department, egged on by organized medicine, forced its withdrawal.[48]

It would be wrong, though, to equate the provider problem with the issue of physicians. New York City was to have problems with all its providers. Only 2400 out of 7500 dentists (32 percent) signed up,[49] 450 out of 1100 optometrists (41 percent), and 450 out of 1000 (45 percent) podiatrists.[50] Indeed, the city was forced to give a three-month extension for signing up,[51] and the state ultimately had to cancel the sign-up requirement. In dealings with hospitals, too, there were problems. Title XIX, as interpreted by the regulations, required that with respect to hospitals Medicaid was to follow Medicare standards for reimbursement—in this case, "reasonable cost." Initially this appeared to be a windfall for the hospitals, or at least the taxpayers of New York. Not only would the voluntary hospitals cease to provide underreimbursed "charity medicine," but New York's massive public hospital system could also be a major beneficiary of federal-state relief. As the financial difficulties of the hospitals were just reaching their climax, there were those who saw Medicaid as a financial savior.

But the hopes of those who saw a transformation of the municipal hospitals were short-lived. Aware of the ramifications of P.L. 89–97 the New York City administration announced its intention of putting the $100 million from federal and state payments for Medicaid care provided at municipal hospitals directly into the City's General Fund. In other words, Medicaid payments were to be treated as a tax windfall. The announcement of this position coincided with a dramatic investigation of the condition of the City's hospitals by State Senator Seymour Thaler (Democrat, Queens), while the Chairman of the Joint Legislative Committee on Public Health and Medicine, State Senator Norman Lent (Republican, Nassau) announced that the greatest danger facing Medicaid was the possible "perpetuation of an in-grown, institutionalized system of neglect in treating the medical indigent."[52] City Council President Frank O'Connor demanded that Medicare and Medicaid funds be "plowed back into an improvement of our health and hospital services, not merely added to general city revenues."[53] Under these pressures the Lindsay Administration reversed itself.[54] The hospital system was to receive the unexpected windfall from Medicaid funding. Nevertheless, the opportunity was not to be taken to use the additional funds in an integrated way to improve all medical care in the city system. More money went into existing inefficiencies.

There were other problems which the hospitals faced with the advent of P.L. 89–97. Payment for care at "reasonable cost" implied that recipients were private patients, rather than objects of institutional benevolence. But the idea that poor patients might have rights was seen by some to threaten both medical education and medical research. Dr. Philip Barnet, immediate past president of the American Hospital Association, noted "the clear probability of the disappearance of the 'ward service' patient—the 'charity patient'—the 'second class' patient—upon whom has rested nearly the whole reliance for graduate medical education and a major part of undergraduate medical education."[55] The research concern was put by the Chairman of the Public Health Committee of the King's County Medical Society, Dr. Philip Cantor, in these terms: "How do you expect [continuing medical research] to be carried out if patients come to a hospital only for medical care and are not interested in taking part in new and as yet unaccepted methods of treatment?"[56] Obviously, Medicaid had psychological hurdles as well as political and economic ones to surmount.

Medicaid: Other States

Only the most optimistic could have asserted by the summer of 1966 that Medicaid was going to be a health program that would sweep equally through all the states. California and New York had provided the most dramatic examples of the potential coverage and the potential costs of Medicaid. But these programs also underscored the independence of each state's responses to the provisions of P.L. 89–97. Each response was colored not so much by the comprehensive vision of federal intent as by local political conditions, prevailing attitudes to welfare, and (perhaps of most importance) the scope of vendor payments already being made in that state.

For some states the trend toward expansion was set before Medicaid, and Medicaid did not so much accelerate it, as more richly underscored it. California and New York could move directly into Medicaid on the basis of decisions already taken in their implementation of the Kerr-Mills program. Connecticut, similarly, received a federal windfall of $30 million in Kerr-Mills funds in five years, through judicious interpretation of that legislation.[57] A progressive package of social welfare benefits was passed by the Connecticut General Assembly in 1965, including provisions for liberalizing the Kerr-Mills program. With an eye to how far the legislature would go, Welfare Commissioner Bernard Shapiro recommended a relatively slow development for Connecticut's already generous program. This meant, of course, a bonus to the state through Medicaid's larger federal subsidy, without a vast additional increase in medical services.[58] The state had nothing to lose. This did not mean there were not consultations. There were.[59] Medical groups, social agencies, and state government departments were consulted. There was considerable consultation with Connecticut's powerful insurance industry, which had extensive experience in dealing with medical claims and whose members were becoming involved as "fiscal intermediaries" and "carriers" under Medicare. Moreover, the Connecticut General group was ultimately made fiscal agent for payments to physicians under the state's Medicaid program.

The Connecticut Medicaid program began on July 1, 1966. It was not an ambitious program for the second wealthiest state *per capita* in the nation. The fiscal limits for a family of four were set at $3800; and it was estimated that some 90,500 families in the state were eligible for the program, 4300 of them being "medically indigent."[60] On the other hand, most of the types of medical coverage permitted by Title XIX were included in the program. Connecticut thus avoided the early disillusion in New York by maintaining relatively low income limits. While the program provided a wide range of services, it was also designed to fit into the state's broader philosophy of welfare: "to help needy persons to achieve their maximum degree of economic independence, and physical, mental and social well-being."[61] In short, Medicaid in Connecticut (as in most other states implementing the program) was one aspect of assisted self-help.

A natural outcome of the low income levels and the administration of the program by the Welfare Department was that the welfare mentality survived. While P.L. 89–97 specifically prohibited holding children responsible for the medical expenses provided to their parents by the state, Connecticut was anxious not to let die an idea which had arrived with the Pilgrims. A bulletin announced that the "Connecticut State Welfare Department policy recognizes that there are many children who feel a moral obligation to provide financial assistance to their needy aged parents if they are requested to do so."[62] Procedures were then laid down to put pressure on the children, including an investigation of their means and a dunning letter from the department itself.[63] The Department later backed off somewhat, but there was little doubt in anyone's mind that Medicaid in Connecticut was the lineal descendant of the Elizabethan Poor Law.

Whereas in Connecticut Medicaid was relatively "safe" in terms of politics during the first year of its operation, in Massachusetts Medicaid became a political cause célèbre in the state elections scheduled for the fall of 1966. It says much for the independent reactions of the states that in Massachusetts the issue was not primarily one of cost or income levels; it concerned the emotional question of children. The state welfare department, with the approval of Lieutenant Governor Elliot Richardson (who had charge of welfare programs in Governor Volpe's administration), proposed, in the summer of 1966, to cover the required categorically needy but not to include medically needy children under 21 who were not eligible through the AFDC category. This last group would eventually be covered, but not until January 1969.

This delay was seized upon in pre-election debates. (Governor Volpe was a candidate for re-election and Richardson a candidate for attorney general.) Thus, curiously, while the New York program was under fire for being too liberal, the Massachusetts program was criticized for not being liberal enough. Faced with charges by Democratic legislative leaders in Massachusetts that the proposed program was "shockingly deficient" and by Senator Edward Kennedy that the state was "failing to take full advantage of the Federal programs enacted in Washington,"[64] the administration capitulated. Massachusetts began its whole program, including all eligible children under 21, in September 1966, two months before election day.

Other states moved into Medicaid with more or less deliberation, and at vastly different speeds. By August, 1966, a full year after the signing of P.L. 89–97, there were 19 Medicaid programs in existence.[65] But it was not always the largest or richest states that proved early entrants into the program; Vermont's program, for example, began in July 1966.[66] For states with limited vendor payment programs in 1965, the establishment of a Medicaid program was slower. Virginia, for example, had only implemented its Kerr-Mills program in 1964, making it one of the last states to participate before that program was overtaken by Medicaid. That state's implementation of Medicaid was thus naturally delayed in comparison with programs in more progressive (or rapacious) states. After the passage of P.L. 89–97, Governor Albertis Harrison appointed an Advisory Committee to study both Medicare and Medicaid.[67] The 1966 General Assembly passed legislation[68] that authorized the State Health Commissioner to submit a Medicaid plan to HEW.[69] The Advisory Committee then produced such a plan, which was approved by the State Board of Health in September 1967.[70] But, although the Advisory Committee recommended that the program be implemented in stages, beginning on July 1, 1968,[71] the General Assembly, sensing no need to rush, postponed the effective date for one year through use of the budget. Virginia's program thus began in 1969.

The programs begun by the end of 1966, however, reinforced the apparently expansionist nature of Title XIX, which was already causing concern in New York. The terms of the federal legislation almost invariably implied some extension in previous vendor payments, either in terms of adding eligibility groups or adding services (or both). Connecticut, for example, added persons over 65 in mental institutions and skilled nursing-home care to patients under 21. Illinois included persons over 65 in mental and tuberculosis institutions, together with needy children under 21, as well as extending services to those groups and to school medical and dental examinations. Idaho included a general category of children under 21. Louisiana added the elderly in mental and tuberculosis institutions and extended services to all groups for emergency-room care and x-ray therapy. Kentucky included additional laboratory and x-ray services. Maine added children under 21 and "caretaker relatives." Utah kept its same eligibility groups but added psychiatric evaluation for those on assistance and increased its maximum number of hospital days (for both the categorically and medically needy) from 20 to 60 days per spell of illness.[72]

Not only did these changes herald far larger programs than had been envisioned, they also stressed the enormous permutations and combinations in eligibility groups and services that Title XIX allowed in the states. Some states covered only the categorically needy; others included the medically needy. And for each group, each state set its own eligibility levels. As the range of services (and, for some states, the amount allowed within types of service[73]) also varied from state to state, the exact nature of the programs at any point in time was difficult to grasp and impossible to assess. But behind the complexity lay the two potent factors of money and state politics. Fear of higher taxes[74] and the absence of money to get the program under way[75] were the most frequent reasons given for delay in developing a Medicaid program. Money had once again taken over as the predominating influence in welfare medicine.

But while costs became the symbol, and the most important political element, of early division over Medicaid, other problems were also becoming evident. Medicaid had begun with one (however vaguely defined) set of philosophies for providing care to the "medically indigent." Implementation was, however, generating its own philosophical difficulties. Did the poor have a "right" to comprehensive medical care at public expense? If so, was this to have a "welfare" element, i.e., was the recipient really to have an entitlement to medical care equal to (or better than) that of the nonrecipient in the private sector? And if this were so, what of the working population above the cut-off line: Did they have no similar "rights," either as potential patients or taxpayers? Besides the rights and expectations of recipients and nonrecipients, there were also questions of professional interest, emphasized by the coming of Medicare. Should health professionals and institutions continue to donate part of the costs of welfare medicine, or did they have a "right" to reasonable fees?

These questions were understandably glossed over in the federal legislation. State reactions were practical and predictable, dependent on balancing various interests. As a working philosophy, decisions were made to extend services to the poor up to a level that would not antagonize the general population and to increase fees to the extent necessary not to antagonize the health professionals. Other problems, however, were bound to emerge.

NOTES

1. *Public Papers of the Presidents: Lyndon B. Johnson, 1966,* vol. 1 (Washington, D.C., 1967), Book I, p. 238.

2. Comprehensive Health Planning and Public Health Services Amendments of 1966, P.L. 89–749; Nov. 3, 1966; 80 Stat. 180.

3. E.g., Senator Robert Byrd's (West Virginia) investigation of cheating in D.C. welfare programs and Senator Russell Long's (Louisiana) various speeches. In respect of the latter, for instance, see "The Welfare Mess: A Scandal of Illegitimacy and Desertion," *Congressional Record,* vol. CXVII (December 14, 1971), p. 49607.

4. N.Y. Soc. Welfare Law, Art. 5, Sect. 11 s366 (McKinney 1966). Annual net income allowable:

Number of persons in household	*No wage earner*	*One wage earner*	*Two wage earners*
1	$2300	$2900	$——
2	3250	4000	4850
3	4350	5200	6050
4	5150	6000	6850
5	6000	6850	7700
6	6850	7700	8550

5. *New York Times,* May 15, 1966, p. 71. The median family of 4 or 5 members had an income of $6371 in New York State in 1959. U.S., Bureau of the Census, *U.S. Statistical Abstract: 1966* (87th ed. 1966), p. 338.

6. *N.Y. State Dept. Health Weekly Bulletin,* vol. 19 (July 25, 1966), p. 118.

7. U.S., Department of Health, Education, and Welfare, *Title XIX Fact Sheets* (1966–67). Among other programs, first-year utilization figures included: California, 5% (1,000,000); Hawaii, 5% (34,000); Illinois, 5% (500,000); Kentucky, 10% (300,000); Maryland, 7.2% (260,000); Michigan, 4% (330,000); Minnesota, 5% (72,000); North Dakota, 2.5% (16,640); Oklahoma, 8% (195,000); Pennsylvania, 6% (583,000); Puerto Rico, 50% (1,200,000); Utah, 4% (40,000); and Wisconsin, 6.3% (262,000).

8. The Governor estimated the comparison as follows (in millions of dollars):

	Total	*Federal share*	*State share*	*Local share*
1965	$429	$ 59	$172	$198
1966	$532	$217	$171	$144

SOURCE: New York, *State Department of Health Weekly Bulletin,* vol. 19 (July 25, 1966), p. 118.

9. *New York Times,* May 19, 1966, p. 49, col. 1; *ibid.,* May 23, 1966, p. 1, col. 2.

10. Dr. Charles L. Hudson, cited U.S., Department of Health, Education, and Welfare, *What Is Medicaid to an M.D.?,* undated.

11. Remarks of Dr. John Carter, Chairman of the Committee on State Legislation, reprinted "Minutes of the Special Session of the House of Delegates, May 26, 1966," *New York State Journal of Medicine* 66 (Sept. 1, 1966), pp. 2329–31. In fact the "freedom of choice" demand was not total freedom of choice. There was a strong suggestion that only those physicians approved by the local medical societies were entitled to be included on Medicaid panels.

12. *Ibid.*, p. 2344.

13. *New York Times*, June 4, 1966, p. 1, col. 2; *ibid.*, June 5, 1966, p. 66, col. 3. On June 10, the Society took out an advertisement in the paper to attack Medicaid. Among other things it was alleged that the traditional doctor-patient relationship would be destroyed by a new bureaucracy. *New York Times*, June 10, 1966, p. 36, col. 1.

14. Benjamin Werne, "Medicaid: Has National Health Insurance Entered by the Back Door?" 18 *Syracuse Law Review* (1966), pp. 56–57.

15. The Associated Industries of New York, Inc., for instance, claiming to represent some 1500 companies in New York, opposed the legislation because it alleged that if most workers would be eligible for public medical care, unions that no longer had to bargain with employers for better medical care would instead demand even higher wages or other forms of benefits. *New York Times*, May 25, 1966, p. 33.

16. *Ibid.*, May 17, 1966, p. 49.

17. They also allowed a former Eisenhower HEW Secretary, Marion Folsom, to call for the dropping of the income ceiling for a family of four from $6000 to $4500. *Ibid.*, May 25, 1966, pp. 1, 38.

18. *Ibid.*, May 25, 1966, pp. 1, 33.

19. *Ibid.*, July 1, 1966, pp. 1, 17.

20. *Ibid.*, July 2, 1966, pp. 1, 7.

21. *Robinson v. Wyman*, 51 Misc. 2d 480, 273 N.Y.S. 2d 450 (S. Ct. 1966), at pp. 481–482 and 451 respectively. In particular, a nominee petitioner argued that he stood "aggrieved by the administrative act, not only as a general taxpaying citizen of New York State, but also as a man who runs his own business in this state; that if this program is allowed, a tremendous tax burden will be placed on both individuals and businesses in New York State and your petitioner frankly believes said burden, as hereinafter set forth, will force him to move his business elsewhere." Justice Koreman held that the petitioner lacked standing and strongly implied that even had that not been the case, there was no valid constitutional challenge available.

22. Social Security Act, as amended, Sec. 1116 (a) (1). The period may be extended "by written agreement of the Secretary and the affected State."

23. *New York Times*, November 16, 1966, p. 56, col. 1.

24. *Ibid.*, January 7, 1967, p. 29, col. 1.

25. U.S., Department of Health, Education, and Welfare, Public Health Service, Margaret Greenfield, *Medi-Cal, The California Medicaid Program (Title XIX)* (Washington, D.C., 1969), pp. 32–33.

26. *Ibid.*, chap. 5.

27. These are set out, *ibid.*, pp. 26–30.

28. Blue Shield was given the task of paying not only physicians but all providers except hospitals, while two other agents handled the hospitals. *Ibid.*, Ch. 6.

29. *Ibid.*, Ch. 7.

30. Again we have relied on R. B. Titus, *New York's Medicaid: A Study of the Development of a State Title XIX Program—Its Problems and Prospects,* 1968 (paper presented at the Yale Law School).

31. The average number of recipients from May to September was 193,470 a month at a monthly cost of $20,321,925. The bulk of these persons were those who were already on other welfare medical programs. *Welfare in Review, passim.*

32. For example:

May 1965	$18,730,688	May 1966	$18,102,616
June 1965	19,430,009	June 1966	20,681,188
July 1965	19,701,527	July 1966	14,951,318

SOURCE: *Welfare in Review, passim.*

33. *New York Times,* Sept. 1, 1966, p. 45.

34. *Ibid.*, Nov. 28, 1966, pp. 1, 31.

35. *Ibid.*, Jan. 28, 1967, p. 28.

36. *Ibid.*, Jan. 20, 1967, p. 88.

37. Art. 5, Title 11, Sect. 365 (c). (McKinney 1966, Ch. 256.)

38. State of New York, *Official Compilation of Codes, Rules and Regulations: Title 18—Social Welfare* (1966 ed.) Reg. 85.10.

39. Remarks of Dr. George Himler, of the Committee to Negotiate with the Governor's Interdepartmental Task Force, "Minutes of the Special Session of the House of Delegates, May 26, 1966," 66 *New York State Journal of Medicine* 2332 (Sept. 1966).

40. *New York Times,* July 5, 1966, p. 39.

41. *Ibid.*, Dec. 18, 1966, Sec. IV, p. E13.

42. *New York Times,* August 6, 1966, p. 10.

43. *New York State Department of Health Weekly Bulletin,* vol. 19 (November 28, 1966) p. 191.

44. *Medical Tribune and Medical News,* Dec. 12, 1966, p. 31.

45. *Ibid.*

46. *New York Times,* December 5, 1966, p. 1.

47. *Ibid.*, Dec. 18, 1966, Sec. IV, p. E13.

48. *Ibid.*, Dec. 31, 1966, p. 8. On this see also Ch. 10.

49. By Jan. 1, 1967. *AMA News,* Jan. 2, 1967, p. 1.

50. By Dec. 1, 1966, *New York Times,* Dec. 5, 1966.

51. *Ibid.*, Dec. 31, 1966, p. 1.

52. *Ibid.*, Oct. 27, 1966, p. 29.

53. *Ibid.*, Dec. 18, 1966, p. 42.

54. *Ibid.*, Jan. 6, 1967, p. 32.

55. *Medical Tribune and Medical News,* Nov. 28, 1966, pp. 1, 17.

56. *New York Times,* Oct. 29, 1966, p. 29.

57. Connecticut's vendor payments, including federal, state, and local funds grew from $16.1 million in 1961 to $28.7 million in 1966. Over half these funds

were spent for nursing-home care. Source: Connecticut State Department of Welfare.

58. Connecticut State Department of Welfare, *Public Welfare Trends*, Oct.–Dec. 1965, pp. 10–11. Writing in 1965, the state Welfare Commissioner had no reservations about why he was anxious to see Connecticut get into the Title XIX program: "Because of the favorable Federal matching under the new Medical Assistance Program . . . it will be possible for the Connecticut State Welfare Department to finance this expanded program to meet the medical needs of these new groups entirely from federal funds without any additional funds from the General Treasury of the State of Connecticut."

59. We here rely on Kate Clair Freeland, *Medicaid in Connecticut: The First Year*, 1969 (a paper presented at the Yale Law School).

60. *Public Welfare Trends, op. cit., supra*, note 58, Oct.–Dec. 1966, p. 12.

61. Connecticut Welfare Manual, *Departmental Bulletin No. 1304*, Sec. 030.

62. Connecticut Welfare Manual, *Departmental Bulletin No. 1796.*

63. *Ibid., Bulletin No. 1872.*

64. Quoted in Martha Derthick, *The Influence of Federal Grants: Public Assistance in Massachusetts* (Cambridge, Mass., 1970), pp. 67–68.

65. *Congressional Record*, vol. CXII, 20267–68 (1966). After New York and California, with estimated expenses for the Calendar year 1966 of $217 million and $210 million respectively, the largest programs appeared to be Pennsylvania ($100 million), Illinois ($40 million), and Minnesota ($39 million). Of these states 3 received federal matching for 1/1/66–6/30/67 at 50 percent; Pennsylvania received 54.38 percent federal support and Minnesota 60.46 percent. U.S. Advisory Commission on Intergovernmental Relations, *Intergovernmental Problems in Medicaid* (Washington, 1968), pp. 16–17.

66. Vermont, Department of Social Welfare, *Biennial Report 1964–66*. Again, though, a combination of factors made this move inevitable. Increasing expenditures on welfare in Vermont were causing concern over the costs falling upon towns and cities in the state; indeed, a comprehensive study of welfare in the state had been authorized by the General Assembly in 1965. Vermont had experience with Kerr-Mills, whose benefits had been welcomed chiefly for subsidizing patients in nursing homes, half of whom were dependent on social welfare payments, and thus relieving local tax burdens in the state. Taking a somewhat similar view, a special session of the Vermont legislature was called in 1966 to enable the state to take advantage of Medicaid by July.

67. Mack I. Shanholtz, "Looking in on Medicaid," *Virginia Medical Monthly*, vol. 97 (April 1970), p. 243.

68. Now 32 Code of Virginia, 30.1(a) (Michie).

69. It was passed unanimously by both houses; 36–0 in the Senate; 86–0 in the House of Delegates. *Virginia Senate Journal, 1964–66*, p. 549; *Virginia House of Delegates Journal, 1964–66*, p. 1090.

70. It appears under the title, Virginia, Department of Health, *Proposed Program and Budget: Medical Assistance Plan Title XIX: 1968–1970 Biennium: Budget Exhibit for Department of Health 1968–70*, mimeograph.

71. Shanholtz, *op. cit., supra*, note 67, p. 243.

72. *Intergovernmental Problems in Medicaid, supra*, note 65, pp. 95, 97.

73. States could still impose limits on services provided under Medicaid, although this practice was far less common than before. For example, Georgia, Louisiana, and Texas limited hospital services to 30 days, Idaho to 20 days,

Iowa to 90 days, Oregon and Kentucky to 21 days, Nevada and Maryland to 15 days (with allowable extensions), Pennsylvania and Utah to 60 days. Some applied the number of days to a spell of illness, some to one admission, some to services given within a year. Washington limited hospital care according to criteria for various types of illness; Wisconsin limited the combination of hospital and in-home care to 45 days; Montana provided care up to $14 a day. Tax Foundation Inc., *Medicaid: State Programs After Two Years* (New York, 1968), pp. 65–66.

74. *Ibid.*, p. 40. The issue of why some states delayed in implementing their programs was taken up a year later by the Advisory Commission on Intergovernmental Relations in its report, *Intergovernmental Problems in Medicaid.* See *supra*, note 65.

75. *Ibid.*, p. 61.

7

Facilis Descensus Averno

The growing problems in the states during 1966 crystallized into specific recommendations in Congress in 1967. In the states the themes for Medicaid were costs and confusion; both stemmed from the lack of foresight built into the initial federal developments. In Congress, the predominant issue was costs; for as state costs rose, so did the federal obligation under the open-ended grant system.

When Congressman Mills proposed his tripartite "solution" for medical care in 1965, HEW had estimated that Title XIX would "increase the Federal Government's contribution about $200 million in a full year of operation over that in the programs operated under existing law," representing a total of approximately $950 million a year.[1] In the closed hearings before the House Ways and Means Committee in 1966, the Chief Actuary of the Social Security Administration, Robert Myers, produced the figure of $3 billion per year as the federal cost of Title XIX under so-called mature conditions,[2] i.e., assuming that the state plans became more like the New York plan in coverage and eligibility. Not surprisingly, these kinds of figures were to provoke an immediate response from fiscally conscious legislators and lead to suggestions for controlling the amount of federal money being channeled to the states. For the first time the traditionally cheeseparing attitudes of the states toward welfare programs could not be relied upon as a sufficient brake on spending; a long pattern of mutual expectations was broken.

Representatives from states with generous Medicaid programs sounded the early warning notes. On Capitol Hill, Senator Leverett Saltonstall (Republican, Massachusetts) espoused the view, also held by some of the New York legislators:

> *There was little discussion of Title 19 which certainly has proved to be the "sleeper" in the bill. I am certain no one dreamed that within*

> *the next five years, "Medicaid," as the program established by that title is called, could come to dwarf Medicare.*[3]

This view was to gain currency in both houses of Congress as New York and California went from one crisis to the next.

Linked to these concerns was the continuing difficulty at both federal and state levels as to what in fact the original legislation had meant. The 1966 report of the Committee on Ways and Means sounded the note that was to be the leitmotif of subsequent events in concluding, "while most of the State plans raise no question at this time, a few go well beyond what your committee believes to have been the intent of the Congress."[4] A more concrete "intent" was destined to develop, culminating in the Social Security Amendments of 1967. The mood was set for continuing Congressional watchfulness of Medicaid in the states.

New York Revisited

Congressional attitudes toward the fiscal, medical, and political problems of Medicaid continued to be dominated by the programs in New York and California, the two largest Title XIX programs. For in different ways their continuing crises, from the winter of 1966 through 1967, shaped the initial demise of the new program at the federal level.

New York's difficulties were both fiscal and administrative. While the cost question plagued legislators in both New York and Washington, the administration of the program was running into serious problems in dealing with health care providers. New York hospitals, which had looked forward to Medicare and Medicaid because they saw themselves being reimbursed more generously for welfare patients, often found themselves sadly disappointed. Medicaid bills were processed so slowly that, by December 1966, the Medicaid administration was forced, in order to keep hospitals cooperating, to advance 80 percent of the hospital's last audited bill,[5] while Governor Rockefeller had to announce a new program involving a subsidy of some $27 million for the 400 or so public and private hospitals that provided care to indigents.[6] It also emerged that New York City had lost some $5 million in state and federal funds because bills were not presented within the 90-day period required by the regulations. Meanwhile, on another front, a Committee comprised of more than 500 pharmacists in New York City threatened to boycott the program unless they were paid more quickly and their fees raised. They also refused to supply generic drugs when drugs were ordered by their brand name (which would have meant foregoing the mark-up on proprietary drugs), alleging that to do so would be "economic suicide."[7] By April 1967, New York City was six months behind in paying physicians, and the program was alleged to be full of red tape. Claims processing was so far behind that a private company began purchasing bills from practitioners, at 90 percent of their face value,[8] and then collecting in full from the administration.

There were also other kinds of fears beginning to emerge. Medicaid was intended to bring better medical care to the inner-city dweller. But were all providers ethically equipped to answer that challenge? Dr. George James, who had been Health Commissioner for New York City from 1962 to 1965, stressed the potential need for utilization and quality controls, for "what is to prevent a doctor from moving into Harlem, offering substandard care, accepting dozens and dozens of patients a day and billing the Government for tens of thousands of dollars?"[9] The fears expressed in 1966 were, sadly, to become the realities of 1967, at least with respect to some practitioners. Yet most general medical practitioners felt the regulations under which they were required to operate were medically unjustified. Under the program, they were not allowed to treat wounds more than 2½ inches long, to deliver babies, or to set broken limbs. To the irritation of what they regarded as totally inadequate fees was added the insult of medical control.[10]

Yet, at the same time, there was evidence that some physicians were falling into the trap Commissioner James had warned about. One doctor was found to be billing Medicaid for an average of 65 house calls a day. Apparently, he waged a personal "preventive medicine" war and examined every member of the house he visited, sick or not.[11] In December 1967, New York City's Social Services Department placed a $5000-a-month reimbursement ceiling on general practitioners, arguing that a doctor working 20 days a month would have to see 800 patients, 40 a day, to justify that sum. While they were prepared to be convinced, the burden was to be on the G.P. There were also moves against squandering hospitals. Spurred by the "reasonable cost" reimbursement formula, some small hospitals discovered that, faced with a disorganized bureaucracy, they could recover from Medicaid anything they spent. Thus some small hospitals were being paid more than $90 a day, while Columbia-Presbyterian Medical Center received only $76.95 for ward care, despite its highly specialized staff and facilities.[12]

Meanwhile, the providers remained dissatisfied. Dentists, who were paid on a fee schedule, protested that, in the words of the Eighth District Dental Society, "fee schedules will be determined by men who sit behind desks who have not been in practice and have no clinical experience."[13] And, as if to show that things had come full circle, the president of the State Medical Society announced that Medicaid "had degenerated into an extended welfare program."[14] Hence, in June of 1967, the city, which acted as the state's agent for the program, gave in to the obvious. It announced that no longer would doctors, dentists, and optometrists be required to sign up to participate in the Medicaid program. (In fact, at that point, some 7000 of the city's 15,000 doctors had signed up, but only 2000 had filed claims.) Moreover, in August it was announced that New York City fee schedules for physicians might be raised above those for the remainder of the state.

The welfare lobbies were certainly not pleased with the way the program was being run, especially in New York City. A Citizen's Committee accused the City Welfare Department of "gross negligence" in the administration of the program and cited its "incomprehensible forms, unnecessary red tape and confused administration."[15] The notion of waste by both providers and recipients had become common currency. These claims were questioned in a sample study undertaken by the state (in August and September 1967) of the two million Medicaid recipients who were "medically needy" rather than being in one of the cash assistance programs. The study found, despite the claims by opponents of Medicaid, that the program was not used by those who could most easily afford to pay their own bills but by low-income and destitute families.[16] The study, however, received little currency. Fraud and waste were much more readily comprehensible.

Such evidence was, moreover, of little help to communities in the state, which were faced by rapidly rising welfare bills patently related to the new program. Franklin County was an extreme, but by no means totally atypical, case. It had the lowest per capita income of any county in the state, and 80 percent of its population was eligible for Medicaid. Roughly a quarter of the County's population signed up for the program, and the original County share of $840,000 had to be augmented by an additional $500,000. Even that appeared to be in danger of being insufficient, and a 2 percent county sales tax was instituted.[17] Suffolk County expected to require an extra $4 million for Medicaid in 1967,[18] and Westchester County an additional $2.5 million.[19] Across the state the same cries were heard. By early 1968, 28 local governments had imposed (or increased) a sales tax, and in almost all 62 counties the real estate tax rose, the alleged chief culprit being Medicaid.[20]

The political climate had been changing too. In Washington, Senator Jacob Javits (Republican, New York) had begun recommending changes that would cut back Medicaid, by abandoning the principles of statewide standards and equivalent services for all eligible groups that had been at the heart of P.L. 89–97. In the November 1966 elections, Representative Stratton made his opposition to Medicaid the basis of his re-election campaign, and he was returned handily. Governor Rockefeller defended the program; and while he won an upset victory, he did poorly upstate, where he had been heckled on the Medicaid issue.[21] It was not surprising then that in his opening address to the legislature the Governor noted that "Medicaid is a new program and therefore may require amendments in the light of experience."

California Revisited

While the sponsor of the New York program was beginning to rethink his position, Governor Brown of California had been voted out, to be succeeded by Governor Reagan, no friend of Medicaid. While Medicaid expenditures in New York continued to exceed those in California ($707 million and $589 million, respectively, for calendar year 1967[22]), the costs of medical vendor payments had risen rapidly in the latter state. With the expansion in services and the transfer of part of the costs of county hospitals to Medi-Cal, per capita payments rose from $10.69 in 1965 to $29.44 in 1967.[23]

It was expected, in the debates over Medi-Cal in the legislature, that the substantial additional costs of the program would be largely absorbed by additional federal matching funds. But in November 1966, after the election of Governor Reagan but before his inauguration, the Administrator of the Health and Welfare Agency hazarded the opinion that Medi-Cal was running out of money and that either the state legislature would have to vote funds or benefits would have to be reduced before the end of the fiscal year. At that time the reasons chiefly advanced were the nursing profession's demand for higher salaries and an unanticipated increase in the number of elderly and disabled persons receiving nursing-home benefits.[24] By the spring of 1967, with bills for services coming in slowly, it was estimated that in the first 16 months of the program the state would be "in the red" to the amount of $130 million, with a further deficit of $80 million for the following fiscal year, half of which would have to be made up from state funds.[25]

It was in this atmosphere that on July 10, 1967, Governor Reagan delivered a televised "Report to the People," arguing that the Medi-Cal program was likely to increase in cost 50 percent each year and that "something must be done before this ill-conceived program bankrupts the state." The premature release of the financial information caught the program administrators by surprise and had the effect of legitimizing the amount of the projected budget deficit and providing ammunition for the Governor's office to castigate the profligacy of the previous Democratic administration. In fact, as we shall see, both the estimate and the multiplier proved to be inaccurate; but they became political facts of life.[26]

In California, staff work on possible cutbacks in the Medicaid program began in the summer of 1967. The problem was to know where to begin, for Medi-Cal had been carefully structured to keep eligibility at a relatively low level.[27] Whereas New York had far more persons classified as "medically needy" than "categorically needy," in California the reverse was true.[28] Moreover, while more than 40 percent of the estimated program expenditures in California were on behalf of the 200,000 persons classified as medically needy, a substantial minority of these were old and disabled persons in nursing homes whose benefits could not be cut off without a resulting public outcry.[29]

To the staff working on the problem, there undoubtedly seemed no alternative but to recommend, instead of a reduction in the number of beneficiaries, the reduction of available services. Specifically, it was recommended that the relatively comprehensive benefits then available, which included such items as family planning services, ambulance services, wheel chairs, some psychiatric care, hearing aids and related devices, drugs, and physical examinations, be cut back to the five basic services at that time required under the federal legislation (inpatient care, nursing home care, physician services, laboratory services, and outpatient clinic services). In addition, other savings were suggested, including a rollback in physician fees to the level of "usual and customary fees" prevailing as of January 1, 1967.

These cutbacks were announced in August 1967 and received widespread public attention. California's crisis joined that of New York as the focus for action at the federal level. In some respects, indeed, the California experience was more important than New York's. For while New York demonstrated the unexpected potential scope of Medicaid as a national program, California went one step beyond: The proposed cutbacks implied that the original concept was a failure.

The proposed cutbacks in California were, however, immediately deplored by an effective alliance between professional organizations in the health field and representatives of poverty groups in the state. The opposition was crystallized in a restraining order obtained the same month by California Rural Legal Assistance (a legal services program funded by the Office of Economic Opportunity) temporarily blocking the cutbacks. Attorneys representing medical, dental, and pharmaceutical groups appeared as *amici curiae*. Despite claims from the state that it would lose $5 million a day if reductions in service were not made, the Superior Court in Sacramento made the order permanent. The state appealed the case, but lost its appeal in November 1967, the California Supreme Court ruling that the Health and Welfare Agency had authority to reduce the program but that the manner in which the reductions were made was *ultra vires* the 1965 and 1967 Medi-Cal legislation: the latter required either elimination of medically needy beneficiaries or a proportional reduction of all services as opposed to elimination of particular services.[30]

Governor Reagan immediately put the question of Medi-Cal before the legislature, then meeting in special session, and warned that he would be forced to remove benefits from the medically needy unless legally acceptable cutbacks could be made; the supposed deficit for 1967–68 was then claimed by the Reagan administration to be $71 million.[31] As the months went by, however, the fiscal situation changed significantly. By the spring of 1968, the deficit had not only disappeared; a surplus of $31 million was allowed for carrying over into 1968–69.[32] But that announcement coincided with the signing of the 1967 Social Security Amendments in Washington. Congress had acted.

Reaction and Response in Washington

Not surprisingly, the checkered course of Medicaid in the states provoked continuing debates on Capitol Hill. Indeed, the publicity given to Medicaid, especially in New York and California, enhanced the probability that the program as envisioned by the 1965 legislation would never be fully implemented. There was no period of relative quiet for routine procedures in HEW to become accepted and to develop. The Medical Services Administration had not been strong enough to control or even shape the crises in the states. Nor, indeed, as we have noted, was this the expected role for a federal welfare agency.

Within MSA itself there were too few staff members to develop basic regulations and guidelines within a meaningful time. Yet brave efforts were made to provide an administrative framework that would both aid and monitor the states. Initially three broad administrative functions were recognized: program planning and development (largely a question of interpreting the law to the states), program management (day-to-day administrative affairs), and program evaluation. While the Office of Program Planning and Development was attempting to codify the law in a series of state letters and in the Handbook of Public Assistance (Supplement D), the Office of Program Evaluation was making an effort to ascertain what in fact was happening in the states and how far the provisions of Supplement D were being met. Lacking any real direction from MSA, however, such efforts were largely peripheral to the actual development of Medicaid in the states. Moreover, the MSA staff was much too small to audit states on a regular basis and to produce annual evaluative reports.[33] Even where such reports were made, there was no guarantee that states would take notice of the recommendations.

The crisis over HEW approval of New York's program in 1966 had presented a typical situation that MSA was not equipped to handle. It had neither the statutory entitlement nor the bureaucratic power. HEW itself inevitably gave priority, insofar as there were clear priorities, to Medicare, which as a prestige operation run by the powerful Social Security Administration as part of the Social Security program was the darling of the politicians and the electorate. Without real power within the Department and without a clearly-defined political constituency, MSA and Medicaid found themselves the whipping boys for rising medical costs and rising "welfare" expenditures for which they were, at most, only partially responsible. Indeed, almost as soon as the state programs were initiated, a remarkable constitutional phenomenon began; administration of the program began ebbing away from HEW towards the powerful committees on Capitol Hill.

Almost as soon as the New York implementing legislation had passed in March 1966, there were efforts to get Congress to "curb" Title XIX, and these efforts soon outstripped in strength the pressures to discourage HEW from approving state plans. It had become clear that HEW had neither the legal authority to alter plans that met the statutory criteria nor the stomach and stamina to battle powerful congressional chairmen. Thus, having failed to persuade Secretary Gardner to veto the New York plan in May, Representative Stratton introduced legislation into the House of Representatives in June 1966 to curb Medicaid. Less than a year after passage, Medicaid was "on the skids."

The Stratton bill proposed three major changes particularly germane to the New York experience. First, the Secretary of HEW was barred from approving any state Medicaid plan that made more than 20 percent of the population eligible for it. Second, the state had to meet the needs of welfare recipients before including other "medically needy" groups. Third, the state had to show that the growth of private medical insurance plans would not be discouraged by the adoption of the state plan.[34] All these conditions would have protected New York's taxpayers and nonrecipients from the threat of high Medicaid eligibility levels. At the same time, the clear endorsements of health provisions through private insurance protected the citizenry from middle-class encroachments by a state. "Welfare medicine" was to be confined to the "less eligible."

In the same month, essentially in defense of the New York plan, Senator Javits introduced a rival bill (S. 3313). This tackled New York's problems from a different direction. Claiming that the controversy over the New York plan resulted from "the fact that federal law . . . has kept [Medicaid] from being more exactly shaped to the need to be met,"[35] the Javits bill called for increased flexibility in state administration. First, the bill would have allowed different eligibility standards in different parts of a state; thus New York City might include many who would be excluded in upstate areas. Second, deductibles would be allowed generally, with beneficiaries being required to pay from $1 to $260, depending on their income, in respect of any medical charge. (As the 1965 legislation had been interpreted, deductibles were permissible only for noninstitutional services provided to the "medically needy.") Finally, the Javits proposal called for flexibility in services provided, so that states might provide different medical services to different age groups. This provision would have tackled the political downstate-upstate dilemma in New York, while allowing the states to make selective service cutbacks.

Senator Javits' endorsement of roll-backs also underlined the general nature of Medicaid's dilemmas, for the Senator had long been an advocate of better health protection to be provided through the states. Congress, however, was concerned with very much more than the problems of New York State. By August 1966, with only 22 out of a possible 52 Medicaid programs in existence, the fiscal outlay for the total programs was running about $500 or $600 million more than pre-Title XIX medical assistance programs, for an annual expenditure of about $1.3 billion.[36] It was during that month that the House Ways and Means Committee began its closed-door hearings on Title XIX.

Addressing itself to the problem of limiting the federal cost of Medicaid, the Ways and Means Committee considered four main solutions. The first was simply to put a ceiling on federal contributions to Title XIX: instead of the traditional "open-ended" federal funding of a categorical program, there would be an appropriation that could not be exceeded. The second was to limit the amount of money going into any one state or to follow the Stratton proposals and limit the program in any one state to a specific percentage of that state's population. Yet another possibility studied was to provide a flexible limit beyond which states might not go, e.g., 90 percent of the average annual earnings of factory production workers in the state.[37] A variation of this latter suggestion would have provided a limit on means-test levels for each state, and it was rumored that New York's limits would be $4150 for a family of four.

Although cost control was the goal, underlying the various approaches was the simple question of equity. Congress could, as one alternative, specify the federal sum to be spent on Medicaid in each state, but there would still need to be some guidelines on how to do that. Such guidelines, as with the other alternatives, required a national definition of "medical indigency." As it was, the variations among state programs were remarkable. For the family of four (with one wage earner), there was a range from $6000 for New York, followed by Rhode Island with $4300, to Utah with $2640 and Oklahoma with $2448.[38] Such variations in per capita incomes and differing welfare commitments were to continue to provide problems not only in Medicaid but also in the negative income tax and its competing programs, which were beginning to surface in this period. It was clear that any nationally mandated means test would either have to be toward the top of the state range (e.g., between $4000 and $6000 for a family) and thus require enormous infusions of additional funds for states currently below that level; or, if specified at a lower figure, would alienate the largest and most powerful states.

The Ways and Means Committee avoided this question by not opting for a flat ceiling, nor even a variable one, on federal funds. Instead, its report called merely for a cutback in federal reimbursement for certain groups generally regarded as having limited political power and appeal. In particular, relatives with whom children lived were to be excluded from Medicaid programs unless they were eligible to receive AFDC payments.

(By the 1960s, AFDC parents were predominantly from minority groups.) As medically needy children were still to be covered, the effect of the Committee's report was thus to take those between 21 and 64 out of the "medically needy" aspect of the Medicaid program.[39] It was estimated that this would cut the federal share of Medicaid in New York State by about 10 percent.[40] Not everyone was satisfied with this solution. Representative Curtis continued to press for a program that would, in his words, clearly distinguish between oranges (catastrophic medical expenses) and apples (routine medical expenses).[41] But while Representative Curtis and others saw the Committee as a step backward,[42] they need not have worried. In October, the Democratic leadership announced that no action would be taken on Title XIX until the Ninetieth Congress convened in January 1967.[43] Both the state and federal problems remained.

The Social Security Amendments of 1967

The opportunity for a new assault on Medicaid's costs came with the introduction of omnibus Social Security legislation in the new Congress: hearings on the 1967 Social Security Amendments began before the House Ways and Means Committee on March 1. As it happened, Medicaid was overshadowed both by proposed legislative changes in the OASDHI (Social Insurance) program and, in political terms, by House-inserted amendments about "mandatory work provisions" and the AFDC "freeze" in the non-medical parts of the public assistance program. Cash assistance itself was under stress and retrenchment, with costs being attacked by a strong back-to-work ethic. Behind the scenes there was no doubt political bargaining with respect to Medicaid. Secretary Gardner was known to be anxious that Title XIX be treated as a broad health care program while Chairman Mills saw the legislation very much as part of the about-to-be reduced welfare program.[44]

It was in this context that HEW compromised by coming to Congress with a bill (H.R. 5710) that tied means-test levels for Medicaid to the means-test levels for cash assistance in each state. This proposal had two political advantages. First, it avoided any federal specification of "medical indigence" levels *per se;* second, it tied Medicaid into the discussions of welfare reform and limitations. The major provision, although it could not cut back on those receiving cash assistance (the categorically needy), cut back on the medically needy by tying their means test to the welfare means test. The bill limited federal sharing under Title XIX to those whose income was no more than 50 percent higher than the categorical assistance maxima in the state.[45] Its provisions thus at least partly reflected Congressional concerns manifested in the previous year.[46]

When the 1967 hearings began, the mood of the Ways and Means Committee was not difficult to fathom, and the House hearings took their predictable directions.[47] The proposed limitations on federal participation in Title XIX were supported by business and insurance groups[48] and opposed by welfare and labor groups.[49] But when all the rhetoric was done, the Committee decided to produce its own "clean" bill (H.R. 12080). It followed HEW's proposals for Medicaid, but the new bill was more restrictive than the administration one. It proposed that federal matching funds not be made available to any family whose income was more than one-third greater than the state's limit on cash assistance payable to a family of the same size by AFDC.[50] For example, if the state's maximum AFDC cash payment to a family of four was $2100, then federal matching would be unavailable for any family of four whose income exceeded $2800. It was made clear, however, that the "spend-down" provision would continue to apply: if this hypothetical family earned $3000, it would become eligible for federal sharing after spending $200 on medical expenses. This limitation was to become a part of the amendments as enacted in 1967.[51]

A second major recommendation also to be incorporated in the law was to give the states greater latitude in choosing which services they would provide to Title XIX recipients. Instead of the required five services, the states could choose any seven of 14 services enumerated in the legislation.[52] Whereas the previous proposal safeguarded federal spending levels, this proposal was designed to alleviate financial problems in the states.

In other respects the Committee generally followed the administration's proposals.[53] The House bill did, however, go beyond the administration bill in areas of cost control and state flexibility. States were to be partially relieved of their Title XIX obligation not to use the new federal money merely to replace other state effort in the field of medical care.[54] At the same time, in the interests of efficiency and to alleviate the difficulties the state agencies had found in certifying providers (hospitals, nursing homes, home health agencies, clinics, laboratories), states were to be required to provide consultative services to provider institutions to help them qualify under Title XIX, keep proper fiscal records, and provide information needed in drawing up fee schedules under Titles XIX, XVIII, and V.[55] States were also adjured to take all reasonable measures to collect fees from third parties who might be liable (for example, due to insurance or tort liability) for the medical care of an eligible recipient of Medicaid. The federal government would in turn receive its share of any such reimbursement.[56]

In one respect, however, the bill moved slightly away from the strict vendor policy of the 1965 statute. In keeping with the increasingly fashionable arguments in favor of educational vouchers and rent supplements, the bill provided that payments for doctors' bills could be made to the recipient, who would then be liable to the doctor. This would apply to the medically needy only, not the categorically needy, and the Committee foresaw no change in fee schedules as a result of this provision.[57] Finally, under pressure from local governments, the Committee proposed that the deadline by which states had to meet the nonfederal share of Medicaid expenditures solely out of state funds (or through an approved tax-equalization formula with the same effect) be moved ahead one year to July 1, 1969. This was done because "the localities in many states should not be subjected to disproportionate burdens any longer than necessary."[58] The bill thus had something for everyone, if "everyone" is defined as federal, state, and local governments. For the recipient, the message was cutbacks in both services and eligibility.

The House bill, introduced under a closed rule as is traditional with Social Security bills, passed in mid-August, and the Senate began hearings at the end of the month. Secretary Gardner attacked the House's limitation on federal participation ("We believe this to be too constrictive a definition of medical indigence"[59]) and the cry was taken up in Undersecretary Wilbur Cohen's detailed evidence.[60] While the inaccurate fiscal projections for Medicaid made in 1965 and 1966 hindered the presentation, Cohen stressed that the House restrictions would be likely to force a cutback in 14 of the 35 states that had Medicaid programs.[61] To a very large extent the testimony before the Senate Finance Committee was similar to that before the Ways and Means Committee. The AMA testimony was sympathetic to Title XIX,[62] while a Medicaid lobby appeared to protest the federal ceiling on cost-sharing,[63] and New York's State Commissioner of Social Services argued that all his state was doing was attempting to meet the "comprehensive services" requirement.[64]

But the House version of the bill, although it was passed with only three dissenting votes, was not without its critics, even on the Ways and Means Committee. Representative Jacob Gilbert of New York, in "Supplemental Views" appended to the Committee Report, was one who argued that the states had acted "in good faith" on the federal commitment implied in the 1965 legislation. Noting the "domestic turmoil through which this nation is now suffering," he claimed it was bad policy to curtail programs that had given hope to the poor, citing the rising costs as proof of the program's success rather than its failure.[65] In two short years, however, his had become the minority position.

The progress of the bill through Congress reflected various differences of opinion. The bill as reported out by the Senate Finance Committee restored (temporarily) the administration's formula of 150 percent of AFDC payments.[66] However, at the behest of Chairman Long, the Committee bill also proposed lowering the federal matching share for payments made on behalf of the medically needy.[67] The Finance Committee accepted the House alternative of any seven out of 14 of the allowable services under the 1965 legislation for the medically indigent, but it required states to continue to provide the five basic services for the categorically needy. It also made mandatory, by July 1, 1969, "early and periodic screening and diagnosis" of eligible persons under age 21, a potentially far-reaching program first proposed in the administration bill.[68] In addition, home health services were also to be mandatory for certain groups by 1970. Finally, the Finance Committee would have allowed direct payments for this medical care, in lieu of vendor payments, to the categorically needy as well as the medically needy, including dentists' as well as physicians' bills in this authorization.[69]

The Senate Finance Committee made other important changes having no corresponding sections in the House bill. Explicitly recognizing that one effect of Medicare and Medicaid had been to accelerate the use of nursing-home facilities, the Committee proposed a lengthy set of standards to prevent abuses by providers of such care. While the House proposals exercised control of costs, the Senate Committee went an important step further in emphasizing control of providers, a role it was to pursue. The requirement included the licensing of nursing homes used by Medicaid recipients and of the administrators of such homes.[70] Closely related was the addition to Title XI ("General Provisions") of the Social Security legislation of a section providing matching funds for "intermediate care facilities."[71] These ICFs were intended to provide a less expensive alternative for persons not needing full nursing-home care. This provision was not at that time formally made a part of Title XIX, and federal matching was to be available only on behalf of cash assistance recipients in the adult categories. Nevertheless, it was anticipated by the Committee that this section would encourage the states to use ICFs rather than unnecessarily place Medicaid recipients in skilled nursing homes, for which matching funds had been available under the 1965 legislation.

To allow closer scrutiny of vendor payments, the Committee added a requirement that the states must enter agreements with each provider to keep and furnish appropriate information and submit to such audits as were deemed necessary.[72] The authority of the General Accounting Office to hold spot checks was underlined. The bill also allowed the states to impose deductibles or coinsurance (on the medically needy only) with respect to inpatient hospital care.[73] In short, while the proposals might vary, the themes of the Senate and House Committees were similar: increased federal management controls, and a re-emphasis on fiscal responsibility at the expense of whatever element of mainstream medicine may have been implicit in the 1965 version of Title XIX. Indeed, the most immediately expansionist provision in an otherwise restrictive bill stands out in stark relief. The Committee added a new category of possible beneficiary—the "essential person," defined as "the spouse of a cash public assistance recipient who was living with him, who was essential or necessary to his welfare, and whose needs were taken into account in determining the amount of his cash benefit."[74]

All of these recommendations were embodied in the usual omnibus Social Security proposals. Thus, while the Senate debates were dramatic, this was chiefly because of the proposed increases in Social Security payments and what many regarded as the repressive changes in cash payments under AFDC.[75] Only two changes were made in the Committee bill with respect to Medicaid,[76] and on November 22, 1967, the bill finally passed the Senate and went to conference. There the Senate version of the bill generally prevailed, with two major exceptions. The House's formula of 133⅓ percent of AFDC payments was adopted, to the exclusion of all other proposed limitations on federal matching for the medically needy; "medical indigency" was thereby tied to cash assistance levels in each state. The conflicting provisions allowing direct payments to recipients for their medical care were compromised to include both dentists' and doctors' bills (Senate version) but were to apply only to the medically needy (as in the House version). Although the House readily accepted the conference bill, because of the AFDC provisions, there was thought to be a possibility the bill might not pass the Senate, but it did, and was signed by the President in January 1968.[77]

The first stage of the history of Medicaid was thus complete. In the space of two and a half years Medicaid had moved briskly from its position as a "sleeper" health program, which optimists at least saw as alleviating medical indigence and standardizing programs within (and among) the states, to a program that many regarded as the paradigm of rising welfare costs, inefficient management, and unfair taxation.[78] The vague notion of helping the deserving poor implied in the 1965 legislation was overtaken by the realities of federal-state administration. The 1967 Amendments recognized those realities. Expansion was replaced by fiscal retrenchment.

Besides administrative questions, however, serious problems still remained. The Congress, in seeking to control federal costs, had rejected Medicaid as a program with national eligibility levels: eligibility was to continue to vary arbitrarily from state to state. The concept of "medical indigency" was thus to be parochial and limited, potentially in conflict with the goals of national legislation. While the goal of comprehensive care remained, there was still no clearer definition of what it meant, and indeed the very concept seemed incompatible with the trends of the 1967 Amendments. Finally, in the 1967 Amendments there were the seeds of coming control over Medicaid providers: a new twist in the search for "mainstream" medicine.

NOTES

1. U.S., Congress, Senate, Committee on Finance, *Social Security Amendments of 1965*, S. Report 404, 89th Cong., Ist Sess., 1965, p. 11.

2. U.S., Congress, House, Committee on Ways and Means, *Limitations on*

Federal Participation under Title XIX of the Social Security Act, House Report 2224 to Accompany H.R. 18225, 89th Cong., 2nd Sess., 1966, p. 8.

3. Remarks of Senator Saltonstall, *Congressional Record* CXII, 20267 (August 22, 1966).

4. *Limitations on Federal Participation, supra,* note 2, p. 1.

5. *New York Times*, Dec. 3, 1966, p. 1, col. 4; *ibid.*, p. 47, col. 2.

6. *Ibid.*, Dec. 4, 1966, p. 1, col. 1.

7. *Medical Tribune*, August 28, 1967.

8. *AMA News*, June 19, 1967.

9. *New York Times*, Dec. 9, 1966, p. 32, col. 5.

10. Michael Petrina, *A Look at Medicaid*, 1969 (a paper presented at the Yale Law School). For an analysis of these developments from the perspective of the New York City Medicaid program, see Chapter 10.

11. The city ruled he was allowed $8 for the first person he examined in any house, but only $5 for subsequent examinations. *Medical Tribune*, June 12, 1967.

12. *Ibid.*

13. *AMA News*, Jan. 2, 1967.

14. Dr. John Lawler, *Medical Tribune*, June 12, 1967.

15. *New York Times*, Jan. 20, 1967, p. 88, col. 1.

16. *New York Times*, December 12, 1967, p. 39, col. 4. The Report found, for instance, that the average gross income of Medicaid families was less than $3200 ($61 a week) and that less than one tenth of the households earned enough to pay New York's deductible. About 56 percent of the households were of one or two persons, with an average gross income of $1900 ($35 a week); the remaining households averaged five persons with an income of $4800 ($93 a week). One quarter of one percent earned $10,000 or more, and each of such households had seven or more persons. Seventy-five percent of those surveyed had no health insurance.

17. *New York Times*, Sept. 17, 1967, p. 1, col. 2; p. 69, col. 1.

18. *Ibid.*, Nov. 11, 1966, p. 28.

19. *Ibid.*, Nov. 13, 1966, pp. 1, 38.

20. *Ibid.*, Jan. 8, 1967, p. 41.

21. *Ibid.*, Jan. 8, 1967, p. 41.

22. U.S. Advisory Commission on Intergovernmental Relations, *Intergovernmental Problems in Medicaid* (Washington, 1968), p. 121.

23. Total medical vendor payments divided by the population of the state. Tax Foundation Inc., *Medicaid: State Programs After Two Years* (New York, 1968), p. 70.

24. U.S. Department of Health, Education, and Welfare. Public Health Service, Margaret Greenfield, *Medi-Cal, The California Medicaid Program (Title XIX)* (Washington, 1968), p. 53.

25. Acton W. Barnes. *A Description of the Organization and Administration of the California Medical Assistance Program: Title XIX*, mimeograph, School of Public Health, Univ. of North Carolina, 1968, pp. 127–28.

26. There was a byzantine series of announcements as to the extent of the deficit that would be carried over into the state budget for 1967–68. One problem involved the use of accrual accounting in recording expenditures, that is, including all outstanding but unpaid obligations rather than using a straight month-

by-month outflow method. The higher figures were ascertained by use of the former method. Eventually, the estimate was reduced to $35.5 million in terms of payments from the California General Fund. But the revised estimate came too late to stem the political action in the state. See Greenfield, *supra,* note 24, pp. 53–60; Barnes, pp. 125–47.

27. Eligibility for service in California was limited until January 1, 1967, to persons considered needy or medically needy under state programs in effect as of December 1965. The initial thrust of the program was a considerable expansion of services to those already eligible, stressing comprehensive health benefits and continuity of care. As of September 1967 the per-month subsistence amounts for medical indigency were fixed at $289 for two persons, plus $26 for each additional person in the immediate family. But even this per-year total of $4092 for a family of four was low compared with New York's initial means test of $6000. See Greenfield, *supra,* note 24, pp. 17–18, 31.

28. Figures for persons for whom payments were made in November 1967 showed the following differences:

	California	*New York*
Categorically needy	518,400	302,200
Others	107,400	481,800

Intergovernmental Problems, supra, note 22, p. 121.

29. Barnes, *supra,* note 25, p. 131.

30. *Morris v. Williams,* 67 Cal. 2d 733, 737; 433 P.2d 697, 700; 63 Cal. Rptr. 689, 692 (1967). While the decision of the Court of Appeal was no doubt far from value-free, Mr. Justice Sullivan sought manfully to insist that law, not policy, had been applied:

> *Our function is to inquire into the legality of the regulations, not their wisdom. Nor do we superimpose upon the Agency any policy judgments of our own. . . .*
>
> [W]*e have concluded that the regulations under review are violative of the pertinent law in two major respects: (1) by restricting physicians' services for recipients of public assistance without eliminating the medically indigent from the Medi-Cal program; and (2) by eliminating certain services entirely in the absence of a showing that proportionate reductions were not feasible to some extent.*

31. Greenfield, *supra,* note 24, p. 59; Barnes, *supra,* note 25, p. 144 and *passim.*

32. Barnes, *supra,* note 25, p. 147. The story is chronicled in detail in Barnes, Chapters 8 ("The Case of the Disappearing Deficit") and 9 ("The Sound and Fury").

33. By 1967 the evaluation process consisted of visits by two or three members of the Office to a particular state, where they would talk not only to the state administrators in the Welfare Department but also the representatives of providers, consumers, and also (where applicable) fiscal agents. From these visits came a written PREP (Program Review and Evaluation Project) report, which had two major purposes. First, it provided evidence of compliance for the state; but second—and what might ultimately have been of more importance—the PREP reports provided a running commentary of Medicaid for MSA. The federal agency could thus act as a channel of communication among the states on current ideas, problems, and practices.

Individuals in HEW also attempted to influence state practices. For example, when the Connecticut State Welfare Commissioner informed Mary Switzer, who was then administrator of SRS (the welfare arm of HEW) that Connecticut was setting an eligibility limit of $3800 for a family of four, she reportedly drew his attention strongly to the $6000 limit in New York; but (as with other suggestions from HEW) such comparisons were ignored. Bisbee, *The Growth of the Connecticut State Department of Welfare, 1953–72,* paper presented at the Yale Medical School, 1973.

34. *New York Times,* June 24, 1966, p. 7, col. 8.

35. Press release for the Office of Senator Jacob Javits, June 16, 1966, p. 1.

36. *Social Security Bulletin,* vol. 29, No. 8 (August 1966), p. 2.

37. *New York Times,* Sept. 8, 1966, p. 27.

38. *Title XIX Fact Sheets,* 1965, 1966, *passim.* Other states' income limits per family of four included: Massachusetts with $4176, Pennsylvania with $4000, California and Connecticut with $3800, Wisconsin with $3700, Illinois with $3600, Michigan with $3540, Kentucky with $3420, Maryland with $3120, Hawaii, Minnesota, North Dakota, and Washington with $3000.

39. *Limitations on Federal Participation, supra,* note 2, pp. 2, 3–4.

40. *New York Times,* October 7, 1966, p. 20.

41. *Limitations on Federal Participation, supra,* note 2, pp. 24–27.

42. Of H.R. 18225, which Representative Mills introduced to implement the Report, Representative Curtis said:

> *This bill which tells States that they will get no Federal matching funds for medical costs of adults in families where there is a medically indigent or "ADC indigent" child, doesn't really help much one way or another. To those who want the Federal Government to relieve the tax structure of State and local communities, it is a step backward. . . .*

Ibid., p. 27.

43. *New York Times,* October 15, 1966, p. 1, col. 8.

44. For a general background to the legislation, see *Welfare in Review,* May–June 1968, p. 1. For detailed comparisons with the earlier law, together with statistics, see U.S., Congress, Senate, Committee on Finance, *The Social Security Amendment of 1967—Public Law 248, 90th Congress: Brief Summary of Major Provisions and Detailed Comparison with Prior Law,* Committee Print, 90th Cong., 2nd Sess., 1968.

45. In addition, the bill would have allowed states to buy into Title XVIII, Part B, not only for those who were receiving cash benefits under public assistance but also for those who were "medically indigent." Moreover, services provided by such "buying-in" procedures were exempted from the "comparability" provisions of the 1965 legislation in the hope that not requiring the states to include the same services for recipients under age 65 as were available to aged recipients would encourage buying-in. In addition, the HEW bill would have increased the scope of the federal 75 percent administrative sharing arrangement, at the same time covering agencies other than the one directing the program. The proposed bill would also have established the free choice of physicians, created a Medical Assistance Advisory Council, and set up certain new programs for children under 21, at the same time linking the program more clearly with Title V (Maternal and Child Welfare).

46. Several restrictive proposals similar to that of Representative Stratton had been made. One, H.R. 18225, had been reported out of the Ways and Means Committee but had died when it became clear that no action could be taken on it by the Senate in the remaining weeks of the session. 22 *Congressional*

Quarterly Almanac 343 (1966). The primary limitation that this bill imposed would have been to eliminate the Medicaid eligibility of adults in AFDC-related families. This restriction would have applied only to the medically needy, not to families actually receiving AFDC cash assistance or to medically needy adults related to the other categories. This bill also would have made some of the same changes that were to reappear in the amendments of 1967, such as further encouragement of Medicaid "buy-in" agreements and limits on the "state effort" requirements of Title XIX. *Limitations on Federal Participation, supra,* note 2, pp. 3–6. In language that was to be repeated, the Committee warned the states that it "never intended that Federal matching under Title XIX would be made in the case of a considerable portion of the adult working population of moderate means" and that the states should "avoid unrealistic levels of income and resources for Title XIX eligibility purposes." *Ibid.,* at pp. 2–3.

47. U.S., Congress, House, Committee on Ways and Means, *President's Proposals for Revision of the Social Security System, Hearings* before the House Committee on Ways and Means on H.R. 5710, 90th Cong., 1st Sess., 1967.

48. Such business and insurance groups included the American Life Convention and Life Insurance Association (who would have preferred dollar limits on federal participation), Blue Cross, Blue Shield, various chambers of commerce, the International Association of Health Underwriters, the National Association of Life Underwriters, various medical groups, and, once again, Representative Stratton (who thought H.R. 5710 did not go far enough).

49. Opposing federal cutbacks were welfare and labor groups, including the AFL-CIO, the Community Council of Greater New York, the International Ladies' Garment Workers Union, the National Association of Social Workers, the National Urban League, the Physicians Forum, and the United Auto Workers.

50. U.S., Congress, House, Committee on Ways and Means, *Social Security Amendments of 1967,* House Report No. 544, to accompany H.R. 12080, 90th Cong., 1st Sess., 1967, at p. 119. This was for states beginning Medicaid programs. For those states with a program already in existence, the proportion would be 150 percent until December 31, 1968, and 140 percent until December 31, 1969. The limitation of 133⅓ percent would apply thereafter.

51. P.L. 90-248. An alternative limitation (not enacted), which would have been used in states where it produced a lower figure, would have set the maximum for a family of four at 133⅓ percent of the state's per capita income. That percentage would have been altered proportionately for larger or smaller families.

52. *Social Security Amendments of 1967, supra,* note 50, p. 121.

53. The states were given added incentives, as in the administration proposals, to "buy in" to Part B of Medicare on behalf of eligible Medicaid recipients, the medically needy as well as the categorically needy. The bill provided that federal matching would be unavailable on behalf of persons whom the states had failed to cover under Part B. In addition the "comparability" requirements would be waived where necessary to permit "buying-in." Other parallels with the administration proposals included the change in the scope of the 75-percent administrative sharing arrangement, the freedom of choice provisions, the links with Title V, and the creation of the Medical Assistance Advisory Council. This MAAC, described in some detail in the bill and in the enacted law, was patterned after the Health Insurance Benefits Advisory Council created by Title XVIII. It was to consist of 21 persons appointed by the Secretary of HEW to 4-year terms and was to present the "views of a variety of individuals interested and knowledgeable about medical administration." *Ibid.,* pp. 120–127.

54. The new provision allowed cash assistance payments alone to be taken into account so that "no state is penalized for limiting its medical assistance program to what it conceives to be sound and proper levels." *Ibid.*, p. 119. This suggestion, too, thus gave more flexibility to the states.

55. *Ibid.*, pp. 120–21.

56. *Ibid.*, p. 123.

57. *Ibid.*, pp. 123–24.

58. *Ibid.*, p. 124.

59. U.S., Congress, Senate, Committee on Finance, *Social Security Amendments of 1967, Hearings* before the Committee on Finance, Senate, on H.R. 12080, 90th Cong., 1st Sess., 1967, p. 217.

60. *Ibid.*, pp. 274–82.

61. *Ibid.*, pp. 279–80. "The House limitation will destroy the concept of medical indigence in a number of States." *Ibid.*, p. 280.

62. *Ibid.*, p. 755. "We recommend, therefore, that any income limit placed on eligibility for Title XIX benefits should not be so rigid as to exclude those who are clearly unable to pay for needed health care, especially those whose need is such that they are already receiving cash assistance. . . ."

63. *Ibid.*, pp. 1591–92. The Chairman of the Citizens' Committee for Medicaid stated that Congress should "make no mistake, if H.R. 12080 passes in its present form, it will strike hardest at those families who have managed to pull themselves up from the lower depths of poverty, who are just beginning to see daylight and learning to become productive members of society. . . . We cannot rationalize the anguish of the medically needy with the unrealistic formula of H.R. 12080."

64. *Ibid.*, pp. 1546–47. George K. Wyman stated, "In fact New York is the only State which has met the 1975 deadline established by Congress in Title XIX which requires all States by that time to have provided comprehensive medical care for all needy persons."

65. U.S., Congress, Senate, Committee on Finance, *Social Security Amendments of 1967*, S. Report No. 744, to Accompany H.R. 12080, 90th Cong., 1st Sess., 1967, pp. 197–98. He also noted that his own state would be penalized more than any other by the limitation on assistance to the medically needy.

66. As a result, the total reduction in costs through 1972 would be $481 million less than would be realized by the House bill. *Ibid.*, p. 177.

67. This would be computed by "squaring" the federal share of payments on behalf of the categorically needy, thus lowering the matching share on behalf of the medically needy to between 25 percent (50 percent squared) and approximately 69 percent (83 percent squared). *Ibid.*, pp. 176–77.

68. *Ibid.*, pp. 181–82.

69. *Ibid.*, pp. 184–85. Other features of the House version which were not substantially changed, included the sections dealing with "freedom of choice" by recipients in selecting providers, "buy-in" agreements with Medicare, expanded federal matching for professional administrative costs, the creation of an MAAC, the alleviation of fiscal burdens on the localities, the requirement for consultation services to providers, the liability of third parties, and the modification of the "state effort" requirements.

70. Various standards relating to the professionalization of staffs were set, and after December 31, 1969, homes were to be required (with some room for waivers) to meet the applicable provisions of the Life Safety Code of the Na-

tional Fire Protection Association or of an approved state safety code. The bill also proposed the creation of a nine-member National Advisory Council on Nursing Home Administration to study and report to the Secretary of HEW on nursing homes and ways to improve their performance, administration, and regulation. *Ibid.*, pp. 185–86, 189–90.

71. *Ibid.*, pp. 188–89.

72. *Ibid.*, p. 187.

73. *Ibid.*, p. 186.

74. There was at least one other expansionist aspect of the 1967 legislation. The "earned income disregard" incorporated into the AFDC program increased the number of persons eligible for cash programs and thus for Title XIX. U.S., Congress, Senate, Committee on Finance, and House, Committee on Ways and Means, *Summary of Social Security Amendments of 1967*, Committee Print, 90th Cong., 1st Sess., 1967, p. 23. Finally, the Committee added a "Christian Scientist" provision to assure that, in general, no person would be required to submit to diagnosis or treatment if he objected on religious grounds. *Social Security Amendments of 1967*, *supra*, note 65, p. 187.

75. Robert B. Stevens, *Statutory History of the United States: Income Security* (New York, 1970), p. 823 *et seq.*; Congressional Quarterly Service, *Congressional Quarterly Almanac*, 1967 (Washington, 1968), pp. 909–16.

76. The provision added by the Committee requiring states to safeguard against unnecessary utilization was augmented by a requirement that the states assure that payments not be in excess of "reasonable charges." And a modification in the "comparability of services" requirement was added to require the states to take into account variations in shelter costs in setting levels of eligibility for the medically needy. This was changed in the conference committee to allow, rather than require, this flexible test of need.

77. *Social Security Amendments of 1967*, P.L. 90–248, 81 Stat. 821.

78. In fairness, however, it should be noted that the 1975 goal of comprehensive services—s 1903(e)—was, despite considerable pressure, retained.

PART III
The Storm

JANUARY 1968–JULY 1970

INTRODUCTION

After the passage of the Social Security Amendments of 1967, Medicaid ceased to be one of the least analyzed programs in the Federal medical care arsenal and became the subject of a series of administrative and legislative inquiries. Data, which had been almost nonexistent, were laboriously produced. Policy, which had not been made by HEW, was gradually developed by Congressional Committees and others. Continuing efforts were made to tighten the administrative operation of Medicaid in its existing framework. These included the development of controls over fees, utilization, and fraud. At the same time, there was a series of projects for drastic reforms in the Medicaid system. These were to range from Governor Rockefeller's strong endorsement of state-run plans of health insurance (to replace Medicaid) to proposals to direct Medicaid funding in deliberate efforts to change the health care system. Fiscal conservatives, including members of the Senate Finance Committee, which was becoming the focus for administrative tightening in Medicaid, and liberal reformers, who would redefine the nature of "welfare medicine," were alike in two important respects. The concerns of both were stimulated by the continuing cost spiral of Medicaid, and the solutions of both demanded increased federal regulation.

Meanwhile, the recipients and the providers grew increasingly unhappy. Recipients, who had rising expectations about the provision of medical care by the state, found themselves increasingly barred from Medicaid rolls. With state legislatures taking on conservative hues, recipients turned to welfare-rights organizations for protection, and they in turn resorted to the courts to seek to stem the tide of reaction. Medicaid thus led to a confrontation on basic questions of services and eligibility.

At the same time providers were faced with the first fruits of massive state intervention into the private sector of medicine. For years, the more conservative providers' groups, led by the American Medical Association, had warned that state medicine would mean state control. P.L. 89-97 had gone through on the assumption that massive federal programs of medical care could be instituted without disturbing traditional patterns of medical practice, including billing. The years 1968, 1969, and 1970 were to illustrate the unreality of that assumption and to confirm the earlier fears of the providers' groups. By June 1970, as the Nixon administration was seeking to develop new health and welfare strategies, Medicaid itself was taking on new guises.

These various processes were to emphasize the shifting sands on which Medicaid was based. The 1967 Amendments injected a note of administrative realism into the program's structure by attempting some fiscal controls and standard-setting. But the Amendments did little to clarify Medicaid's underlying goals and objectives. Lacking a clear mandate to provide health services to nationally-defined groups of recipients, the agencies administering Medicaid were inevitably sensitive to the immediate anxieties of powerful groups. The development of Medicaid in these years reads, as a result, as a saga of institutional pronouncements and power plays rather than of concern with the recipients of medical care. There was at the same time a continuing search for scapegoats, who could be blamed for Medicaid's administrative ills.

To develop these issues, we look first at the problems of administration as seen from the standpoint of HEW. Its overall administrative problems in dealing with Congress, the states, providers and recipients are examined by looking particularly at the issue of nursing homes (Chapter 8). We next look at the problems in the states, focussing mostly on California and New York—and particularly on the attempts of New York City to implement the state's legislation (Chapter 9). We then turn to the costs of medical care, the efforts to curb the price spiral, and the efforts during these years to isolate the villains (Chapter 10). Finally, in this Part, we examine the competing social policies which were emerging in the final years of the Johnson and the initial years of the Nixon administrations (Chapter 11).

8
The Scene in Washington

The 1967 Amendments established, in one stroke, a set of principles by which Medicaid was to be judged, while most state programs were still embryonic or in their infancy.[1] It had become clear that effective control over the costs of the program could be exercised only through Congress. As assistance grants are part of Social Security legislation which also includes the raising of Social Security taxes, this meant the beginnings of health care regulation through Congress's major tax committees.

General Implications of the 1967 Amendments

One principle was clear. Eligibility for the "medically needy" was to be tied to eligibility levels for cash assistance in each state. For states whose Medicaid plans were approved prior to July 1967, income eligibility levels for the medically needy were, by July 1968, to be limited to 150 percent of the maximum AFDC payments authorized by the state and, by January 1970, to reach the specified 133⅓ percent. (States could retain higher eligibility levels, but no federal matching funds would be forthcoming.) All other states had to move directly to the 133⅓ percent levels. Within these limits funding remained open-ended.

As the AFDC eligibility levels were notoriously uneven from state to state, this meant not only a rejection of any broad national criterion of "medical indigency" for Medicaid but that one rocky system of grants-in-aid had been attached to another. A committee of federal and state legislators, reporting in 1968, put the matter succinctly: "The effect of linking the limit to AFDC is to make this federally sanctioned eligibility standard no more consistent among the States than the level of actual AFDC payments on which it is based."[2]

In one sense the 1967 Amendments heralded stronger federal controls. In the proposals for stricter standards over the quality of nursing-home care and for better systems of management and audit, Congress was taking upon itself a watchdog function over economy and efficiency, a function which was to expand in 1969 and 1970. The inclusion of compulsory health screening for all eligible children under 21 also promised more standardization imposed by the federal government. Yet, at the same time, some federal criteria were weakened. The substitution, at least for the medically needy, for the initial five basic services of a choice of seven out of 14 moved away from the 1965 requirement of a common base of services that would be expanded into "comprehensive care" in each state by 1975. In the interests of cost control, the goal of comprehensiveness was slipping toward abandonment.

One further aspect of Medicaid was also becoming evident. The rising costs of medical care made Medicaid important as both a cause and a symbol of such increases. In January 1967, before the passage of the restrictive Social Security Amendments, the President's budget predicted total federal and state medical vendor payments of $2.25 billion in fiscal 1968, with 48 states participating. The actual expenditures for that year, with only 37 states having operating programs, were $3.54 billion. For fiscal 1970, the estimated expenditures were $5.5 billion, of which the federal share was $2.8 billion.[3] Between 1965 and 1970 federal expenditures had undergone a fivefold increase, with similar increases on the part of the states. Nor was there any sign of a lessening of the cost acceleration.

The dilemmas of Medicaid were evident. As a service program attached to a system of cash assistance benefits, Medicaid lacked the financial controls of other aspects of public assistance. As a system of the public purchase of services in the private medical sector, Medicaid had little or no authority over medical care providers who were by then, in many instances, receiving self-determined fees.

The role of HEW was limited, with almost total devolution of programs to the states; and the states had a major interest in maintaining good relations with providers. There was no unified national policy toward Medicaid emanating from the executive. Thus the only institution capable of dealing with the growing budgetary problems was Congress. Powerful spokesmen such as Representative Mills and Senators Russell Long, Jacob Javits, and Clinton Anderson brought the experiences in their own states back for renewed committee consideration in the House and the Senate.

This, then, was the Medicaid context as states grappled with the 1967 amendments and MSA moved to attempt a new series of administrative interpretations. The problems of Medicaid were not of any one organization's making; rather, they were inherent in the system itself. They were expressed in terms of Medicaid's spiralling and uncontrollable costs, but they were at root problems of goals, authority, and administration.

Medicaid and Other Health Programs

No doubt many politicians hoped the Medicaid problems would just go away after the 1967 Amendments were signed into law in January 1968. But they did not, for many reasons. First of all, the medical needs and expectations of the poor and the near-poor did not evaporate. While, politically, a conservative reaction was developing in 1968—culminating with the election of President Nixon in November—the memory of past events was still fresh in the minds of those who felt themselves oppressed. As black riots erupted (perhaps for the last time) after the assassination of Martin Luther King in the spring of 1968, the identification of poverty with racial inequality was stressed. The "deserving poor" could no longer be patronized because they were little old ladies or thin-boned children. These poor were able-bodied and militant. While there still seemed no generalized sympathy for such developments, if the (Kerner) Riot Commission Report[4] was to be believed, the problems of poverty and inequality had at least reached a new phase of public awareness. Deficiencies in health care were part and parcel of this consciousness. Indeed, poor health services in the black urban ghetto were described in the Kerner report (and elsewhere) as contributing to poor health conditions, which in turn contributed to the summers of violence in major cities in the mid-1960s.[5]

The proliferation of federally supported health programs for the poor in the years of the Johnson Administration also stressed the special needs of low-income groups, with the underlying assumption that these should be met. An HEW report, *Delivery of Health Services for the Poor,*[6] prepared at Secretary Gardner's request and published in 1968, emphasized that there were 45 million low-income Americans. Expenditures for federal grants and payments for health care for the poor had risen from $1.6 billion in fiscal 1966 to an estimated $5.1 billion in fiscal 1968.[7] But most of this (about $4 billion) was represented by payments on behalf of the poor through Medicaid and Medicare. The remainder was scattered in an array of programs for specific groups, such as migrants, for special problems such as venereal disease, and in demonstration or experimental grants providing comprehensive care (e.g., the OEO Comprehensive Health Services Program and Children and Youth project grants available through the Children's Bureau). These various programs were estimated to assist in providing care for only 10 to 12 million of the 45 million low-income persons. Moreover, the programs themselves, notably Medicaid, provided services that were often partial and fragmented.

The clear acceptance in HEW's *Delivery of Health Services for the Poor* that Medicaid was one of HEW's array of health programs marked a new consciousness of federal involvement in the program. If Medicaid were to be regarded as a major federal program, any attempt to rationalize existing programs in HEW would naturally include it. The HEW report, while coming out strongly for an expansion of health services to the poor, made it clear that federal monies would be more usefully directed if they were focussed more efficiently. Comprehensive health centers for low-income areas were suggested, emphasizing preventive services, continuity of care, and "family-oriented health care resources." Other programs were recommended to improve the effectiveness of existing sources of care to the poor, such as outpatient clinics, and to provide appropriate manpower for the programs.

Irrespective of the form of these recommendations, what was implied was a new way of considering federal funding—not merely in terms of subsidizing states in order that they might subsidize medical vendor payments, but in terms of at least a limited restructuring of the organization and provision of medical care. The seed was sown for later recommendations under the Nixon administration for revamping Medicaid and, more generally, for redirecting federal funds into the establishment of organized health care systems. Indeed, out of all this was to come an Administration commitment to a federal subsidy for health maintenance organizations.

But there were other forces at work, too, in 1968, which kept Medicaid at the forefront of legislative interest. One of the problems in evaluating Medicaid up to this point had been the lack of virtually any reliable information. The authors of Secretary Gardner's report had been forced to admit, rather lamely, that they were unable to ascertain "with any degree of certainty" such elementary questions as how large a proportion of the medical costs incurred by potential Medicaid recipients were in fact being covered by the programs or what percentage of the medically indigent were covered by or made use of Medicaid services.[8]

Information, Interests, and Expectations

Information was, however, beginning to be gathered outside HEW. Indeed, the first major attempt to describe Medicaid was undertaken by a private institution, the New York-based Tax Foundation, Inc., an independent research organization. Questionnaires had been sent in the fall of 1967 to private and public agencies in the 50 states; the ensuing report was published in June 1968.[9] It provided the first detailed critique of the program and at the same time provided information on problems currently being experienced by different states.

A second study was generated by the states. As the 1967 Amendments moved through Congress there had been, not surprisingly, an increase in interest in the state legislatures about the future federal role in Medicaid. A meeting of the National Conference of State Legislative Leaders in December 1967 reflected this concern and led to a formal request to the statutory Advisory Commission on Intergovernmental Relations to undertake an analysis of the Medicaid program, a request granted in February 1968. Because the membership of the Commission included public figures at all levels of government,[10] any report it produced was likely to command considerable attention.

One of the standing functions of the 26-member Commission was to "recommend, within the framework of the Constitution, the most desirable allocation of governmental functions, responsibilities and revenues among the several levels of government. . . ."[11] Medicaid offered a fertile field for such considerations. Moreover, the Commission's staff moved fast. In addition to a questionnaire, information was gathered from MSA, from the data collected by the Tax Foundation, and from other relevant sources; and a draft document was prepared that focussed mainly on the policies affecting the federal, state, and local sharing of responsibility for financing Medicaid.[12] The report was issued in September 1968.

Yet a third report was brewing,[13] this one called for by President Johnson during the Conference of Governors of the States and Territories in February 1968. The President took the occasion to remark upon the high cost of Medicaid and the need for its improvement. In typical Johnsonian style, he noted that "We in the Federal Government have inadequate information on which to predict what the States will do," and concluded: "Let us try to arrive at a solution together."[14] The result was a special State-Federal Task Force on the Costs of Medical Assistance and Public Assistance, officially established in March 1968. The resulting report came out in October. Focussing on costs, the report pulled together budgetary information and made specific suggestions on budget procedures and cost information in the states.[15]

Thus by the fall of 1968 there were for the first time a basis of information, a survey of problems, and specific recommendations on Medicaid. Moreover, the three 1968 reports in large part intermeshed. The Tax Foundation report outlined the implementation of the various state programs, including the various services provided and the eligibility levels, and gave an overview of fiscal operating experience. Respondents in the states complained, in particular, about the sharp increase in medical care costs and, where fee schedules were maintained, about the unwillingness of some providers to serve Medicaid patients because of low fees. These comments underlined the general lack of efficiency in the provision of medical care. One respondent noted: "Title 19 has scraped raw what has been bothering us so long."[16]

The Advisory Commission's report took these themes further. Medical care prices had risen 6.6 percent in 1966 and 6.4 percent in 1967, compared to rises of 3.3 percent and 3.1 percent in the over-all consumer price index.[17] The Commission concluded that Medicaid had contributed to these cost increases, out of all proportion to the number of persons served, by rapidly stimulating consumer demand. The implication of this conclusion, interpreted by a body which was weighted toward state and local interests, was twofold: first, that there was a need to slow down the development of state Medicaid programs and second, that increased funding should be sought from nonstate sources. The Commission recommended keeping to the 1975 goal of comprehensive care (noting that the goal applied to "substantially all" the needy and medically needy, a phrase of some potential latitude), but it suggested that Congress and the Administration examine the feasibility of involving the private sector in this, including "some form of employer-employee contributory health insurance."[18] These themes were to be important in subsequent debates. The states were saying, in effect, that without extra funding they would have to cut services; but that an acceptable alternative would be to abandon Medicaid in favor of a publicly regulated (nonstate-funded) insurance system. Thus Medicaid, rather than providing an alternative to health insurance, began to appear as a direct incentive for such a program, at least to hard-pressed legislators in the states.

The Commission also made other recommendations to help the states. These included deferring the date when federal assistance for vendor payments would be withdrawn from states without Medicaid programs from January 1970 to January 1972 (thus slowing up Medicaid's implementation). Governor Rockefeller was among the dissenters from this proposal. While the Commission endorsed the principle of tying eligibility levels to AFDC, although recommending that they be at the 150 percent level, it urged that federal matching continue to be on an open-ended basis. But there was also a stronger commitment to providing medical services than was evident in the Congressional Tax Committees. The Commission recommended, for example, including the large number of childless needy persons aged 21–64 in Medicaid, presumably on Governor Rockefeller's recommendation.[19]

A series of recommendations sought to give states more flexibility in Medicaid administration, for example, in revenue raising and in allocating medical services among needy groups in the states. Finally the Commission made recommendations for increased economy and efficiency in medical services. These ranged from abolition of the "reasonable cost" reimbursement for hospitals to encouraging the expansion of prepaid group practice of health care through eliminating the legislative barriers then existing in many states. Taken as a whole these recommendations encapsulated the problems of Medicaid. On one hand were proposals for expansion, including making Medicaid a more efficient medical service; on the other, proposals for limitations on the basis of cost considerations.

The third report appearing in the fall of 1968, that of the special State-Federal Task Force on the Costs of Medical Assistance and Public Assistance, concentrated on improving administrative arrangements within the existing system, a theme of particular Congressional interest. Gross deficiencies were found in available management information, both in terms of budget and in terms of service utilization; indeed, some of the underlying problems overflowed into the recommendations. One major conclusion, for instance, was that the states and HEW "should work more closely together and should fully share their budgetary knowledge . . . ,"[20] a pointed reflection on the then current state of affairs. An information system was proposed that included regular sampling studies in each state, and the general thrust was to improve both state and federal forecasting abilities.

Thus, at the same time that the states were implementing the 1967 Amendments, new proposals for change were emerging. These ranged from relatively minor administrative changes to major overhauls. What came out clearly in these efforts was the fiscal strains of the Medicaid program and the impossibility of undertaking any more than a Band-Aid approach without more general changes in federal-state responsibilities and, inevitably, in the health care system itself.

Meanwhile, Back in HEW . . .

Increased federal responsibility would ultimately devolve on HEW. But here lay another source of difficulties; the unwieldiness inherent in the congeries of empires making up the nation's major social-policy agency was in danger of becoming an American tradition. Despite a series of departmental reorganizations in the 1960s, even the nation's top health official, the Assistant Secretary for Health and Scientific Affairs, had "effective control" over only 22 percent of HEW's health budget; and Medicaid was not included in that fraction.[21] Medicaid, as we have seen, was run by the Medical Services Administration, an arm of the Social and Rehabilitation Service,[22] the old Welfare Administration. Any attempts to use Medicaid as a lever for regulating the health system promised to founder in HEW's piecemeal organization.

To these difficulties was added continuing understaffing at the federal level. By mid-1969, the renamed and nominally upgraded Medical Services Administration, as part of the Social and Rehabilitation Service, still had only 76 positions (including secretaries) in Washington and 24 in the regional offices, yet MSA staff were responsible for communicating with 44 states' Medicaid programs, for guiding program planning and development, and for providing program evaluation. The lack of staff in MSA must be counted as a major contributing factor in the "Medicaid Crisis." Title XIX, as passed in 1965, was so vague that only a well-staffed department could have implemented it effectively.

As it was, mandatory dates were not met; for example, Arizona and Alaska failed to meet the December 1969 deadline for producing a state plan for Medicaid, and cut-offs in state funds (which could, for instance, be imposed on those several states that had not met utilization review requirements) were not only not made but never considered seriously. Despite the fact that each year Medicaid took an increasingly significant share of the federal budget, the issuing of regulations—the very core of an effective federal-state grant-in-aid program—proceeded remarkably slowly. Indeed, the basic regulations for administration of the program were not issued until 1969.[23] MSA just made the 1970 deadline mandated by the 1967 legislation for establishing federal standards for the licensing of nursing-home administrators and for the development of a definition of a skilled nursing home,[24] and this burst of speed was partially achieved by co-opting representatives of the industry to undertake the drafting.[25] Even then, regulations were often provisional, with the result that regional offices and state welfare departments treated them with some suspicion, lest the offices and departments commit limited resources to implementation only to discover the regulations withdrawn.

The Medical Services Administration also had difficulties in making use of its representatives in the regional offices. The Title XIX staff in the regional offices was inadequate to handle the work load and ill-equipped to deal with the medical profession (and sometimes the state health departments). To add to the difficulties, the Associate Regional Commissioners for Medical Services were not subordinate to the MSA staff in Washington but were responsible to regional SRS Commissioners, who were in turn responsible to the SRS Commissioner in Washington (MSA's chief). This circular line of responsibility encouraged administrative confusion and put additional burdens on offices that were already short-staffed. In Boston, for instance, in 1970, a staff of three professionals and one secretary handled Medicaid for the six New England states. The coming to power of a Republican administration in Washington in 1969, committed as it was to devolution of federal programs to the regions (and states), only served to deepen the problem. Getting messages from MSA in Washington to MSA regional personnel required almost as many clearances as those required of a desk officer in the State Department in getting a signal to an embassy overseas.

Until the advent of the Nixon Administration, regional offices had not played a significant role. The work of the regional office was an advisory and auditing one: the Boston office, for example, mediated the dispute between the ophthalmologists and optometrists under the Rhode Island program. The staffs of all regional offices joined the Washington staff in a bienniel or trienniel review of each state's program. Often, however, regional offices saw themselves as defenders of "their" states against Washington. The over-all result was considerable conflict between Washington and the regions.[26] With the leadership in HEW pressing for further devolution of policy-making through the Associate Commissioners of SRS in each of the ten regions, the earlier parochialism was shored up with potential power. But the relationship between MSA and the regions remained (as it does today) largely undefined and unclear.

The 1967 Amendments had given the Washington office a blue-ribbon advisory council which might have been used to publicize administrative problems and staffing difficulties. But no fruitful relationship materialized. The Medical Assistance Advisory Council earned the reputation of being "one of the least-used panels in HEW's large stable of advisory councils," partly because it was uncomfortably attached to Medicaid after the program had been in existence for two years, partly because it was given no effective secretariat, and partly because it was thought not to have the support of the Democratic HEW Secretary.[27] Even the Nixon Administration, however, seemed disinterested in using the Council. The Council was not consulted when Dr. James Haughton was appointed to review Medicaid's reimbursement procedures for physician, dentist, and other health professional services; and this event was reported as "bruising the already battered feelings" of the Council.[28] Administratively, nothing attached to Title XIX, so it seemed, worked.

Federal Administration: A Case Study of the Nursing-Home Industry

Nothing better illustrates the problems encountered in the administration of Medicaid than its difficulties in dealing with the nursing-home industry. The issue of nursing homes and their control was, in some respects, wider that MSA or Medicaid. The modern nursing-home industry had begun with the Social Security Act of 1935 when, as part of the attempt to stamp out the poor-farm and the workhouse, it was provided that federal matching funds under Title I (OAA) were not to be available to those in "public institutions."[29] The private sector responded, and boarding houses for the elderly and nursing homes *per se* began to appear. The most dramatic growth in the nursing-home industry, however, occurred with Kerr-Mills and reached its zenith with the introduction of Medicare and Medicaid.[30]

Total expenditures on nursing-home care in the United States rose from $1.4 billion in fiscal 1966 to $3.4 billion in fiscal 1971; and of this latter $3.4 billion, as much as $1.7 billion was met through Medicaid and related assistance programs.[31] Medicaid alone was disbursing more money on nursing homes in 1971 than had been spent in the entire industry five years earlier. As most nursing homes in the United States were profit-making institutions,[32] a number owned by doctors,[33] there was an obvious need to develop and enforce controls to ensure that public money was being appropriately spent.

The initial Medicaid legislation, P.L. 89–97, made "skilled nursing-home services" one of the basic requirements of a state Medicaid plan. Exactly what these skilled services were was not initially defined. Nursing homes come in all shapes and sizes, and their staffing and functions vary. Some are places for elderly persons to live with minimal medical and nursing supervision, some convalescent or rest homes, some sophisticated nursing and treatment centers. Prior to Medicaid, each state had developed its procedures of recognizing nursing-home care for the purposes of payment. The passage of Medicaid, however, crystallized the absence of any nationwide definitions.

Medicare included nursing-home benefits under the new rubric of "extended care," i.e., care provided in a nursing home following a period of hospitalization. The limited nature of these benefits meant that Medicare had a much smaller fiscal impact on nursing homes than Medicaid, but the need for federal guidelines for an "extended care facility" (ECF) forced an appraisal of the whole industry, so that standards for participation could be established.[34] Indeed, during the 18-month period between the passage of the legislation in July 1965 and the implementation of the extended-care provisions in January 1967, as many as 122 persons from the Social Security Administration (SSA) and the "health" side of HEW were involved developing appropriate conditions of participation for these Medicare providers.[35] The ensuing regulations for ECFs were detailed.[36] As befitted the purpose of Medicare's nursing-home benefits, they defined the ECF as a facility capable of serving elderly sick patients who were transferred directly from a hospital bed. The regulations, promulgated from Washington, were made the responsibility of state health agencies for the purposes of initial certification for Medicare and subsequent compliance.

Skilled nursing-home (SNH) benefits under Medicaid, on the other hand, were not limited to posthospital care, nor indeed to the elderly, although the elderly formed the bulk of the recipients. But MSA was in no position in its early days to carry out the kind of supervision SSA was able to develop for ECFs. Even in 1970, when MSA was additionally responsible for carrying out the requirements imposed under the 1967 Amendments, there were only three members of the staff of MSA in its nursing-home unit spending an estimated one half to one third of their time on the development of standards.[37] But over and above this, it was not clear where the Medicaid responsibility for standard-setting appropriately lay. Was it the federal government's responsibility as a condition of grants to states to develop federal guidelines or should standard-setting, like licensing, be delegated entirely to the states?

In the first flush of Medicaid, the MSA staff had attempted to link the nursing-home requirements to those being developed for Medicare.[38] But there were problems in this definition from the very beginning. The American Nursing Home Association protested on two counts: first, on principle, that the legislation "clearly fixed the responsibility of establishing standards with the state agency";[39] second, on grounds that the ECF definition would provide only one level of nursing-home care and in so doing would disregard the needs of over 50 percent of the welfare patients.[40] And that,

of course, would have the effect of forcing states to provide welfare payments that might be spent in unaccredited facilities.

The linking of skilled nursing homes under Medicaid with ECFs under Medicare naturally carried a restrictive definition. Critics of the SSA regulation might complain that the standards for ECFs left too much discretion to the state surveyors[41] and that SSA had abandoned the Congressional concept that ECFs would be special convalescent extensions of hospitals in favor of a looser definition.[42] The facts were, however, that the original conditions of participation proved much too high for most of the existing nursing homes. Faced with the choice of retaining high standards but depriving people of needed care or developing lower standards and thereby making facilities more accessible, SSA moved toward the latter position.[43]

Here was no crutch on which to lean, and MSA rapidly dropped the effort toward parity with Medicare as it slowly developed its thoughts about skilled nursing homes. While MSA was not prepared to capitulate entirely to the states, in March 1967 less stringent requirements were issued for homes participating in Medicaid. Notably, the standard for a charge nurse was changed from the requirement that an RN or LPN be on duty at all times to the requirement that the charge nurse could be a licensed practical nurse who need not be a graduate of a state-approved school but was serving as a charge nurse as of July 1, 1967, and had completed training satisfactory to the state licensing authority. Other requirements tended to be worded vaguely. Staffing, for example, was to be "sufficient in number and qualifications to meet the requirements of the patients. . . ."[44] Even these limited requirements did not have to be fully met until January 1969.

The requirements satisfied no one. They avoided the issue of what was a "skilled nursing home" in terms of the patient needs to be served. If it were one rung removed from hospital care, there was no apparent reason why the standards for nursing homes under Medicaid should be demonstrably lower than those for ECFs under Medicare. If, on the other hand, the needs were different, how were they different? Patients in so-called nursing homes ranged from the sick and bedridden to those who could cope with day-to-day living provided supporting services were available (but usually they were not). Senator Frank Moss (Democrat, Utah), chairman of the Special Subcommittee on Long Term Care, summed up the important question in testimony before the Senate Finance Committee in its consideration of the 1967 Amendments: "Too often patients entering nursing homes are simply left there for the rest of their days."

State health departments were concerned with standards of physical plant and equipment but not with patient care; welfare departments, too, while determining eligibility for the program, were usually not concerned with the patient's medical care or social casework problems; and physician visits were "infrequent and often perfunctory."[45] While nursing home regulation was largely left to the states, which were specifically required under Title XIX to establish or designate an authority responsible for "establishing and maintaining standards" in medical care institutions,[46] the states had no clearer definitions of nursing homes by standards of patient care than did HEW.[47] Meanwhile, a series of audits of welfare payments to nursing homes by the General Accounting Office (at the request of the Moss Subcommittee on Long Term Care) highlighted the problems inherent in the lack of basic standards against which to measure "appropriate" care. A 1967 study of the Cleveland area was typical. The nursing-home operator, it was reported, "has no financial incentive to improve the level of care but does have an incentive to keep costs as low as possible."[48]

As a result of Senator Moss's efforts, outline standards for care and safety in skilled nursing homes under Medicaid were finally incorporated into legislation in the 1967 Social Security Amendments.[49] States were also required as a condition of receiving federal Medicaid funds to have a professional medical audit program for skilled nursing homes, under which periodic medical evaluations would be made of the appropriateness of care being provided to Medicaid beneficiaries,[50] and to license nursing-home administrators according to standards developed by a new National Advisory Council on Nursing Home Administration.[51]

Two other important provisions of the 1967 Amendments rounded out the legislative basis on which more effective nursing-home regulation could be based. The first was the specification that, effective July 1968, no federal matching funds could be granted to a nursing home that, even though licensed, did not meet requirements.[52] This section paved the way for the current ruling (June 30, 1972) that MSA can selectively refuse to pay federal funds to identified institutions that do not meet required standards.[53] Potentially these developments could provide MSA with "clout." Second, in large part to settle the problems inherent in a single relatively high standard of nursing home care, the 1967 Amendments included the new nursing-home classification of Intermediate Care Facility (ICF),[54] which would also be entitled to federal assistance. In theory, at least, the question of what would happen to patients who did not need such highly skilled nursing care could thereafter be answered; they would receive long-term supportive care in nursing homes other than skilled nursing homes and in other types of facilities.[55]

This package of provisions provided the ammunition for federal regulation of the nursing-home industry. But, as history has made abundantly clear, the passage of legislation does not necessarily mean that it is effectively implemented. These provisions were dropped into the lap of MSA at a time when, having already backtracked once on standards, it was ill-prepared to deal with them. MSA thus did nothing; there followed a long period of procrastination.[56] Senator Moss protested bitterly:[57]

> *It is difficult to tell exactly what has been going on within the Department. It is as though a protracted quarrel has been taking place behind closed doors. From time to time a door is opened and one hears commotion and a confusion of raised voices. Then the door swings closed and all is quiet again. We know with certainty only that there has been little practical result from our legislative efforts.*

Finally, in June 1969, regulations were published to implement the basic standards for nursing-home care,[58] only to run into immediate criticism, chiefly from consumer groups, because of the continuing vagueness of the definitions. Nursing care was again the major point at issue. Instead of strengthening the existing guides for nurse staffing, the new regulations appeared to weaken them. Despite the 1967 Amendments, the new regulations were less demanding than those proposed under the 1965 legislation. Senator Moss, the author of the amendments, called special hearings to discuss the "crisis" caused by the regulations.[59]

The combined impact of private and Congressional complaints about HEW's inability to produce acceptable regulations provided a salutory jolt to HEW administrators. There was much dissatisfaction when it emerged that the regulations had been drafted by an HEW consultant who was concurrently a consultant to the American Nursing Home Association.[60] With unprecedented speed, a special task force was appointed,[61] the various criticisms were reviewed, recommendations made and accepted, and revised and somewhat stronger regulations were published in April 1970,[62] two years after passage of the original legislation and 15 months after the legal deadline for implementation.

Thus Congress dragged MSA, reluctantly, into regulation of one aspect of the health care system, a major extension in welfare administration. While nursing homes were a special case, most of their beds being filled with Medicaid recipients, the principle was far-reaching. Purchase of care through vendor payments could be used as a means of affecting health delivery.

The Congressional Reactions

While the implications of the 1967 Amendments were being assessed and implemented, a process aided by the publication of the various Medicaid reports, Congress itself was not standing still. More Medicaid changes were projected. The Chairman of the Senate Finance Committee, Senator Russell Long, reintroduced his earlier plan for reducing the federal share of Medicaid payments for the "medically indigent." This would have lowered the matching formula from the range of 50 to 83 percent to the range of 25 to 69 percent for those optional groups a state included in its plan. Such a measure was expected to save $310 million in fiscal 1969.[63] The effect on states that had made the effort to include the nonwelfare groups would have been profound: $129 million would have been cut from New York, $27.5 million from California, $40 million from Massachusetts, $16 million from Minnesota, and $30.5 million from Pennsylvania. All told, 23 states and the District of Columbia, but no southern states, would have been affected. Yet with little debate—and articulated opposition only from Senator Case of New Jersey—the amendment was passed by the Senate, 44 to 25, as part of the socalled Christmas Tree Tax Reform Bill.

After passage, however, there was an outcry both from HEW and the states.[64] Senator Long's goals of reduced federal spending could not be reconciled with the goals of better health care for the poor and alleviation of the burdens of state taxation. While Senator Long argued that the states "with the connivance and cooperation (of HEW) have found ways to make all kinds of people eligible," Wilbur Cohen, by then Secretary of HEW, responded that "it is absolutely unrealistic to expect states to put up $500 million additional this year to keep the Medicaid program at its present level." Senator Long, however, was more concerned with deficient budgetary estimates: "The Federal share of Medicaid is $700 million more than they said it would be in December. . . . That is getting pretty badly off on a program of this size." While the earlier Senate vote was characterized by Senator Mondale as a "hasty and unwise decision,"[65] the protest was registered. Senator Long, however, eventually capitulated, and the amendment was withdrawn.[66] This little flurry was thus ended.[67]

Continuing cost crises in the states, together with the publication of the various reports on Medicaid, however, ensured a continuing concern in Congress, particularly in the tax committees. This concern increased still further in 1968, when HEW was discovered to have made an error in estimates of nearly $1 billion.[68] As it was not politically feasible to cut federal grants, there appeared a vital need to ensure that existing expenditures were regulated. Senator Long thus continued to be sharply watchful both of the administration of Medicaid and of fiscal control of the program. As Chairman of the Finance Committee, he held highly critical hearings on Medicaid and Medicare in both 1969 and 1970. Meanwhile, the Finance Committee staff began a probing analysis of Medicare and Medicaid, whose results, published in 1970, provided the most detailed review as of that date of management practices and cost deficiencies in these programs.[69] Tougher federal controls were indicated, as the corollary of federal accountability.

At the same time, a general concern over health care costs in Congress was leading to other proposals for federal health care regulation. Hearings entitled *Health Care in America* were held before Senator Abraham Ribicoff's Subcommittee on Executive Reorganization of the Committee on Government Operations in April and July 1968 and they underlined the relationship between the costs of care and the organization of medical services.[70] The Subcommittee concluded that government expenditures of all kinds ought to be used to further an integrated federal health policy and that this policy should attempt to influence and improve the system for providing medical care.[71] Rather similar conclusions were being generated by other Congressional groups also concerned with the costs and implications of Medicaid. A Report of the Special Committee on Aging noted the fragmentation and impersonality of medical care for the elderly, the lack of organized services to keep people well, the continuing stigma of relief attached to Medicaid, the fears by old persons of losing their life savings, difficulties in understanding the programs and its requirements, and (perhaps above all) the over-all "crisis" in health care organization.[72] Medicaid could not be considered in isolation.

But while health care programs as a whole were coming under attack, so too was the other system on which Medicaid hung: welfare programs were attracting increasing criticism. Indeed, many of the same criticisms were levelled at both systems.[73] In fact, neither health nor welfare was a "system"; each was a patchwork of programs developed at different times for different needs and different groups; each provided uneven levels of service to different members of the population; each was costly; and each was demonstrably inadequate in more than one respect. The replacement of state welfare programs by a negative income tax was increasingly widely discussed. The notion of federal responsibility for funding income maintenance programs, through national criteria, was taking root. This concept was to receive a considerable boost with the publication of the Heinemann Commission Report in 1969,[74] and it was not long before the idea of a national family assistance program became an integral part of the social policy proposals of the new Nixon Administration. Efficiency and comprehensiveness were attractive to the new Republicanism.

On three major fronts, therefore, Medicaid was under the Congressional gun. Its problems of cost estimation provoked one set of potential controls. Meanwhile, there was a need for major reforms in both the health and the welfare systems.

Beginning the Nixon Administration

As the Nixon Administration took office in 1969, these various movements toward federal control were becoming evident. Each had both "conservative" and "liberal" elements. Welfare reform could be seen in terms of both rationalization and service expansion. The federal role in health could be used to stimulate the private as well as the public sector. No one argued that better budgeting for Medicaid was unnecessary. Robert Finch, a former Lieutenant-Governor of California, became Secretary of HEW; and it was expected that the administrative emphasis of HEW would be on economy, while policy-making would be pragmatic.

Economy was, however, the major priority with respect to Medicaid. In March 1969, the *Wall Street Journal* noted that "Whether HEW submits legislative proposals this year probably depends on how much the costs rise and on the extent of the pressure from Congress."[75] This did not, however, rule out major changes in the health and welfare systems; indeed, the "pragmatists" were soon to develop proposals for sweeping changes. At the same time, the stage was set for greater control of the vendors of medical care in order that costs could be contained. The theme of controls in Medicaid (and Medicare) was to become a watchword of the Nixon Administration.

Nearer at hand, however, some immediate actions were taken. In March 1969, regulations for utilization review, required in the 1967 Amendments, were finally issued, to "safeguard against unnecessary utilization."[76] In April, HEW announced that physician and dentist payment schedules would be established for Medicaid.[77] Although the original proposals were later amended, the message of increasing control was clear. The message was amplified by a request to HEW from the Senate Finance Committee, also in April, for a list of all practitioners who received $25,000 or more from Medicaid in 1968. The Finance Committee itself was preparing for its hearings in July, with its own message similar to that of HEW's new leaders: "The administrative laxity in medicaid is omnipresent. There is very little effective control of the program at either Federal, State, or local levels with respect to costs and utilization."[78] It was evident that one major area for controls was regulation of the providers of care.

Such sentiments emphasized both the prevailing mood in Washington and the growing role of the Senate Finance Committee as an overseer of federal spending on medical care. Other, more immediate concerns were also evident. Senator Clinton Anderson (Democrat, New Mexico), a member of the Finance Committee, began to push for specific changes in Medicaid that were of immediate concern to his state. New Mexico's program had begun in December 1966 and had almost immediately run into financial difficulties. While having no program for the medically needy, New Mexico offered 19 services to those in the welfare categories: the basic five, plus 14 additional services. While receiving a relatively high federal subsidy under the Medicaid formula, the expansion of the program had imposed additional strains on state and local government.[79] As with other states, New Mexico was in a lockstep. It could not reduce its services, by law; and the single most expensive service, hospital care, was tied to reimbursement at "reasonable cost." As hospital costs escalated, so did the cost of Medicaid.

In February 1969, Senator Anderson introduced his first (unsuccessful) bill to limit payments under Medicare and Medicaid for inpatient hospital care, as well as for extended care and skilled nursing-home care. Above a specified baseline, cost increases would have been limited to general cost rises reflected in the Medical Care Price Index.[80] The second proposal introduced by Senator Anderson (in April 1969) took a different approach: freedom of a state to provide limited services. S 1829 aimed at eliminating section 1902(c) of the Social Security Act, which required states to include all health services in the Medicaid program provided under the most liberal medical assistance programs prior to Medicaid. The Anderson bill also postponed the deadline of 1975 for "comprehensive care" mandated under Section 1902(c). In presenting the bill the Senator struck a responsive chord: "We are frequently paying too much for too many kinds of care for too many people";[81] more practically, he conceded that the bill would "relieve my state of New Mexico of virtually unbearable fiscal pressure."[82]

The Chairman of the Committee, Senator Long, preferred to look at the amendment in different terms. He called it a "technical correction" to express the original intention of Congress that basic cost maintenance payments not be reduced as the result of the introduction of Medicaid.[83] But whatever the rationalization, the Committee gave the proposal importance by attaching it as a rider to a convenient tax bill whose primary purpose was to extend the suspension of duty on shoe-copying lathes. The Committee duly reported that the rider only made the original intention of Congress "unequivocably clear."[84] But in order to justify a cutback in state Medicaid services, the new section required that over-all spending for Medicaid in the state not be decreased in cutting services, that the state comply with provisions for cost control and utilization review, and that the cutbacks not be for the purpose of increasing payments to providers in the remaining services.

On the question of deferring the "comprehensive services deadline" provided by section 1902(e), the Finance Committee implied that it was recognizing a reality: states were not "making efforts in the direction of broadening the scope of the care and services available under the plan and in the directions of liberalizing the eligibility requirements," as they had been required to do under the 1965 legislation. While the Senate liberals and the AFL-CIO fought to retain a deadline, all but one of the state governors polled was in favor of a suspension. The ultimate goal of comprehensive care was retained, but 1975 became 1977 and the bill was passed in both the Senate (in June 1969) and the House (July).[85]

An important breathing space was thus gained for the states and Congress to reconsider the potential and the costs of "comprehensive care." On the House Floor Representative Wilbur Mills had argued that the proposals did not represent a move away from the original concept of health care for all.[86] But it was becoming clear that the notion of giving states a greater freedom to determine their own programs was opening the door to retrenchments.

Meanwhile, other forces were emphasizing Medicaid's chameleon nature. Having been rather clearly relegated again to the sphere of welfare by the

1967 Amendments, Medicaid became caught up in the various suggestions for the over-all reform of welfare. On this count there was more legislative ferment in 1969 than there had been in 1968. The administration was known to be developing what became the Nixon Family Assistance Program, and liberals seemed anxious to force the President's hand. For instance, Senator Goodell's Federal Public Assistance Bill,[87] designed as a total overhaul of the nation's welfare programs to bring all families up to the poverty level, provided among other things that all needy persons would have been included in Medicaid after 1972. Additionally the bill would have paid 75 percent of the costs of each state's plan. But whereas the Goodell Bill would only have raised the maximum for Medicaid eligibility to 150 percent of AFDC payments, several House liberals introduced bills to repeal the 1967 Medicaid limitations altogether.[88] Other less sweeping expansions were also proposed.[89] None of these proposals was reported out of committee, but they added to the complexity of threads already weaving around Medicaid.

It was in this context that in July 1969, the same month the Finance Committee held its hearings on Medicare and Medicaid, an HEW Task Force was appointed under Walter McNerney, President of the Blue Cross Association, to examine the deficiencies of Medicaid. In November the Committee's responsibilities were broadened to include the long-term methods of financing the nation's health care. The Task Force made an Initial Report in November 1969[90] and submitted its Final Report in June 1970.[91] By this time, it was clear that Medicaid, at the national level, could not be profitably considered outside concurrent proposals for the better organization of health services in general and the fate of welfare reform in particular. Meanwhile, the states were left to struggle within the confines of the 1967 Amendments.

NOTES

1. By January 1968, 37 states had established Medicaid programs, but some of these were barely off the ground: Texas, Georgia, Missouri, and South Dakota initiated their programs in September and October, 1967. U.S., Advisory Commission on Intergovernmental Relations, *Intergovernmental Problems in Medicaid* (Washington, 1968), p. 19.

2. *Ibid.*, p. 63.

3. U.S., Congress, Senate, Committee on Finance, *Medicare and Medicaid: Problems, Issues, and Alternatives*, Committee Print, 91st Cong., 2nd Sess., 1970, pp. 4, 42.

4. U.S., *Report of the National Commission on Civil Disorders* (Washington, 1968).

5. *Ibid.*, pp. 136–37.

6. U.S., Department of Health, Education, and Welfare, Office of the Assistant Secretary, *Delivery of Health Services for the Poor, Human Investment Programs* (Washington, 1967).

7. *Ibid.*, pp. 4–5.

8. With a bow to bureaucratic custom, the report noted that "the Social and Rehabilitation Service has initiated studies which will provide this information." *Ibid.*, p. 37. Indeed, as early as June 1967 a large study had begun under a contract made with Columbia University School of Public Health and Administrative Medicine to study the effects of Title XIX on low-income families (HEW Contract No. WA-406 1967). But lacking results, quite apart from any useful routine information, HEW was in the embarrassing position of not knowing much about one of its largest "health" programs.

9. Tax Foundation, Inc., *Medicaid: State Programs After Two Years* (New York, 1968).

10. The Commission included *inter alia* Spiro Agnew (then Governor of Maryland), Ramsey Clark (U.S. Attorney General), Senator Edmund Muskie (Democrat, Maine), Governor Nelson Rockefeller, and Jesse Unruh (Speaker of the California Assembly).

11. *Intergovernmental Problems in Medicaid, supra,* note 1, p. iv.

12. The Commission also had a public hearing in San Francisco, inviting representatives from local, state, and federal governments.

13. U.S., Department of Health, Education, and Welfare, *Report of the State-Federal Task Force on the Costs of Medical Assistance and Public Assistance* (Washington, 1968).

14. *Ibid.*, p. 2.

15. Its special consultant was Robert Myers, Chief Actuary of the Social Security Administration.

16. Arthur Jarvis, Director, Division of Hospital and Medical Care, State Health Department, Hartford, Connecticut. Tax Foundation, Inc., *Medicaid: State Programs After Two Years* (New York, 1968), p. 56.

17. *Intergovernmental Problems in Medicaid, supra,* note 1, p. 57.

18. *Ibid.*, pp. 60–61. This was based on Governor Rockefeller's proposals for health insurance in New York—a way to alleviate the state's burdens.

19. In November 1967, a total of 153,000 persons aged 21–64 who were not "categorically related" (e.g., they were not parents of AFDC children) were receiving Medicaid. Of these, 133,000 were in New York State. Because no federal matching was available for this group the costs were borne entirely from state and local sources. *Ibid.*, p. 94.

20. *Report of the State-Federal Task Force on the Costs of Medical Assistance and Public Assistance, supra,* note 13, p. 1.

21 The Assistant Secretary was (and is) responsible for the U.S. Public Health Service, which contains the Health Services and Mental Health Administration (a sprawling complex of different programs with a budget, at that period, of nearly $12 billion), the National Institutes of Health ($1.4 billion), and the Consumer Protection and Environmental Health Service ($0.2 billion). These three divisions are supposedly the Department's major health foci. Yet Medicare (with $7.3 billion in the trust funds for Part A and Part B), because of its organization as part of the Social Security System, was administered by the well-entrenched and secure Social Security Administration, a separate arm of HEW.

Medicaid ($2.7 billion in federal funds) was run by the Medical Services Administration (MSA), a division of the separate Social and Rehabilitation Service (SRS), that part of the Department which used to be the Welfare Administration.

22. SRS is also responsible for an array of health programs for children ($0.2 billion) run through the Children's Bureau. Altogether the HEW health budget in fiscal year 1970 was almost $13.5 billion, out of a total federal health budget of nearly $18.8 billion. Medicaid thus represents 20 percent of the HEW health budget and 14.4 percent of all federal health expenditures.

23. Reg. 250.20, "Utilization review of care and services," was eventually made in March 1969. 34 *Federal Register* 3745 (1969). Other regulations published by that time were: Reg. 250.21, *Ibid.*, at 14,649 (September 1969); "State Plan Requirements; agreements with providers" Reg. 250.30, "Reasonable charges," *ibid.*, at 1244 (January 1969), revised, 35 *ibid.*, at 10,013 (June 1970); Reg. 250.13, "Payments for medical services and care by a third party," 34 *ibid.*, at 752 (January 1969) revised, *ibid.*, at 6322 (April 1970).

Two further regulations, representing interim policy, were issued during this period. Reg. 250.71, "Information reporting requirements, Internal Revenue Code," *ibid.*, at 3898; Reg. 250.80, "Fraud in the medical assistance program, 34 *ibid.*, at 19,775 (1969). There was one further proposed regulation—251.10—on "Interrelations with State Health and State vocational rehabilitation agencies, and with title V grantees." 35 *ibid.*, at 8664 (June 1970). For two related regulations see Reg. 250.120, "Staffing for administration of medical assistance programs, Federal financial participation," and Reg. 250.210, "State financial participation; State plan requirements." 34 *ibid.*, at 205 (1969).

The regulations covering this period were codified at 45 C.F.R. §250 *et seq.* 1970.

24. Interim regulations were issued on February 28, 1970. See 35 *Fed. Reg.* 3968 (1970). For an outline of regulations on state licensing, see *Medical Tribune,* July 17, 1969.

25. For the somewhat strange role of the MSA in the implementation of §1908 see Sullivan & Byron, *Nursing Home Administrator Licensing Under Section 1908 of the Social Security Act,* 1970 (paper presented at the Yale Law School).

26. On these generally see K. Gideon, *The Role of the HEW Regional Office in the Administration of Medicaid,* 1970 (paper presented at the Yale Law School).

27. *Washington Report on Medicine & Health,* March 10, 1969.

28. *Ibid.*, May 19, 1969.

29. Glenn R. Markus, *Nursing Homes and the Congress: A Brief History of Developments and Issues,* Library of Congress, 1972, p. 5.

30. For a study of the rise of the nursing home in New York State, see William C. Thomas, Jr., *Nursing Homes and Public Policy: Drift and Decision in New York State* (Ithaca, New York, 1969).

31. U.S., Department of Health, Education, and Welfare, Office of Research and Statistics, *Compendium of National Health Expenditure Data* (Washington, 1973), pp. 15, 57.

32. In 1969 there were 18,910 nursing homes in the United States, of which 11,484 provided nursing care and were thus potentially eligible for Medicaid. Of these, 9321 were profit-making ("proprietary") institutions, providing a total of 521,000 beds out of the total nursing-care beds of 704,000. U.S., Department of

Health, Education, and Welfare, National Center for Health Statistics, *Health Resources Statistics 1971* (Washington, 1972), p. 327. A number of nursing home chains had "gone public," and so rapid was the profit rise of such stocks that by 1969 financial journals were reflecting concern; e.g., "Unhealthy Growth? The Nursing Home Business Is Expanding at a Feverish Pace," *Barron's*, Feb. 10, 1969, p. 3; "Nursing Homes: Caution Signals," *Magazine of Wall Street*, June 21, 1969, pp. 19–21. Since 1969 the growth appears to have slowed.

33. *Medical Economics* advised physicians in 1969 that the "extended-care facility" (Medicare's phrase for a skilled nursing home) was a profitable investment, "eminently suited to doctor ownership and investment," but noted that cash requirements for a franchised facility in one of the big chains were in the order of $100,000 for a 60-bed facility. However, up to 90 percent of the investment could be financed, and profits of 10–14 percent a year might be expected. A. I. Schutzer, "New Profit Potential in ECF Investments," *Medical Economics*, vol. 46, No. 3, 1969, pp. 21–33.

34. The conditions cover administrative management, patient-care policies, physician services, nursing services, dietary services, restorative services, dental care, social services, diagnostic services, patient activities, clinical records, transfer agreements (between hospitals discharging patients and nursing homes receiving them), physical environment, housekeeping services, disaster plans, and utilization review. *Code of Federal Regulations*, Title 20, Part 405. For much of this we rely on Kathryn Meyer, *Federal Regulation of the Nursing Home Industry*, 1972 (paper presented at the Yale Law School).

35. U.S., Congress, Senate, *Trends in Long-Term Care, Hearings* before the Subcommittee on Long-Term Care of the Senate Special Committee on Aging. 91st Cong., 2nd Sess., 1970, p. 629.

36. Thus the ECF had to have a 24-hour nursing service, including at least one full-time registered nurse and an R.N. or L.P.N. on duty at all times, to provide that every patient was under the supervision of a physician (and was actually visited once a month) and that a physician was available for emergency care, as well as offering a full range of rehabilitation and social services.

37. *Trends in Long-Term Care*, see note 35, p. 636.

38. Temporary approval would also be given, provided the facility showed promise of meeting the ECF requirements by January 1968. U.S., Department of Health, Education, and Welfare, Welfare Administration, Bureau of Family Services, *Medical Assistance Programs under Title XIX of the Social Security Act*, Handbook of Public Assistance Administration, Supplement D, Sect. D-5151, Item 4. A statement in Supplement D for June 17, 1966, defined a skilled nursing home quite clearly as a facility (or a distinct part of a facility) which was both licensed by the state, and was qualified—effective January 1967—to participate in Medicare as an extended-care facility.

39. Under P.L. 89–97, Section 1902 (a) (9).

40. American Nursing Home Association, *Public Assistance Payments for Nursing Home Care*, May 1968, pp. 27–28. See also Markus, *op. cit., supra*, note 29, pp. 64 *et seq*.

41. Since they used language such as "is desirable," "may be based," "with discretion." See, for example, U.S., Office of the Comptroller General, Report to the Congress, *Problems in Providing Proper Care to Medicare and Medicaid Patients in Skilled Nursing Homes*, No. B-164031 (3), May 28, 1971.

42. Claire Townsend *et al., Old Age: The Last Segregation* (New York, 1971), p. 41.

43. In order to certify as many homes as possible two categories of approval were recognized which were below full compliance. "Substantial compliance" implied that a facility had deficiencies neither hazardous to patients nor in violation of statutory requirements, which the facility was attempting to correct. "Conditional compliance" was granted to a facility that lacked a qualified registered or licensed practical nurse for each tour of duty because there was a nursing shortage. And these wider definitions in large part succeeded in increasing the supply of nursing home beds. By July 1967, 4160 homes had been certified as ECFs for Medicare, but only 740 of these were in full compliance. U.S., Congress, Senate, Finance Committee, Report, *Medicare and Medicaid* (1970), p. 94. As of June 1970, 3382 out of Medicare's 4800 ECFs were still only in "substantial compliance." Townsend, *op. cit., supra,* note 41, pp. 44–45. The Senate Finance Committee stated flatly in 1969 that "the majority of extended care facilities participating in the (Medicare) program do not meet the standards set in the law and regulations." *Trends in Long-Term Care, supra,* note 35, p. 36.

44. *Handbook of Public Assistance Supplement D, supra,* note 38. See D-5141, revised, 3–2–67.

45. U.S., Congress, Senate, Committee on Finance, *Social Security Amendments of 1967, Hearings* . . . on H.R. 12080 before the Senate Committee on Finance, 90th Cong. 1st Sess. 217, 1967, vol. 2, p. 894.

46. P.L. 89–97, Sect. 1902 (a) (9).

47. State licensing of nursing homes is largely a product of the Social Security Amendments of 1950 (P.L. 81-809; 64 Stat. 477), which required that each state have a licensing program as a condition of participation in Old Age Assistance. The licensing statutes, which developed from the 1950s, were not required to distinguish among different types of nursing home care in terms of the types of services given. Massachusetts, for example, licensed long-term care facilities under five categories—rest homes (without nurses), nursing homes (with nurses), charitable homes for the aged, town infirmaries, and public medical institutions—but these categories were only indirectly related to any functional requirements of patients for long-term care. In 1966, the Council of State Governments reported as general opinion that "very few jurisdictions approach the possession of a complete nursing home statute, adequately administered." See Robert K. Byron, David W. Calfee, Peter Hiam, "A Model Act for the Regulation of Long-Term Health Care Facilities," *Harvard J. of Legislation,* vol. 8: 54, pp. 54–122. This conclusion was also implicit in the 1965 hearings, held in various parts of the country by Senator Moss's Subcommittee on Long-Term Care. In his opening statement, Senator Moss stressed the need to guarantee both safety and "proper care." U.S., Congress, Senate, Subcommittee on Long-Term Care, *Conditions and Problems in the Nation's Nursing Homes, Hearings* . . . part 1, p. 1, Indianapolis, Indiana, Feb. 11, 1965.

48. Reported in *Medical Tribune,* April 26, 1967, p. 8.

49. The standards required states to meet environmental, sanitation, and housekeeping requirements at least equivalent to those applied to ECFs under Medicare, to "have and maintain an organized nursing service" under a full-time registered nurse, to provide proper conditions for meal planning, medical record-keeping, and arrangements with hospitals for diagnostic and other services, and (by no means least) to meet the provisions of the Life Saftey Code of the National Fire Protection Association. Title XIX, sec. 1902 (a) (8), added under P.L. 90-248. Under this subsection, nursing homes were also required to file with

the state licensing authority details of ownership. This subsection was replaced by a new subsection in the Social Security Amendments of 1972, for all practical purposes assimilating the requirements for certification of skilled nursing homes to those of extended-care facilities under Medicare. Section 1861 (j).

50. Sect. 1902 (a) (26).

51. Sect. 1908. Administrator licensing also grew out of the Moss Committee hearings of 1965–66, but while Senator Moss concentrated on improving standards by requiring states to regulate nursing homes more effectively through the leverage of federal funds, the idea of licensing of administrators was developed by Senator Edward Kennedy. The original proposals appeared as two separate bills in 1966 (S. 3436 and S. 3384, 89th Cong., 2nd Sess.), and both were incorporated, as amendments, in the 1967 Social Security legislation. Brian D. Sullivan, Robert K. Byron, *Progress Report on Nursing Home Administrator Licensing under Section 1908 of the Social Security Act,* 1970 (paper presented at the Yale Law School).

52. Sect. 1902 (28) (c).

53. In general public assistance categorical funding was on an "all or nothing" basis—i.e., HEW could withhold federal funds for an entire state program, but not for selected aspects of the program. Because such massive withholding was, to say the least, politically almost impossible to enforce and in any event practically undesirable (as good programs would be penalized along with the bad), the revision was to be of enormous administrative importance. See Gilbert Y. Steiner, *Social Insecurity* (Chicago, 1966), *passim.*

54. The American Nursing Home Association supported the Moss Amendments as part of an over-all package that would also include "intermediate care." Public Assistance Payments for Nursing Home Care, *supra,* note 40, p. 28. ICFs were introduced by the Miller Amendment. For details, see Markus, *op. cit.,* note 29, p. 106 *et seq.*

55. Under P.L. 92–223. Federal assistance to ICFs was initially handled through the cash-assistance arm of SRS but was handed to MSA when ICFs were made part of Medicaid in January 1972.

56. Interim policy statement #19 was issued on Nov. 5, 1968, to implement the Moss amendments on a temporary basis. However, these did little more than state the statutory provisions. Meyer, *Federal Regulation of the Nursing Home Industry, supra,* note 34, p. 20.

57. "Whatever Happened to the Moss Amendments," *Congressional Record,* vol. 113, col. s 5872 (1970).

58. *Federal Register,* June 24, 1969. Regulations for periodic health screening for eligible youths under 21 and for intermediate care facilities (also implementing the 1967 Amendments) were published at the same time. See Markus, *op. cit., supra,* note 29, p. 102 *et seq.*

59. Opening Statement of the Chairman, Hearings . . . *Trends in Long-Term Care, supra,* note 35, p. 1. One critic noted that in his own state (Connecticut) there were more stringent standards for the care of poodles. Statement of Paul de Preaux, President, Connecticut Association of Nonprofit Homes and Hospitals for the Aged, *ibid.,* p. 31.

60. *Medical World News,* September 26, 1969; *Hospital Practice,* December 1969. And see Markus, *op. cit. supra,* note 29, pp. 88 *et seq.*

61. Under Miss Charline Birkens, Director of the Colorado Welfare Department. According to Senator Moss, the report was a "stinging rebuke to HEW's stand." *Congressional Record,* vol. 116, pp. 11193–11196 (1970).

62. A small battle was won in nursing provisions. After July 1, 1970, only licensed practical nurses who were graduates of approved state schools of practical nursing could serve as charge nurses, and until July 1970 only those LPNs of unapproved programs who had been charge nurses on July 1, 1967, could continue in these positions. *Federal Register*, April 29, 1970.

63. *1970 Staff Report, supra,* note 3, p. 202.

64. Liberals in the Senate—particularly those from states hardest hit by the cutback (led by two liberal Republicans from New York, Senators Goodell and Javits)—threatened a "minibuster." *American Medical News*, Oct. 7, 1968.

65. For further details of his views, see 24 Congressional Quarterly Service, *Congressional Quarterly Almanac 1968* (Washington, 1969), p. 633.

66. *New York Times*, Oct. 12, 1968, p. 1, col. 2.

67. Indeed the only legislation relating to Medicaid passed during 1968 was a provision in the Revenue and Expenditure Control Act of 1968 (P.L. 90–364, Sect. 303; 82 Stat. 274) extending the time during which states might sign up Medicaid patients under Title XVIII (Medicare) Part B without losing matching funding. For details see Congressional Quarterly Service, *Congressional Quarterly Almanac 1968* (Washington, 1969), p. 265.

68. Congressional Quarterly Service, *Congressional Quarterly Almanac 1969* (Washington, 1970), p. 203. It should be noted that the estimating process has been fraught with some unavoidable difficulties. These have included the difficulty of estimating accurately the size of the potentially eligible population and the rate of enrollment, estimates of service utilization by the population, problems of assessing the amount of funds transferred to Medicaid from other state and local programs, lack of adequate estimates of the combined effect of both Medicare and Medicaid on the medical-care economy as a whole, and the lack of controls over provider participation and charges. Inaccurate budget estimates were a reflection of the more general administrative deficiencies in the programs and of inadequate mechanisms for cost controls.

69. *1970 Staff Report, supra,* note 3. The staff also published a report of background information for the 1969 hearings. U.S., Congress, Senate, Staff of Senate Committee on Finance, *Staff Data Relating to Medicare-Medicaid Study,* Committee Print, U.S., Congress, Committee on Finance, 91st Cong., 1st Sess., 1969.

70. U.S., Congress, Senate, Committee on Government Operations, Subcommittee on Executive Reorganization, *Hearings* on *Health Care in America,* 90th Cong., 2nd Sess., 1968.

71. U.S., Congress, Senate, Committee on Government Operations, Subcommittee on Executive Reorganization, *The Federal Role in Health,* 91st Cong., 2nd Sess., 1970.

72. U.S., Congress, Senate, *Developments in Aging 1967,* A Report of the Special Committee on Aging, pursuant to S. Res. 20, Feb. 17, 1967, 90th Cong., 2nd Sess., Report No. 1098, 1968. Both this Committee and Senator Ribicoff's Subcommittee took evidence and discussed alternative forms of health care, including group-practice arrangements.

73. U.S., Congress, Joint Economic Committee, Subcommittee on Fiscal Policy, *Federal Programs for the Development of Human Resources,* 90th Cong., 2nd Sess., 1968.

74. U.S., *Poverty Amid Plenty: The American Paradox* (*The Report of the President's Commission on Income Maintenance Programs*), November 12, 1969.

75. *Wall Street Journal,* March 31, 1969, p. 4, col. 3.

76. 34 *Federal Register* 3745 (1969).

77. See Chapter 10.

78. Statement of Jay Constantine, Professional Staff Member, U.S., Congress, Senate, Committee on Finance, *Medicare and Medicaid, Hearings,* before the Committee on Finance, 91st Cong., 1st Sess., 1969, p. 45.

79. State and local contributions for medical vendor payments in New Mexico more than doubled from 1966 to 1967 alone. In calendar year 1967 the state-local share was $3.0 million and the federal share $7.1 million. *Intergovernmental Problems, supra,* note 1, p. 91.

80. *Congressional Record,* vol. 115, at 4829, 4842, S. 1195 (1969).

81. *Congressional Record,* vol. 115, at 9512, 9523, 10621, S. 1849 (1969).

82. *Congressional Record,* vol. 115, at 17703 (1969).

83. *Ibid.*

84. U.S., Congress, Senate, *Temporary Suspension of Duty on Certain Copying Shoe Lathes,* Senate Report No. 91–222 (Finance Committee, May 29, 1969), at p. 4.

85. P.L. 91–56.

86. Representative Burton (California) called it "a step backward." He added, "I would hope that we will not find ourselves in future sessions agreeing to further retrenchment. . . ." *Congressional Record,* vol. 115, col. 20528–30 (1969).

87. S. 1806 (April 15, 1969). A similar bill was introduced into the House: H.R. 13274 (Representatives Hastings and Smith, New York; August 1, 1969).

88. H.R. 618 (Ryan, January 3, 1969); H.R. 1352 (Scheuer, January 3, 1969); H.R. 3272 (Gilbert, January 14, 1969); H.R. 8283 (Farbstein, March 5, 1969).

89. Bills by Senator Percy and Representative Erlenborn would have ended the requirement (42 U.S.C. § 1396a (a) (17) (D)) that the resources of the parent of a blind or disabled child be taken into account in determining his eligibility. S. 1251 (Percy, March 4, 1969); H.R. 6752 (Erlenborn, February 17, 1969). Representative Burton proposed that Medicare and Medicaid monies be available for persons under 65, as well as over 65, in mental institutions. H.R. 14377 (Burton, October 16, 1969). A bill by Representative Garmatz would have allowed the states to include in their programs institutional services in intermediate care facilities. H.R. 13122 (Garmatz, July 28, 1969). Two bills in the House would have extended for a short period the temporary provision (42 U.S.C. § 1396b (c)) that the federal share of Medicaid payments for a state be at least 105 percent of the federal share of medical expenditures under public assistance programs in 1965. H.R. 10762 (Watts, April 30, 1969); H.R. 12707 (Perkins, July 8, 1969). Finally, Representatives Rarick and Zion introduced separate bills which would have allowed payments for doctors' services either to a recipient on the basis of an itemized statement of charges or directly to the doctor, whether or not the patient was receiving welfare payments. H.R. 1336 (Rarick, January 3, 1969); H.R. 13695 (Zion, September 9, 1969).

90. Not published. Cited as *McNerney Interim Report.*

91. U.S., Department of Health, Education, and Welfare, *Report of the Task Force on Medicaid and Related Programs,* 1970.

9

The Scene at the State and Local Level

The 1967 Amendments, and later the 1969 Amendments, brought some comfort to the states. But, by 1968, state Medicaid programs had developed their own momentum, and their own problems. No matter how many persons were lopped off the Medicaid rolls by lowering eligibility standards in the states, the cost of Medicaid still seemed to rise. And as if that were not enough, a new newspaper sport was developing, the discovery of fraudulent medical providers. The Tax Foundation Report listed "Profiteering" (i.e., pushing up fees) by doctors, hospitals, and other providers as a factor in a sharp rise in fees and charges by eight states and "racketeering" (e.g., reporting payments for doctors' visits never made) in one.[1] In the states, as well as in Washington, the political pot was on the boil.

The Effect of the 1967 Amendments

The impact of the 1967 Amendments in the different states was considerable. By July 1968, 37 states were operating Medicaid programs. Twenty of these states had had their state Medicaid plans approved prior to July 26, 1967, and made some provision for the medically needy.[2] These 20 were effectively required to limit their "medically needy" income levels to 150 percent of the top AFDC level by July 1, 1968; to 140 percent by January 1, 1969; and to 133⅓ percent by January 1, 1970. Three other states also included the medically needy but were approved after July 1967; these had to adhere directly to the 133⅓ percent guidelines, as did new approvals. The other states included services only for the categorically needy and were thus not affected by this cutback. Strictly, of course, the legislation did not mandate any cuts in eligibility levels. States were always free to go on with existing levels of Medicaid eligibility, but no more federal matching funds would be forthcoming. Alternatively, they could raise AFDC eligibility levels. The chances of state legislatures appropriating extra monies where these were required were remote in almost every state.

A questionnaire survey in 1968 found eight states with medically needy tests in excess of 150 percent of AFDC levels[3]—states accounting for over 60 percent of the federal share of Medicaid. Seven of these cut back their programs by the July 1, 1968, deadline.[4] Pennsylvania, the eighth state, solved the problem by increasing its maximum AFDC payment. By January 1, 1969, Connecticut and Illinois were expected to order cutbacks, because their programs exceeded the 140 percent limits. Some ten states, while including the "medically needy," set the limit at or below the magical 133⅓ percent of AFDC limit.[5] Governors of nine states whose eligibility levels were cut back and 25 without cutbacks were polled in the summer of 1968. Six of the former and 19 of the latter considered the cutbacks desirable, on grounds that the limits were realistic and reasonable, or that the limits would force states to raise public assistance levels, and that this would keep the wealthier states from taking an undue share of available federal money.[6]

But cutbacks did not prevent fiscal crises. While such dramatic financial events as those in California and New York were generally avoided, budgetary crises, if on a lesser scale, occurred in other states. Medical payments represented less than one third of state welfare budgets in 1965. By 1969 medical payments had risen to well over 40 percent of the welfare budgets.[7] It was reported that one out of every three states had been forced to raise its taxes, at least in part because of Medicaid.[8] California, Michigan, and New York had run into fiscal difficulties even before the end of the 1967 fiscal year. By 1968 three other states, Maryland, Nevada, and Oklahoma, were running ahead of their budgets. Except for Nevada, categorical coverage in these states was quite broad. In Maryland, Michigan, and New York, moreover, substantial proportions of the Medicaid payments were being made for nonwelfare cases.

In Oklahoma, in fiscal 1968, the Welfare Department's cash reserve became so low that the state was forced to draw federal funds in advance to make monthly welfare payments; as a result, services under the Medicaid program were cut for all persons receiving aid (predominantly for payments to hospitals and physicians) and the number of people classed as medically indigent was reduced.[9] In that state, some 145,000 on welfare were eligible, together with 35,000 of the medically indigent. The cutbacks were made primarily among the providers and included, among other things, limiting physicians to one hospital visit per day and two nursing home visits per month. But for recipients, hospital stays were limited to ten days, and recipients were exposed to an information program "urging them to carefully use the benefits available."[10]

In Maryland, which initially offered services to all the categorical groups eligible for federal cost sharing and to the medically indigent aged 21 to 64 (from state and local funds), medical vendor payments were running, three-quarters of the way through 1967, at a rate nearly four times that of calendar year 1965. Some 70 percent of payments were being made on behalf of the "medically indigent."[11] To pay for the unexpected costs of the program (which were ascribed to increased costs of hospital care) in 1968, a transfer of money was made from the 1969 capital construction fund. In this state, as elsewhere, there was growing concern over where Medicaid money was going.

In July 1968 Governor Spiro Agnew cut eligibility for a family of four from $3120 to $3000 and for a single person from $1800 to $1500, in the expectation of cutting 22,000 persons out of the Medicaid program.[12] In addition, for the "medically indigent" (who received a special card to distinguish them from other "indigents") a $40 deductible for each admission to hospital was imposed, together with a 21-day maximum stay, while partial charges were imposed for use of dental services and emergency rooms, for drugs, and for visiting a physician. The program was designed, in the words of the *Maryland State Medical Journal,* to "weed out certain persons" and not to affect "the legitimate indigent."[13] Meanwhile, the state medical society resolved at its 1969 meeting that Medicaid services for hospital inpatients and outpatients should continue to be reimbursed at the usual and customary levels until the budget was depleted; thereafter physicians would give care without charge.[14] Even this apparently generous gesture was insufficient. By the end of 1969, hospital officials claimed the state owed Baltimore hospitals more than $6.3 million in unpaid bills.[15]

State legislatures were increasingly mirroring the hostility of Congress to the Medicaid program. New Mexico, which did not even cover the "medically indigent," was faced with a legislature which refused to allocate enough funds to pay even for a barebones Medicaid program.[16] Nevertheless, as a result of rapidly rising hospital and other medical charges, medical vendor payments in the state rose from $5.4 million in 1965 to $16.9 million in fiscal year 1969.[17] A series of budget cuts was made in 1968, including a reduction of 25 percent in physician fees. Other attempted belt-tightening included limiting payments to nursing homes to situations when care was certified by a physician and limiting drugs to listed items.[18] But these measures were not enough. A meeting of the New Mexico legislature on April 11, 1969, ordered the state to withdraw from its relatively liberal Medicaid program and re-enter with a reduced program, a procedure contrary to federal regulations. (Indeed, it was this move which prompted Senator Clinton Anderson to sponsor a relaxation in the federal requirements and led directly to the 1969 Amendments.) New Mexico became the first (and so far the only) state to close down its Medicaid program (on May 1, 1969); the program was reinstated after nine days, although remaining chronically under-funded.[19]

The experiences of Oklahoma, Maryland, and New Mexico were not atypical. The state welfare department of Nebraska was forced to seek a $1 million deficit appropriation in 1969, three-fourths of which was allegedly attributable to Medicaid.[20] In August 1968, Louisiana retrenched, cutting inpatient stays, drugs, and payment of co-insurance under Medicare's Part B;[21] even then there were demands for further cutbacks.[22] In Connecticut, after the eligibility levels were actually raised slightly in 1967, they were reduced in 1969.[23] Meanwhile Massachusetts reduced eligibility by executive order,[24] after seeing its Medicaid program costs rise dramatically compared with earlier programs.[25] The effects on state budgets, not to mention state politicians, can be readily surmised.

Various other states which instituted the program well before the December 1969 deadline had begun their program parsimoniously, and for these there were diminishing prospects of any eventual program expansion. The "poorer" states (for example, Mississippi) and the more fiscally conservative (for example, New Jersey) delayed action until the last moment and in general put in modest plans.[26] Florida, a relatively wealthy state, lived in fear of "spending millions on indigents"[27] and, as a result, its program did not begin until January 1970. Although some states had never included the "medically indigent," other states—for example, Iowa in January 1969—began the process of dropping them.[28]

Typical of the vicissitudes of the period are those of Virginia. A moderately wealthy state, it had spent two years planning its Medicaid program with the assistance of the State Medical Society when in 1968 the legislature authorized the Commissioner of Health, subject to certain safeguards, to institute a Medicaid program. Although the Advisory Committee had suggested the program start on July 1, 1968, for the categorically needy (i.e., welfare recipients) and on January 1, 1969 for the categorically related medically needy (i.e., the medically needy), the legislature postponed both dates for a year.[29] Services were to be relatively limited—the five services required (at that time) by federal law together with prescription drugs, home health care, and special prosthetic devices.[30]

Yet, even with this limited program, problems began almost at once. The Department of Health had made no provision for the bills outstanding from prior medical assistance programs. Moreover, 117,000 people signed up for Phase One. Twenty-four days after the program began, the *Richmond Times-Dispatch* reported "Medicaid Benefits Cutback Is Hinted" (the story saying recipients might be required to pay a part of their drug bill).[31] Even before it began, the income limits for Phase Two were cut to $1700 for an individual and $3000 for a family of four. In this way it was expected to cut the number of eligible "medically indigent" from 282,000 to 182,000.[32] Ultimately, on July 1, 1970, these limits were increased slightly, to $1900 for an individual and $3300 for a family of four.[33] The whole Virginia story, however, was a warning that nothing in Medicaid may be taken for granted.

Everywhere state welfare budgets were being strained, with payments for medical care competing and in some cases threatening to overrun funds for direct cash assistance. This situation ensured increasing political unpopularity for Medicaid, especially in terms of requiring additional taxes on those lower-income groups whose own medical care was not always adequate. There thus seemed to be no alternative to an attempt to cut back coverage and tighten payments to providers. State retrenchments therefore joined retrenchments by the federal government.

Some sense of the impact of the 1967 Amendments in the states may be gleaned from the reactions in California and New York. California's plight during its period of apparent deficit and service reduction had a major impact not only on subsequent concern in Washington but also on political reactions to Medicaid in other states which in the event were not so fortunately situated. New York had similar visibility and national importance. Taken together, in the fall of 1967 the two states accounted for 49 percent of payments to medical vendors and for 37 percent of all recipients of medical assistance in the country. The experiences in these two states thus continued to be of particular importance to the general development of Medicaid programs.[34]

California

In California the 1967 Social Security Amendments had less direct effect on the eligibility levels than in many other states. In order to reflect the new ceilings, the financial limits for a family of four were reduced from $3900 to $3600 in January 1969,[35] but some ceilings—although not in fact this one—were raised again in August 1970. But the effects of this were not dramatic. Indeed, between 1966–67 and 1970–71 the numer of persons eligible for Medi-Cal rose from 1,298,200 (6.8 percent of the population) to 2,294,500 (11.3 percent of the population).[36]

The earlier California cutbacks, instituted in August 1967, had been restrained by the courts and, before the legislature had an opportunity to pass cutback legislation which might meet with the courts' approval, the projected financial catastrophe had evaporated, and the pressure for change was gone.[37] All this had become clear by December 1967, although Governor Reagan, in his State of the State Message in January 1968, still called for controls in Medi-Cal in order to prevent the state from being plunged into bankruptcy.[38] One of the tragic long-term effects of the financial crises in Medi-Cal was that it became a political football for any California politician short of issues. Suddenly during 1968, everyone was investigating Medi-Cal: the Governor's Survey of Efficiency and Cost Control, the Assembly Committee on Public Health, the Senate Finance Committee, the

Attorney General, the Los Angeles City Council, and the Senate-Assembly Joint Committee on Medi-Cal.[39]

Many of the hearings held were largely for political purposes and provided few insights or improvements. The Governor's Survey was the main weapon in the Reagan armory for the over-all re-examination of state government. Although heavily weighted with businessmen, some of whom were not particularly friendly to state administration, the team investigating Medi-Cal turned out to be reasonably sympathetic. The Committee called for a new Task Force on Medi-Cal and a new state Department of Health Care Services. Much of its effort was directed towards the fiscal agent system (i.e., the use of Blue Cross–Blue Shield to make Medicaid reimbursements) and the need for competitive bidding in such contracts, as well as better administrative procedures in paying claims. There were other recommendations for preventing recipient abuse and for controlling provider quality and utilization. It was indicative of general trends that many of the recommendations, such as the mandatory use of generic drugs and control of dental work, were likely to alienate provider organizations rather than Medicaid recipients.[40] The Report appeared in November 1966 and its recommendations were pressed in early 1967, but when the huge predicted 1967 deficit gradually changed to an acceptable surplus, the impact of the Report faded.

The report of the Assembly Committee on Public Health (February 1968) also addressed the issue of providers. Although it was a somewhat erratic document, some of its recommendations were to have considerable effect on Medi-Cal and on other Medicaid programs. For instance, the Committee's report emphasized the desirability of using prepaid contracts for Medicaid recipients. Such contracts would pay vendors a set amount, in advance, for specified services; they would thus protect the state from the inflation inherent in the regular post-payment system in which a provider largely called the shots. Among other proposals, most of which did not become law, was an important one enacted in 1968, that prior authorization for care under Medicaid should be expanded to include elective medical and surgical procedures.[41] Generally, the tone was for a much more directive state role than before with respect to value received for money spent by Medicaid.

The Attorney General's Report, which appeared in the fall of 1968, went a step further in its account of fraud by Medicaid providers and received wide publicity. In November 1967, the California Department of Justice had held hearings in Los Angeles and, while it gave the nonprofit hospitals a clean bill of health, it found that over-servicing, kickbacks, and duplicate billings "seem to be predominant in physician-owned hospitals."[42] The Attorney General's Report a year later showed that $8 million had been "drained" from Medi-Cal by unethical means. Hospitals, doctors, the fiscal agents, and almost all providers came in for attack.[43] The same month, the

Senate-Assembly Joint Committee on Medi-Cal began hearings, with a heavy emphasis on fraud by providers. As in other states, concern over effective administration was swamped by a glad seizing on some apparent villains who could be blamed for Medicaid's deficiencies. Allegations of fraud by physicians, pharmacists, dentists, and others were reaching epidemic proportions. The October 1967 issue of *Parade* had charged that during the first eighteen months of Medi-Cal, 1200 physicians had been paid an average of nearly $70,000 each.[44] Although the president of the California Medical Association denied that there had been abuse by providers and claimed that instead Medi-Cal had saved taxpayers millions because of effective utilization review,[45] there was increasing evidence that some providers, at least, had not been particularly restrained in their billing.

But California, with an administrative system which seemed superb compared with New York's inept activities, at least attempted to be innovative. Assembly Bill 1140, passed in 1967, gave the Bureau of Health Care Services authority to provide medical care in the most efficient manner possible. As a result of this authorization, two prepayment pilot projects were begun: the San Joaquin Foundation Pilot Project and the Foundation for Medical Care of Sonoma County. Blue Shield also advanced a proposal to cover all the categorically needy in a prepayment program.[46]

One thing, however, remained constant, the rising Medi-Cal budget. Excluding administrative costs, the 1966–67 budget of $507.5 million rose to $563.4 million in 1967–68, and then seemed to take off. Expenditures for 1968–69 were $754.8 million, for 1969–70 were $987.5 million; and for 1970–71 were $1056.1 million, i.e., over $1 billion. In a 5-year period, the Medi-Cal budget had doubled.[47] (The budget for 1972–73 was $1.58 billion.) The costs were, to put it mildly, dramatic.

New York

In New York, too, there were immediate problems of costs exceeding budget estimates. Initial estimates stated that during fiscal 1967 the Medicaid program would raise public assistance costs by $36 million; this was to be accompanied, as a bonus, by expected increased federal funding of $114 million and a decreased state and local share of $78 million. In fact, costs increased sharply for all three levels of government. Original total outlays of $350 million were expected for fiscal 1967; the actual expenditures reached $461 million, and further deficits were expected for fiscal 1968.[48] By fiscal 1969 New York State was spending $426 million from state funds alone; the total cost of the program (federal, state, and local) was $1.29 billion.[49]

Although Governor Rockefeller had joined Mayor Lindsay in urging that President Johnson not sign the bill which became the 1967 Amendments, once it was law the Governor was faced with a need to raise an extra $150 million in connection with the different welfare changes made. Where was this to come from? Already, many municipalities had raised their sales tax and counties their property tax, most alleging the "Medicaid problem." Politically, Governor Rockefeller had no choice but to admit that his early enthusiasm about Medicaid had been mistaken. In his budget message to the legislature he called for cutbacks in the program, and he hurriedly appointed a committee to advise on how to cope with the new federal legislation. Aided by a firm of accountants, the committee concluded that "the Program would have to be curtailed to avoid intolerable increases in state and local expenditures." The Governor was blunter still: "We are simply going to have to revamp our Medicaid program to reduce its cost." Although he held out some form of State Health Insurance as the long term panacea, for the short term the answer was a cutback.[50]

The New York State Senate, controlled by the Republicans, cut back the program with little debate. In the Democratic-controlled Assembly, Speaker Travia tried to keep the bill bottled up in committee, but eventually a group of upstate Democrats forced him to release it, fearing a taxpayer revolt in their districts. After an emotional 3-hour debate, the bill was passed, Travia declaring it a "day of infamy" when the needy ill were sold for "a few paltry pieces of silver." Although the bill made greater cuts than he requested, Governor Rockefeller signed the bill almost as soon as it reached his desk—some said in the hope of obtaining conservative backing for his Presidential bid. The cost of the state's Medicaid program would, it was estimated, be cut by some $300 million (although experience did not bear this out), while the new eligibility levels—down to $5300 from $6000 for the family of four[51]—were expected to remove roughly a million persons from the nearly three-and-a half million who had by that time enrolled. Mayor Lindsay claimed that New York City would lose $120 million a year and have to curtail services. (He also argued that Washington and Albany had flunked the first test posed by the National Advisory Commission on Civil Disorders.) But even at $5300, New York's was still the most generous Medicaid program in the nation.[52]

The medical care needs of the people cut off the rolls in New York City, as elsewhere, of course did not suddenly go away. Mayor Lindsay's estimate that the eligibility cuts would mean a loss of about $100 million in state aid to municipal and voluntary hospitals alone[53] and could mean closing public health facilities, suggested that part of the costs would be shifted from one public pocket to another. To help those dropped from Medicaid, the New York City Department of Hospitals was forced to cut its own fees in municipal outpatient departments.[54] The situation thus aggravated the already perilous financial status of the city hospital system. As there was no adequate resource to pick up the services and patients that Medicaid dropped—"charity" having been largely eliminated—the medical care available to the many thousands of poor in New York City who were no longer eligible for assistance was worse in 1968 than it had been before Medicaid was enacted.

Yet the cutting was not yet ended, for Medicaid was only one of the inflated tax programs of the 1960s causing fiscal crises in state capitals. When the New York state legislature met in January 1969 with the task of producing a state budget by the new fiscal year, April 1, there was a demand for further cutbacks.[55] Governor Rockefeller called for a 5 percent cut in the proposed budget across the board, which would cut $104 million in educational spending and $51 million from the welfare budget (including Medicaid), together with big cuts in school and welfare budgets for fiscal year 1970–71. But the reaction in the legislature, in general, reflected outrage about the educational cuts and lack of concern about the welfare cuts. As Mitchell Ginsberg, the New York City Human Resources Commissioner, put it: "the poor have no constituency."[56]

Education had not only millions of parents but, in New York City especially, a very powerful teachers' union. Thus the welfare budget was pared down, with the net result that $128 million was cut from the welfare budget but only $30 million was cut from the education budget. As the basic justification was that the projected cuts for 1970–71 should be implemented in 1969–70, the heaviest inroads in the welfare budget were to be in the area of Medicaid. The assault on Medicaid took place on various fronts—reducing eligibility, requiring co-insurance, and curbing providers. When it came to the crunch, Medicaid had a low state priority.

The Medicaid limit for a family of four in New York, originally $6000, had been reduced to $5300 in 1968; reducing it still further to $5000 in 1969 was predicted to save $19 million,[57] by removing a quarter of the "medically needy."[58] Opposition by New York City's Department of Health on the ground that it would in the long run force more people onto the welfare rolls[59] was in vain; the cutback was implemented. By June 1969, New York City was mailing out "Certificate of Continued Eligibility" cards to some 200,000 families to see if they were caught by the new cuts. Those who failed to return this card, even if they did meet the new standards, ran the risk of being dropped from the program.

In terms of numbers enrolled the cutbacks worked. The State Department of Social Services reported that average monthly utilization in the state was 958,236 in 1969, with 427,326 being "medically indigent." By 1970, the average monthly utilization by the "medically indigent" was 278,777, a 35 percent decline.[60] The figures in New York City were even more dramatic. In March 1968, some 2.4 million persons were enrolled for Medicaid, two thirds of them being "medically indigent" rather than cash assistance recipients. As a result of the 1968 changes, the enrollees fell to 1.7 million by December 1968—a decline of 30 percent, all presumably in the "medically indigent" category. With the 1969 changes there was another drop in enrollees.

The effect on recipients was predictable. In August 1969 the *New York Times* published an article entitled "Medicaid Shift Causes Bewilderment," accompanied by a photograph of a line of persons outside a medical center waiting "to clarify their status."[61] The legislature had achieved its goal. By December 1969, only 1.46 million persons were enrolled in New York City, with only 28 percent being in the "medically indigent" category. By June 30, 1970, of the 1.45 million enrollees in the City, only 370,138 (26 percent) were not also on public assistance. But while, in terms of numbers, Medicaid had become predominantly a program for cash recipients, payments on behalf of the medically indigent, who were by definition in need of medical care, continued to absorb a large part of the budget. For the first six months of 1970, 43 percent of the $343.9 million spent on Medicaid in New York City went for services to the medically indigent.[62] For those cut off the rolls no information was available.

Providers were also affected by the parsimonious reactions of the legislature. As in California, the providers were becoming Medicaid's apparent villains. Reimbursements to hospitals were frozen and a general cutback of 20 percent in fees ordered effective as of June 1, 1969. When servicing the medically indigent (but not those on welfare), doctors, dentists, and pharmacists were to collect 20 percent of bills directly from Medicaid recipients.[63] On behalf of users of the program, U.S. District Judge Constance Baker Motley in New York City issued a temporary restraining order against the putting into effect of the regulation for compulsory contributions from the medically indigent,[64] although this stay was dissolved after a hearing before a three-judge court.[65] But another three-judge federal court in Brooklyn struck down Medicaid reimbursement restrictions on hospitals in New York, on the ground that they violated federal law.[66] The eligibility levels, however, stuck, as did the restrictions on nonhospital providers, and Albany's efforts to curb the state Medicaid budget continued.

The growing toughness in the legislature reflected both a stand against rising taxes and a desire to reduce the status of recipients. Rockefeller had asked for a 1 percent increase in the sales tax to finance even the pared budget. But upstate Republicans, led by Senator John Hughes, were not prepared to grant him this unless the consumers were also taxed for Medicaid. The conservatives demanded that the medically indigent, unless they were actually in hospital, pay 20 percent of their medical costs; there was a tendency to label the medically needy as "freeloaders." Debate was bitter in both houses, the Democratic leader in the Assembly, Stanley Steingut, opining that "The Republican Party and the Republican Governor . . . make Ronald Reagan and Barry Goldwater look like pipsqueaks."[67] But the mood of retrenchment prevailed. Despite Administrator Ginsberg's view that a co-insurance provision affecting some and not others might be unconstitutional or at least in violation of federal regulation,[68] the 20 percent "use tax" was voted. The Governor also probably had some doubts, especially after the state had been forced to rescind its earlier attempts at co-insurance, but he finally signed the bill, a signal for the litigation to begin.

New York City: The Impact of Decisions in Albany

The exigencies of balancing state budgets to cope with the combined impact of the 1967 Amendments and continued increases in medical costs provided the major theme in Medicaid retrenchments in 1968 and 1969. But, as we have noted, the mood of austerity toward Medicaid reflected in Albany, Sacramento, and other state capitals was also in part provoked by more conservative views of welfare, which were in turn a reaction to the array of Great Society programs of the mid-1960s. The War on Poverty had not, in one fell swoop, decimated the ranks of welfare recipients. Rather, the reverse was clearly true: The more money spent on welfare, the greater the welfare rolls. It was only a step from here to the view that welfare cutbacks would in some way reduce poverty by forcing those unable to get public funds back into the labor market where they would have to struggle along "like everybody else." Here was the old argument of the "undeserving" as well as the "deserving" poor, clearly visible in the "workfare" aspects of the 1967 Social Security Amendments, with respect to cash assistance recipients.

New York City, with a million persons on cash assistance, was a major national target in the implementation of such views. With respect to Medicaid, there was the apparent suggestion from the state level that cutbacks evolved in Albany would reduce problems in Harlem or the Bronx. And there was also the assumption that providers' fees could be controlled without the program collapsing altogether. Indeed, all the problems at the state level were magnified when the implications of state legislation had to be implemented locally.

The Medicaid program in New York City was run by the City. (The New York State Department of Welfare, which became "the single state agency" in New York for the administration of welfare, was required by state law to operate through local welfare departments.) The New York City Medical Assistance Program, with its 2.4 million enrollees in March 1968, was, indeed, larger than those in almost every state. At its height, almost $1 out of every $4 spent for Medicaid in the United States was spent in New York City, and the City had almost one out of every five Medicaid patients enrolled. The operation of this vast system was thus obviously nationally important.

It was, moreover, complicated by the internecine struggle between the city's health and welfare agencies, the former taking a much more liberal view of benefits than the latter. The program was initially run, with respect to both eligibility and standards, by the Welfare Department. In 1967, however, the Health Department set up an organization to handle the standards and evaluation processes: the Bureau of Health Care Services. Once established, the Bureau became an aggressive exponent of the idea that Medicaid ought to be a medical care rather than a welfare program. But by this time "the Welfare tail was wagging the health dog. . . . (The) Welfare (Department) . . . contended that Medicaid could not be separated out from other welfare activities."[69] And while the Health Department has continued to insist that "Medicaid is not welfare," the program has been run by the Welfare bureaucracy.

But although the aggressive administration of the New York City Health Department was denied the right to run the program—there were, for instance, bitter protests that the Department of Social Services rather than itself was allowed to have the Medicaid computer—the Department turned its talents instead to the issues of standards and evaluation. If it was not to be responsible for buying the services, it could at least ensure that health care was available, at a reasonable cost and of an appropriate quality. Hence, from 1967 on, the Health Department, vested with the power under Title XIX to suspend errant providers, was concerned with twin problems—encouraging professionals to participate and detecting possible frauds. The Executive Medical Director of New York City's Medicaid program, Dr. Lowell Bellin, became a prolific publicist of the department's activities. On the one hand, then, the welfare department was cutting back on Medicaid eligibles; on the other, the health department was attempting to improve the medical services and the choice of services for recipients. In some respects these restrictionist and expansionist movements were in conflict. Providers, too, were soon to be subject to restriction, as state-imposed fee cuts took effect.

By 1968, any effort to encourage providers to "sign up" for Medicaid had been abandoned.[70] But while the cuts in Medicaid imposed by the legislature were reducing the number of enrolled recipients the number of participating physicians and dentists increased rapidly.[71] Because there were fewer eligible patients, the cost of physician services fell by 14 percent between the first and the fourth quarter of 1968 and that of dental services by 56 percent.[72] At the same time, as we have noted, the state was also moving to save funds by cutting professional fees, a move that would deter providers as well as recipients. Under existing regulations, local communities had the option of setting professional fees lower than those recommended by the State Department of Health. Ironically, only New York City, where customary fees were higher than in any other part of the state, had exercised that option.[73] The Governor's decision in his 1969 budget message to cut all fees to providers by 20 percent—a move estimated to save some $25 million annually[74]—not surprisingly led to an especially hostile reaction in New York City, with its already low fees and high Medicaid population.

Dr. Lowell Bellin announced that the cuts would cripple physician participation in New York City.[75] Gone was the earlier notion that physicians were willing to give free services to the poor. The President of the New York State Medical Society, Dr. Edward Hughes, complained that the measure was a "real push to get something for nothing."[76] And the squeals were equally loud from the other providers. Leaders of the State Dental Society said they planned to withhold their services.[77] In New York City, some 400 dentists who, although representing only 5 percent of the City's dentists, did 60 percent of the city's Medicaid dental work, refused to accept new Medicaid patients. In 1968, these 400 dentists had averaged approved gross payments of $124,500 from Medicaid,[78] and they claimed the new scales would cut almost 75 percent from their net incomes.[79] The President of the Dental Society of the State, Dr. Robert Montgomery, explained the high costs of the dental component in Medicaid in terms of the fact that the poor had so long neglected their teeth that extensive treatment was necessary. (Dental costs under Medicaid had gone from $10.9 million in fiscal year 1966–67 to $124.4 million in fiscal year 1968–69.)[80] All the dental good done would now be undermined.

The pharmacists were outraged. Their fees were to be cut twice, as they provided not only services but a product as well. A 20 percent cut in fees together with a requirement of collecting 20 percent of the cost from some recipients would, said Bernard Weitzman, cochairman of the State Pharmaceutical Society's Emergency Medicaid Committee, make life impossible.[81] Senator Norman Lent had even suggested an end to the mark-up system altogether and the payment of the wholesale cost of the drugs plus a (presumably small) professional fee.[82] The pharmacists resorted to direct action. Roughly half of the New York City pharmacies began boycotting the program on June 22, 1969, and Weitzman claimed there was a virtual 100 percent boycott in the low-income areas where Medicaid patients lived.[83] As an emergency measure, the city hospitals began dispensing drugs to Medicaid patients until the boycott was called off on July 1, when negotiations about fees began between state officials and leaders of the State Pharmaceutical Society.[84]

The 20 percent reduction in fees effective June 1, coupled with the other retrenchments, cut the annual expenditure to health professionals by 15 percent compared with 1968 and, with the exception of podiatrists and chiropractors, cut the number of such providers participating.[85] During the first half of 1970, there was a 6 percent drop in payments to providers compared with the first 6 months of 1969. (Although with the cutbacks the percentage of the "medically indigent" dropped to 26 percent they still, as noted, consumed 43 percent of expenditures, suggesting the health plight of this group.)[86] At least, however, the decline in the number of providers participating was halted. But the amounts paid to most providers, and especially dentists because of the curbs on dental procedures, fell. The only increases in payments were to physicians, podiatrists, and chiropractors.[87] There were problems of matching recipients and providers. Brooklyn had 43 percent of the public assistance recipients, but only 31 percent of the participating providers, and the Bronx had 28 percent of the public assistance recipients but only 15 percent of the participating providers.[88] Implementation of state programs at this City level was a source of continual heartbreak.

New York City: Regulating Providers

The series of confrontations with providers over fees, by no means confined to New York City, formed a strong and continuing element in Medicaid's development, pervading all governmental levels. Providers had joined recipients in the eyes of legislators as "exploiters" of the program. But in one respect, New York's regulation of providers was unique. Although the City Health Department fought vigorously during these years to encourage providers to participate, it also developed the most effective system of standard-setting in the nation.[89] A series of advisory committees was developed, and extensive programs of quality care were organized—there was even a program for setting standards for dispensing hearing aids to children covered by Medicaid.[90] While the Medical Services Administration in Washington gingerly approached nursing-home regulation, New York City was imposing (and attempting to exact) quite stringent standards of professional behavior as part of Medicaid's day-to-day operation.

The development of such programs was not always easy, especially with the "less professional" groups of providers.[91] Negotiations were, for instance, particularly intricate with respect to chiropractors, who were included in the New York Medicaid program. In addition to being looked on with some skepticism by other groups of providers, the group itself was severely fragmented. Thus, when the New York City Medicaid program appointed a chiropractic consultant to advise it, the Chiropractic Association of New York hailed the appointment as a brilliant one; the New York State Chiropractic Society was dissatisfied with the appointment, alleging a "conflict of interest"; while the Federation of Licensed Chiropractors alleged a "sell-out" and referred to the consultant as a "Judas Goat."[92]

Perhaps the most important program developed for physicians and dentists[93] was peer audit performed by an on-site office visit. But the attempts to monitor the services of other practitioners in New York's extensive program were in many ways more interesting. There was considerable participation in the program by paraprofessionals, about whom little was known. In 1968, the average podiatrist in New York City was paid $6500 by Medicaid; a program was set up whereby podiatrists billing at the rate of more than $3500 a month were audited. (The parallel "red flags" for other professions were for physician general practitioners $5000 a month, for dentists $5000 a month, for optometrists $4500.) But the concern was not solely financial. The department worked out, with the Lewi College of Podiatry, a program of quality control. At the same time prior authorization programs were developed for some procedures.[94]

Bringing pharmacists into Medicaid and ensuring quality and audit controls also posed problems. Medicaid primarily took over the former welfare system of pharmacy reimbursement, but, as with other providers, an Advisory Committee on Quality Pharmacy was established. Fortunately, pharmacies were generally willing to participate in the program (there was an average 70 percent participation), although as has been seen there were various disputes between the pharmacists and the Medicaid Administration over reimbursement. In the early days of the program, for instance, there were delays of up to 6 months in reimbursement and a significant number of claims were rejected because of an invalid Medicaid number. But at least the potential battle between the City Health Department and the pharmacists about the mandatory substitution of generic for prescribed proprietary drugs was averted because the State Health Department determined that this change, mandated by the City Administration, would violate state law. This left, as the chief administrative battle, the method of payment of pharmacists.[95]

Under the pre-1965 systems of welfare medicine, there had been programs of welfare optometry, but they were erratic and quality control was virtually nonexistent. After Medicaid, there was a high level of participation by optometrists (64 percent by December 1968), and nonparticipation was at least partly due to the fact that some optometrists were thought by the City Health Department not to be fully qualified. Although the Medicaid administration allowed considerable professional latitude to optometrists, certain procedures were mandated. There were also audit reports and peer-review procedures; and there were efforts to ensure that the optometrists participated in continuing education programs.[96]

Compulsory continuing education in fact became one of the main goals for the Executive Medical Director of the Medicaid administration. Dr. Bellin took the view, now increasingly accepted among leading professionals, that licensure alone was not enough to guarantee quality care.[97] As early as 1966, Dr. Howard Brown, who was to become Health Services Administrator when New York City's health super-agency was formed in 1968, announced that Medicaid practitioners would be required to take a specific number of hours of continuing education. For example, 50 hours a year in three years was prescribed for general practitioners and half that amount for dentists, optometrists and podiatrists. Local medical societies were incensed. They were not opposed to continuing education; indeed they urged it on their members, but they were not about to have it forced on their members by the Medicaid administration.[98] The medical societies appealed at once to the State Health Department, where they had appreciably greater influence than with the City Health Department; the latter Department ordered a stay.

The City Health Department pressed on with its demand for a program of compulsory education, while the physicians, led by the King's County Medical Society, strongly denied the Department's right to make such demands. But at least the threats by the City's Health Department led many GPs to join the American Academy of General Practice, which the City recognized as the equivalent of participating in its own compulsory education program. The City's program ran into one roadblock after another; it was, for instance, accused of discriminating against black physicians. The fact that Title XVIII (Medicare) had no effective methods of evaluating participating providers made it very difficult for Medicaid to demand the development of effective standards.

The Bellin Blitz

Dr. Bellin, however, was indefatigable. In a speech given to various county medical societies, he pressed the basic question: "How is the Medicaid program to deal with the health care professional who has not responded to voluntarism and whose knowledge of medical advances continues to derive almost exclusively from drug house detail men or *Time* magazine?" But physicians were not alone in receiving Dr. Bellin's attentions. The State Dental Society was as opposed to the compulsory education program as was the State Medical Society. Rather surprisingly, the State Optometric Association endorsed the program. Statewide, the podiatrists also favored compulsory continuing education, although in the City there was dissent from this position. The pharmacists remained neutral.

So much for the inital skirmishing. In January 1968, Dr. Bellin finally threw down the gauntlet and announced that guidelines for compulsory continuing education would be issued by the City Health Department; providers who did not comply would be dropped promptly. The State Health Department at once moved to head Bellin off; and the City's Commissioner of Health agreed. In October, the 2nd and 10th District Dental Societies moved the courts for a temporary injunction to prevent the implementation of the regulations. A six-month temporary stay was granted. Thus nothing was done about dentists, and the State Health Department was clearly backing away from any urge to demand compulsory education.

Indeed, with the cutbacks in professional fees decreed by the legislature, the State Health Department took the position: "How can we insist on educational standards and simultaneously cut fees by 20 percent? Practitioners will withdraw from the program." While Dr. Bellin persevered with the optometrists and podiatrists, the die had really been cast. As Dr. Bellin produced one move, the State Health Department undercut his position. The general response was, "perhaps we should look at these things later,"[99] As far as Medicaid was concerned standards beyond the basic license were not to be pressed.

But although Dr. Bellin looked on compulsory continuing education as the center of his program, in fact the New York City Medicaid administration became best known for its attempt to curb fraudulent providers or providers who violated basic standards of quality care. Here the confrontation was selective, and the purpose a more obvious form of taxpayer (as well as recipient) protection. The City Health Department put a significant segment of its staff to work on the anti-abuse program, including 134 professionals, 60 paraprofessionals and 143 clerks—a larger staff, one should note, than the Medical Services Administration at that time had in Washington.

The work of this department rapidly revealed three major areas of provider abuse: fraud, where the provider charged for a service he had not in fact performed; unsatisfactory quality, where the service performed failed to meet Medicaid standards; and overutilization, where the provider undertook a superfluous service. To detect all of these, the Department undertook inspection in the providers' offices, much to the chagrin of professional organizations. But the extent of fraud seemed to justify the inspections. On the pharmacy side, for instance, various fraudulent practices were discerned. "Kiting" involved escalating the quantity of medication prescribed, by the adding of "x's," while "shorting" was the term for supplying fewer tablets or capsules than the prescription called for.

According to Drs. Bellin and Kavaler, "The Medicaid fee-for-service mechanism is an implicit fiscal incentive for overutilization." Thus it came as no surprise to the administration that there was promiscuous mutual referral between some physicians. For example, in a group pràctice in a predominantly Medicaid area, it was discovered that the intake group pediatrician routinely referred every child to the otolaryngologist. (The Medicaid fee for this was $20.) But "ping-ponging," as this arrangement was called in the trade, was far more widespread than this. In Medicaid areas, cross-referrals were widespread; yet the medical consultants to the Medicaid administration had their time cut out developing adequate quality review.

Dentistry, however, received the accolade for the highest degree of overutilization. Dentures were subject to prior authorization for Medicaid, and during 1968 the dental staff of the City's Medicaid program cut proposed dental treatment plans from an aggregate $110 million to $83 million. Throughout the system, though, overutilization was discovered. The department came to suspect relationships in cases such as one in which all the prescriptions for a nursing home were filled by one pharmacy, especially when that pharmacy was some distance away from the home. Podiatrists had also apparently worked up such profitable relationships with nursing homes that the Health Department was forced to lay down a rule that one podiatrist be assigned to each nursing home and be reimbursed on a session basis; the cost of the fee-for-service arrangement for clipping the nails of each person in such a home had become prohibitive. But podiatrists had other overutilization techniques outside the nursing homes, chiefly the prescribing of nominally therapeutic shoes, which had to be paid for by Medicaid. The "patients" also urged on the podiatrist the need for therapeutic shoes as specific welfare grants for clothing were cut or eliminated. This abuse became particularly widespread since the podiatrists did not have to pay a "kickback" to the shoe store, while he normally "reimbursed" nursing homes for being allowed to cut nails.[100]

Some sense of the problem of the quality of care can be obtained from the department's examination of the work of dentists. Some 1300 patients were examined after work had been done by private dentists about whom the department had some questions. Nine percent of those examined showed poor quality dental work and a further 9 percent showed a discrepancy between work performed and work claimed. More alarming were the results with a group of 500 patients who had received optometric services. Some 72.2 percent had received satisfactory care, and 17.2 percent unsatisfactory care; fraud appeared to be involved in 2.4 percent of cases. Over-all, by September 1969, of the full-scale investigation of providers undertaken, 207 had been sustained in full and 64 had not.[101]

General Issues

Administrative regulation of providers stressed the evident need for sophisticated programs of audit and quality control, whether in New York City or in the states, yet administration in the states had been an endemic problem. While the choice of welfare departments made to run Medicaid by the majority of states was partially encouraged by HEW—a disappointment to those who hoped the 1965 legislation was a move away from the welfare image—[102] these departments were not skilled in medical audit techniques. More important still, welfare departments were often thin in top-level talent and rarely had the political influence to buck powerful lobbies such as the providers of medical care in their state. State health departments were, however, rarely headed by physicians of sufficient prestige to stand up to leaders of the professions or the legislators.

And in terms of nonmedical personnel, they were probably no stronger than welfare departments. The problem of attracting good bureaucrats is even more evident in state government than it is in federal service. There was thus no firm base for implementing legislative retrenchments.

The results were predictable. Congress mandated cutbacks on the states, and state legislators moved to cushion the blow by their own restrictive legislation. But as the circle widened, the fiscal aspects of such restrictions were dissipated. When cutting back on the costs of a program, state legislatures rarely added into the budget money for additional staffs to carry out the cutbacks. This omission is a question not merely of oversight, but of strategy: welfare rights organizations and a vigilant press would naturally seize upon the irony of an enlarged state bureaucracy at the apparent expense of welfare recipients.

In the event, it was relatively easy, if eligibility levels were dropped, to remove recipients from the rolls, as Medicaid automatically required the administration of an individual means test by social caseworkers already attached to the department's local offices. Dealing with hundreds or thousands of providers was inevitably much more difficult, particularly since the initial posture of state agencies had been a careful wooing of providers so that they would participate. Not surprisingly, as the Senate Finance Committee staff revealed, a "number of States have yielded to demands that they reimburse skilled nursing homes on the more generous basis under which extended care facilities are paid under Medicare."[103] It seemed natural (if regrettable) to state welfare and health departments that, in most states, when cuts were made in Medicaid programs, recipients rather than providers were the first ones to be axed.[104] States frequently failed even to live up to the minimum requirements laid down from Washington. Thus, while Supplement D stated that Title XIX agencies should also participate actively in community planning for facilities where they were substantial purchasers, for example in the case of skilled nursing home care, this was honored only in the breach. Professional advisory committees, too, where they have been effective, have tended to reflect majority interests.[105]

In theory, state bureaucracies could have been protected against excessive pressures from providers by the use of private fiscal agents to administer the program. No doubt in some states, especially the smaller ones,[106] use of the fiscal agent has helped develop a buffer against provider lobbies. In Vermont, for instance, use of the New Hampshire–Vermont Blue Cross–Blue Shield program as fiscal agent for most services undoubtedly made life bearable for civil servants in the Department of Social Welfare. Yet, in some states, the multiple fiscal agent arrangements were (and are) so complex, they almost defy description.[107] Although the fiscal agent procedure was a useful political device in the early years, as a long-term delegation of fiscal decision-making to a private body (often related, as in the case of Blue Cross and Blue Shield, to the providers themselves) it may be inherently unsatisfactory.

In some respects, too, the use of fiscal agents encouraged the already piecemeal nature of cost reimbursement. The use of fiscal agents was similar to the use of fiscal intermediaries and carriers under Medicare,[108] and it might have been supposed that the opportunity would be firmly grasped in the states to run both programs on a similar basis. But, in at least one state which expected such intermeshing of administration, the levels of usual and customary fees for physicians as determined under Medicare were held by the carrier to be confidential information and were not released to the Medicaid administrators, and the situation is thought to have been similar in other states. Finally, the use of fiscal agents added to the confusion in available information about Medicaid in all the states; the California budget crisis of 1967 was merely the most spectacular example. Budgetary confusion was compounded by the problem of whether the amounts "tossed out" from time to time were the total costs of all payments for medical care to welfare recipients and the medically needy, whether state costs alone were being quoted, whether the costs of services to welfare recipients and the medically needy were separated, and so on.

Sometimes even the most elementary statistical data were lacking. The welfare departments in smaller states were hard-pressed enough in accounting to their legislatures for expanding welfare budgets and at the same time explaining the limited provision of services to welfare rights organizations, let alone in proposing expensive new systems for data collection and analysis. A 1969 Report to the Governor of Vermont noted: "There is a regrettable lack of meaningful statistical data available on the operation of the Medicaid Program in Vermont. For example, as recently as April of this year, the Department had no reliable statistics on how many persons were receiving Medicaid benefits."[109] Although some states like California made great efforts with statistical data, even that had its limitations.[110] In effect, across the country huge multimillion-dollar programs were established without the basic mechanisms of program accountability; and the tradition of inadequate statistical data in the welfare programs was carried through into Medicaid.[111]

Growing problems of administration, high costs, and fraud were not of course necessarily related, but they became so in the eyes of the press, as concern over all three mounted simultaneously. The line between inept management on the part of administrators and fraud on the part of providers is never clear. The existence of fraud was, however, the most flagrant administrative deficiency, and on a major scale the easiest to identify. Moreover, as time passed, the rumors of fraud were being shown to have more than a core of truth. In early December 1968, the Attorney General of Maryland announced he was investigating frauds by physicians, dentists, and pharmacists.[112] By the end of the month, providers in Massachusetts were under attack (one dentist was said to have grossed $164,000 from Medicaid in 1968[113]), and the prosecution of ten physicians for fraud had begun in Maryland.[114] Fraud was by then an established part of the Medicaid way of life—so established in fact that the Senate Finance Committee took over responsibility for investigating it.[115] The moment for re-examining vendor payments had arrived.

NOTES

1. Tax Foundation, Inc., *Medicaid: State Programs After Two Years* (New York, 1968), p. 42.

2. U.S., Advisory Commission on Intergovernmental Relations, *Intergovernmental Problems in Medicaid* (Washington, 1968), pp. 31–34.

3. *Ibid.*, p. 34.

4. California, Delaware, Kentucky, Maryland, New York, Oklahoma, and Rhode Island.

5. Hawaii, Kansas, Massachusetts, Michigan, Minnesota, Nebraska, North Dakota, Utah, Washington, and Wisconsin. Of the three states (Iowa, Kansas, Vermont) which had instituted programs after July 1967 and were therefore required to reach the 133⅓ percentage by July 1, 1968, in fact only one—Iowa—was affected by the provision.

6. *Intergovernmental Problems in Medicaid, supra,* note 2, p. 34.

7. Vendor payments for medical care from state funds amounted to $1.52 billion in fiscal year 1969; total state funds for federally subsidized public assistance amounted to $3.47 billion. Taking all funding sources together (federal, state, and local), nine states and Puerto Rico spent more than half of their welfare funds on medical care. U.S., Department of Health, Education, and Welfare, Social and Rehabilitation Service, *Sources of Funds Expended for Public Assistance Payments* (Washington, 1969), Tables 2, 3, 8.

8. Data Presented by Staff of Senate Finance Committee. U.S., Congress, Senate, Staff of Senate Committee on Finance, *Staff Data Relating to Medicaid-Medicare Study,* Committee Print, U.S. Congress, Committee on Finance, 91st Cong., 1st Sess., 1969. The Tax Foundation survey noted, however, that state tax increases were associated with expansions in more than one government program. There was some evidence that Medicaid was being used as a convenient scapegoat. *Medicaid, supra,* note 1, p. 40.

9. *Medicaid: State Programs After Two Years, supra,* note 1, p. 38.

10. *American Medical News,* June 24, 1968.

11. *Medicaid: State Programs After Two Years, supra,* note 1, p. 36.

12. The 22,000 were restored to the rolls in January 1969. *AMA News,* Jan. 29, 1969.

13. Details from *AMA News,* July 8, 1968, and Oct. 14, 1968. There were still deficit problems. See *ibid.*, Oct. 17, 1967.

14. *Ibid.*, May 5, 1969.

15. *Ibid.*, Jan. 19, 1970.

16. *Ibid.*, June 24, 1968.

17. *Medicaid: State Programs After Two Years, supra,* note 1, p. 70; U.S., Department of Health, Education, and Welfare, Social and Rehabilitation Service, *Medicaid, Fiscal Year 1969* (Washington, 1969), Table 4.

18. *AMA News,* Feb. 19, 1969.

19. *Ibid.,* April 28, 1969, and July 7, 1969.

20. *Ibid.,* April 7, 1969.

21. *Ibid.,* Sept. 2, 1968.

22. *New Orleans Times-Picayune,* Dec. 28, 1968; *ibid.,* Dec. 29, 1968.

23. For details see *CCH Medicare & Medicaid Guide,* par. 15,566. For some of the political implications, see Editorial, *New Haven Register,* Sept. 24, 1969, p. 22, col. 1.

24. *AMA News,* Feb. 2, 1969, and March 3, 1969.

25. Samuel Levey, "A Perspective on Medicaid," *New England J. of Medicine,* vol. 281 (1969), pp. 297–298. The bill for chronic-hospital care had been $11 million in 1966; in 1967 it was $22 million. Out of a total budget of almost $127 million in 1967, $52.6 million went for nursing homes.

26. See, e.g., on New Jersey proposals, *AMA News,* July 22, 1968.

27. *Miami Herald,* June 2, 1967.

28. *CCH Medicare & Medicaid Guide,* par. 15,586.

29. *Richmond Times-Dispatch,* Sept. 12, 1967.

30. In addition to developing professional backing, the Commissioner had warned—for example in a speech to the Richmond Academy of Medicine—that it was impossible to estimate the real cost of the program. *Ibid.,* Nov. 15, 1967. And, as an extra caution, Governor Mills Godwin warned providers to exercise restraint as the day for implementation drew near, warning that the success of the program would depend largely on doctors. *Ibid.,* April 3, 1969. After competitive bidding, the Department of Health contracted with Blue Cross–Blue Shield to serve as carrier for the program. Because they had advanced data-processing equipment and had close relations with providers—they were fiscal intermediaries for Medicare—it seemed a logical choice. *Ibid,* Sept 10, 1968. By June 1969, the Department of Health had certified 1045 physicians, 691 pharmacies, 123 hospitals, and 52 nursing homes as eligible to provide Medicaid services. Meanwhile the Department of Welfare and Institutions had certified 49,379 families (100,668 persons) as eligible for Phase one (categorically needy only). *Ibid.,* June 25, 1969. With HEW approval granted on June 18, what may have been the nation's most cautious and carefully planned Medicaid program began.

31. *Ibid.,* July 24, 1969.

32. *Ibid.,* Nov. 28, 1969.

33. Limits on real and personal property have remained constant. These are: (1) The recipient may own income-producing property if the equity is less than $10,000; (2) He may own a house; (3) He may own life insurance whose face value is less than $5000; (4) Liquid assets of $600 for an individual, $900 for two, and $100 for each additional dependent are allowed. Virginia Department of Health, *State Plan for Virginia Medical Assistance Program. CCH Medicare & Medicaid Guide,* par. 15652.

34. *Medicaid: State Programs After Two Years, supra,* note 1, p. 35. Even with expanded programs in other states, New York and California continue to

dominate Medicaid. In fiscal year 1969 New York accounted for 28.1 percent of all medical assistance expenditures, and California for 17.1 percent—a total of 45.2 percent. *Medicaid Fiscal Year 1969, supra,* note 18, Chart I.

35. *CCH Medicare & Medicaid Guide,* par. 15560.

36. C.M.A., *Socio-Economic Report,* vol. 10, No. 10, p. 3.

37. See Chapter 7.

38. Acton W. Barnes, *A Description of the Organization and Administration of the California Medical Assistance Program: Title XIX,* mimeograph, School of Public Health, University of North Carolina, 1968, p. 146.

39. *Ibid.,* p. 149.

40. An outline of the report is provided in *ibid.,* pp. 153–176.

41. Predictably, the report also called for far greater flexibility in determining groups to be covered and services to be provided.

42. *This Week for Hospitals,* Nov. 15, 1967.

43. *AMA News,* Dec. 2, 1968.

44. *Ibid.,* Nov. 13, 1967.

45. *Medical Tribune,* Nov. 6, 1967.

46. State of California, *Budget Report 1969–70,* p. 920.

47. California Medical Association, *Socio-Economic Report,* vol. 10, No. 10, October 1970, p. 2. State of California, Annual Budgets, *passim.*

48. These deficits occurred in spite of the fact that less than half of the estimated eligible population applied for participation in the program in fiscal 1967.

49. *Sources of Funds Expended for Public Assistance Payments, supra,* note 7, Table 8. Out of this New York spent $54 million (including $14 million in state funds) on administering the program, including determining eligibility. U.S., Department of Health, Education, and Welfare, Social and Rehabilitation Service, *Public Assistance Cost of State and Local Administration, Services and Training, Fiscal Year ended June 30, 1969,* Table 8.

50. New York State, Department of Social Services, *No one can stop it—Except us,* 1967 Annual Report, p. 16.

51. In certain cases counties could lower eligibility still further. The new state legislation also disqualified working persons between 21 and 65, except in cases of catastrophic illness where medical cost exceeded more than 25 percent of a patient's annual income.

52. For a study of the politics of reduction in New York, see Michael Petrina, *A Look at Medicaid,* 1969 (paper presented at the Yale Law School).

53. *New York Times,* March 15, 1968, p. 35, col. 1.

54. The standard fee was to be $16, graduated down to $3 a visit for a family of four with an income of $5300. The department took the step reluctantly, after pressure from house staffs and from the HEW Regional Office.

55. Jo Ann Silverstein, *Medicaid in New York State: A Play in One Act,* 1972 (paper presented at the Yale Medical School), p. 8 *et seq.*

56. *New York Times,* March 28, 1969, p. 1, col. 3.

57. *Ibid.,* February 7, 1969, p. 1, col. 1.

58. *Ibid.,* April 4, 1969, p. 21, col. 2.

59. *Ibid.,* February 20, 1969, p. 55, col. 4.

60. *Ibid.,* May 18, 1970, p. 23, col. 1.

61. *Ibid.*, August 13, 1969, p. 33, col. 5.

62. City of New York, Department of Health, *A Compendium of Selected Medicaid Data 1968–1970*, mimeograph, 1970, *passim.*

63. *New York Times,* June 24, 1969, p. 20, col. 3; *ibid.*, August 13, 1969, p. 33, col. 5.

64. *AMA News,* July 21, 1969.

65. *O'Reilly v. Wyman,* 305 F. Supp. 228 (S.D.N.Y. 1969). Despite its success, the state decided to delay implementation. *New York Times,* Oct. 28, 1970, p. 53, col. 7.

66. See Chapter 15.

67. *New York Times,* March 29, 1969, p. 1, col. 1. The Assembly did not pass the bill until 11:58 p.m. on the last day of the legislature (83–65), and it had cleared the Senate an hour earlier (35–22). *Ibid.*, March 30, 1969, p. 1, col. 8.

68. *Ibid.*, March 31, 1969, p. 1, col. 1.

69. Raymond Alexander, "Administrative Dynamics in Megalopolitan Health Care," *American J. of Public Health,* vol. 59 (1969), p. 815, 86.

70. The data used here are taken from City of New York, Department of Health, *Materia Medicaid: New York City: A Compendium of Selected Medicaid Data 1968–1970* (Florence Kavaler, Lowell Bellin, David Lieberman, Zipporah Haber, Arnold Rabby, Haydoo Inclan).

71. Thus in March 31.7 percent of the city's physicians gave some Medicaid services; by December 44.3 percent. For dentists the parallel figures were 57.9 percent and 66.0 percent. There were slight rises for podiatrists (67.2 percent by December), optometrists (63.8 percent by that date), ophthalmic dispensers (18.7 percent), and pharmacies (71 percent). Chiropractors joined the program on June 1, and by December 26.1 percent had given Medicaid services. *Ibid.*, Table A.

72. *Ibid.*, Table E.

73. *New York Times,* March 12, 1969, p. 35, col. 1.

74. *Ibid.*, Feb. 7, 1969, p. 1, col. 1.

75. *Ibid.*, February 20, 1969, p. 55, col. 4.

76. *Ibid.*, February 11, 1969, p. 28, col. 3.

77. *Ibid.*, March 12, 1969, p. 35, col. 1; *ibid.*, May 23, 1969, p. 32, col. 6.

78. Siverstein, *op. cit.*, note 55, *supra,* p. 18.

79. *New York Times,* July 1, 1969, p. 21, col. 1.

80. *Ibid.*, July 9, 1969, p. 28, col. 4.

81. *Ibid.*, June 23, 1969, p. 1, col. 2.

82. *Ibid.*, July 9, 1969, p. 28, col. 4.

83. *Ibid.*, June 25, 1969, p. 95, col. 3.

84. Silverstein, *op. cit., supra,* note 55, p. 20.

85. *Materia Medicaid, supra,* note 70, p. 18. During 1969 37 physicians (including 22 specialists) earned more than $71,000 from Medicaid; 2 osteopathic physicians were in this category; 7 optometrists; 114 dentists; 6 podiatrists; 27 pharmacies. *Ibid.*, Tables 31–39.

86. *Ibid.*, p. 46.

87. *Ibid.*, p. 48.

88. *Ibid.*, p. 24.

89. E.g., Lowell E. Bellin, "*Realpolitik* in the Health Care Arena: Standard-Setting of Professional Services," *American J. of Public Health,* vol. 59 (1969), p. 820.

90. *Ibid.*, pp. 822–823.

91. "Certain professional groups became instantly franchised as publicly funded providers of care. For them Medicaid meant new dignity, new money and an opportunity to gain newly found power through negotiations with city and state government." Lowell Bellin, *The Inception of Publicly Funded Chiropractic in New York Medicaid.* Mimeograph, undated, p. 3.

92. *Ibid.*, p. 18.

93. Florence Kavaler, "People, Providers and Payment—Telling It How It Is," *ibid.*, p. 825.

94. Norman Schuman, Florence Kavaler, Lowell Bellin, David Lieberman, Benjamin Watkins, Zipporah Haber, "Publicly Funded Podiatry: The New York City Medicaid Experience," *Medical Care,* vol. 9 (1971), p. 117; see also *Podiatry Today,* vol. 51 (1969), p. 437.

95. Florence Kavaler, Lowell Bellin, Alex Green, Elihu Gorelik, Raymond Alexander, "A Publicly Funded Pharmacy Program under Medicaid in New York City," *Medical Care,* vol. 7 (1969), p. 361. In New York this is calculated by paying a 66⅔ percent markup on base cost, rather than by paying a straight professional fee.

96. Raymond Alexander, Lowell Bellin, Florence Kavaler, Harold Najac, Jess Rosenthal, "The Participation of Optometrists in New York City's Medicaid Program," *Public Health Reports,* vol. 84 (1969), p. 1008.

97. See, for example, Rosemary Stevens, *American Medicine and the Public Interest,* New Haven, 1971, pp. 534–535.

98. *New York Times,* Oct. 8, 1966, p. 1, col. 1.

99. Lowell Bellin, "Compulsory Continuing Education for Licensed Health Care Professionals Participating in Medicaid: A Case History," Mimeograph, 1969.

100. Lowell Bellin and Florence Kavaler, "An Inventory of Medicaid Practitioner Abuses and Excuses vs. Counter-strategy of the New York City Health Department" (A paper presented at the 1970 APHA meeting: mimeograph).

101. The investigations had led to three suspensions, 17 temporary suspensions, 12 referrals to the State Board, 100 warnings and restrictions, and 86 fiscal readjustments.

102. See, e.g., American Public Welfare Association, *Survey of State Public Welfare Directors Regarding Problems in Implementing the Provisions of Title XIX of the Social Security Act 15* (1969).

103. *1969 Staff Report, supra,* note 8, at 30.

104. E.g., cutbacks in the Louisiana program, where physicians' usual and customary fees were protected, *AMA News,* September 2, 1968.

105. Connecticut, for example, set up a medical advisory committee to assist the welfare commissioner in reviewing claims for payment to physicians. The committee consisted entirely of physicians—15 selected from a list of nominees submitted by the state medical society and eight others added by the commissioner, the later including university medical school representatives and medical administrators from three major insurance companies.

106. R. Girard, *The Use of Fiscal Agents in Medicaid: Who Does What, Why and How* (1970) (paper presented at the Yale Law School).

107. In Alabama inpatient, outpatient, and emergency hospital services, together with skilled nursing home services were reimbursed through Blue Cross–Blue Shield of Alabama as fiscal agent. Laboratory and x-ray services outside these categories, physician services, eyeglasses, and optometric services were reimbursed through the Equitable Life Assurance Society. Prescribed drugs and non-legend drugs were reimbursed through the State National Bank of Alabama. *CCH Medicare & Medicaid Guide*, par. 15,550; *Staff Report, supra*, note 9, p. 285, also notes that Blue Shield (and not Equitable) is carrier for Medicare Part B, while Blue Cross and Mutual of Omaha are carriers for Part A. *Ibid*., pp. 262, 267.

108. On the functions of such intermediaries under Title XVIII, see P.L. 89–97 § 1816 (1965): "Use of public agencies or private organizations to facilitate payment to providers of services" under Part A; and *ibid*., § 1842, "Use of carriers for administration of benefits" under Part B.

109. State of Vermont, *Report of the Governor's Committee Investigating Social Welfare*, 1969, p. 74.

110. Officials in California made more strenuous and imaginative efforts than most states to set up statistical reporting methods; information including the type of procedure and primary diagnosis was coded by a clerk in the offices of the fiscal agents, together with other information such as the date and type of service, amount of payment, claim and check number, and identification of recipient and vendor. Each month the agents sent the resulting tapes to the state Department of Health, which was the responsible agency until September 1967 (when responsibility was shifted to the Welfare Agency). Such information was, however, limited in its usefulness. It referred only to bills paid (and there was an initial allowable time lag of up to seven months between service and payment) and comprised relatively crude data, as it was derived from claim forms carried over from the time of hand-processing and providing far from specific information about service utilization. A former head of the Medi-Cal Surveillance Unit later remarked, "The possible uses of computers within the new health care programs have scarcely been touched." See Henry Anderson, "Statistical Surveillance of a Title XIX Program," *American J. of Public Health*, vol. 59, 1969, pp. 275, 289.

111. For instance, states reported a total sum of $172 million spent on the costs of administering medical assistance payments in fiscal 1969, of which 52 percent was from federal funds (and nine percent from local funds). *Public Assistance Cost of State and Local Administration, Services and Training, supra*, note 49, Table 8. Much of this, however, was being funneled to pay the salaries of social workers and supporting welfare offices, in the expensive process of determining a potential recipient's eligibility, rather than in ensuring the efficient operation of the whole system. As a result, the administrators of the Medicaid programs (and other interested groups, including the recipients themselves) had little ammunition to defend the operations or to justify the rapidly increasing expenditures.

112. *AMA News*, December 2, 1968.

113. *Ibid*., Dec. 9, 1968.

114. *Ibid*., Dec. 30, 1968.

115. In one further respect state experience became more generalized. Increasingly, all states were brought into the litigious side of Medicaid. California and New York were by no means the only states to have Medicaid issues brought before the courts. In *Lee v. Laitinen*, 448 P. 2d 154, 1968, for instance, the

Supreme Court of Montana upheld the right of the Montana Board of Public Welfare to use a flat rate for the payment of nursing homes and refused to compel the payment of "usual and customary" charges. More common was litigation about eligibility. In *McNiff v. Olmsted County Welfare Department* (176 NW 2d 888, 1970) the Supreme Court of Minnesota had no difficulty in holding that a resident of a nursing home was not entitled to Medicaid when it construed a trust document as evidencing an intent that she should share in a trust worth $22,000. The Appellate Division of the Connecticut Circuit Court, in *Hunt v. Shapiro,* 5 Conn. Cir. Ct. 505 (1970), refused to hold that a hearing terminating the plaintiff's right to Medicaid was either illegal or unconstitutional when the state financial limit for the family was $4400 and it was stipulated plaintiff earned $5142 (App. Denied, 257 A 2d 44. S.C., Conn., 1970).

In general the state courts seemed sympathetic to the administrative burdens of welfare departments and the fiscal stringency faced by legislatures. On all of this see Chapter 13.

10
Costs, Successes, and Scapegoats

If the beginning of Medicaid can be called the period of expansion and the years 1967 to 1969 the period of retrenchment, by 1970 the wheel had turned again to a new period of management. The first phase had been expansionist in terms of both recipients and providers. The second had led to restrictions primarily on recipients. The third was to concentrate on the vendors of care; for, as a series of Senate Finance Committee Staff charts dramatically highlighted, though eligibility levels were reduced, the health care providers continued to gain. Vendor payments for medical care had risen from $0.5 billion in 1960 to an estimated $5.5 billion in 1970.[1]

These cost increases had far outstripped expansion in the number of persons served; for instance, the Finance Committee staff noted a 57 percent cost increase for Medicaid between 1968 and 1970, but only a 19 percent increase in the number of recipients. Medical vendor payments had also grown as a proportion of both state and federal welfare costs:[2] Almost half of the state and local costs of welfare were filtering into medical care. Hospital rates had climbed from an average $45 a day in 1967 to $62 in 1970 and were continuing to rise rapidly, while the level of physician fees was well above expectations. The staff of the Finance Committee felt the message was clear. The combined impact of Medicare and Medicaid, which together were injecting about $14 billion into the health care system in fiscal 1971,[3] had been to create additional demand, to push up costs, to stimulate overutilization and unnecessary services, and to encourage an "alarming growth in chain operations in the nursing home field,"[4] leading in all areas to inefficiencies. In Congress, as in the states, the providers appeared to be the major villains. Better management appeared to be the answer, from cost estimation to day-to-day administration.

Cost Estimation

The difficulty of making accurate cost estimates for the federal share under Medicaid continued to be a focus for sharp criticism in Congressional hearings in 1969 and 1970, as in earlier years. One problem was that, according to the Chief Actuary of the Social Security Administration, Robert Myers, the initial additional cost for Medicaid for noninstitutionalized recipients was originally estimated as $238 million in the first full year of operation, calendar year 1966, but this figure was misleading. By excluding the costs of patients in institutions, who were to form an important group for the purposes of Medicaid payments, as well as excluding the new Medicaid category of medically indigent children (the so-called Ribicoff Amendment added during the passage of the 1965 act), the figure gave only a partial notion of Medicaid's costs. Altogether it was estimated that additional costs would be $353 million. Moreover, these had to be added to the previous medical vendor payments through the categorical assistance and MAA programs (an estimated $678 million), which were transferred to the Medicaid program. The total cost of Medicaid was thus expected to be over $1 billion.[5] Although this annual figure was much lower than actual costs were to prove, it was much higher than the $238 million which some legislators assumed was the total estimated costs.

It was hardly surprising that there was both initial and continuing confusion. First, it was not always clear whether figures referred to total costs or just the federal share. But second, Medicaid involved substantial shifts of money among the previous categories, a process at which states were increasingly adept. As states moved into Title XIX, their vendor payments under OAA, MAA, AB, APTD, and AFDC were absorbed into the states' new Medicaid programs. In December 1969, for example, 45 jurisdictions were receiving payments under Title XIX (a total of $342.8 million in that month), and another nine were still working through previous arrangements (a total of $17.7 million).[6] Not surprisingly, there was confusion as to what were the costs of "Medicaid." This was reflected in questions by Senator John Williams to Undersecretary Wilbur Cohen in the Finance Committee hearings on the 1967 amendments:

> *Your first estimate on the cost of Title XIX was $238 million, if I understand it correctly. Then you were before the committee a year ago and were shocked to find it was going to cost a billion and a quarter. Now, what is the estimated cost of this Title XIX as it stands, about $3 billion or more, is it not?*[7]

Although Undersecretary Cohen reiterated the explanation of the partial and additional nature of the $238 million, the initial obfuscation hindered all later HEW attempts to explain the early estimates. The basic fact remained that the total federal share of medical vendor payments had been consistently underestimated, and this was a critical factor in growing

Congressional concern. This situation was clearly underlined in evidence to the Finance Committee in the 1969 Hearings. The estimate for fiscal 1969, made in December 1967, was $1.58 billion in federal funds; a month later the estimate was enlarged by $450 million; by January 1969 it had had another $200 million added to it; and in the revised budget three months later another $40 million appeared. The resulting estimate was thus almost 50 percent greater than the initial estimate.[8]

The problems of cost estimation were not confined to Medicaid. Caught in the same medical price spiral, the Medicare program, too, consistently underestimated its fiscal needs. Little more than a year after the Medicare program started, Congress increased Medicare taxes by some 25 percent to meet unexpected hospital cost increases under Medicare's Part A. The contributory premium paid by the elderly under Medicare's Part B for physician services was also increased from the initial $3 a month to $4 a month, and later to $5.30 a month, effective July 1, 1970, each sum being supplemented by parallel increases in federal matching funds.[9] Both parts of Medicare are, however, self-limiting in that they have indentifiable contributions into national trust funds, with income matched to expenditure. Medicaid, even with the 1967 retrenchments, continued to be relatively uncontrollable, because its financing was open-ended.

In both the public and the private sector, health care costs were rising rapidly. Estimates of total public and private health expenditures for fiscal 1969 reached $60.3 billion.[10] This represented additional expenditures of $18 billion over fiscal 1966, and in total accounted for 6.7 percent of the gross national product. Increased public expenditures represented no mean part of the increase. In fiscal 1966, the public sector funded about 22 percent of total expenditures for medical care; three years later the proportion had risen to 36 percent, most of the additional funds being funneled to private practitioners and institutions. Because of accelerating prices, even Medicare's major contribution to financing health care for the aged had not been sufficient to reduce the need for other public programs. Instead, then, of Medicaid acting as a relatively limited backstop to a social insurance program, it appeared to have an important and continuing financial responsibility; but the nature of the responsibility was such that Medicaid was blamed for failures cased essentially by the inadequacies elsewhere in the health care system.

When there are problems it is convenient to have someone to blame. But within both Medicare and Medicaid at least some of the blame was to be reassigned. It was to be one of the curiosities of these large public programs that blame for inefficiency was laid at the door of the private sector. Medicare was predicated on the assumption that government money could be pumped through private intermediaries and carriers (normally insurance companies) into the pockets of private health care institutions and independent professionals, with relatively little governmental control.

Yet there were in this system no checks and balances to provide alternative forms of regulation. Hospitals and professionals submitted bills, which were paid by the intermediaries and carriers, who were then reimbursed (and paid processing costs) by the Social Security Administration from one or other of Medicare's two Trust Funds. As the 1970 Report of the Senate Finance Committee staff noted, the result was "inefficiency subsidized."[11]

Medicare estimates, like those for Medicaid, rose higher and higher, with few effective controls. Indeed, the whole structure appeared inflationary: the more insurance money available, the more money spent.[12] The estimate made in 1965 for Medicare Part A costs in 1970 was $3.1 billion. This was steadily revised upward to $5.8 billion. Part B costs meanwhile doubled between fiscal 1967 and fiscal 1971.[13] For the first three years of Medicare there was, moreover, little attempt by the Social Security Administration to exert influence over the fiscal intermediaries and carriers or to ensure that hospitals, which were required by the 1965 law to establish utilization review committees, were in fact attempting to audit Medicare costs and use.

There were obvious political reasons for beginning a new program by creating as few administrative waves as possible; indeed, the relatively smooth implementation of Medicare could be accounted a success.[14] With the attending cost increases in services, however, the success was soon discounted. The Senate Finance Committee staff's probe in 1970 revealed, inter alia, that it cost one carrier (Delaware Blue Shield) more than $6 merely to process a physician bill.[15] Delays in payment, spotty performance, and reluctance to provide appropriate information all added up to a negative view of private enterprise, which was in turn to lead to a climate in which the general regulation of health insurance carriers began to seem inevitable.

The Hospitals

The hospitals, too, became labeled as villains under Medicare and Medicaid.[16] As hospital costs rose, so did government expenditures. In the calendar year 1970, public funding (from all sources) contributed almost $14 billion to the nation's hospitals (the equivalent of $67 for each person in the United States) out of a total of $28 billion spent on hospital care.[17] About $7 billion, i.e., one fourth of all hospital expenditures in the United States, was derived from Medicaid and Medicare.[18] This alone would have raised questions of where and how Medicaid and Medicare money was being spent. But there was more at stake. While Medicare and Medicaid were undoubtedly the precipitating factors in rising hospital rates after 1965, these rates were not limited to recipients in those programs: They applied to all hospitalized patients. Thus Medicare and Medicaid had a generalized impact on hospital expenditures.

Hospitals, like insurance agencies, soon found a critical eye upon them. Both the House Ways and Means Committee and the Senate Finance Committee had looked to utilization review as a means of limiting the use of expensive hospital facilities.[19] Not surprisingly, therefore, there was sharp criticism following the report by the Social Security Administration of a survey in 1968 that almost half of the hospitals were not reviewing any admissions, although this was a statutory requirement.[20] Hospital costs appeared to be rising without any attempt by the hospitals themselves to keep costs down. Thus the way was open to greatly increased public controls over hospitals in the future. From the state point of view one of the most frustrating aspects of dealing with providers was that hospital costs were the least subject to control at the state level. Yet they represented the largest and most rapidly rising costs of care.[21] Indeed, the primary reason for rising health care expenditures lay in the costs of providing inhospital and nursing home care. Total expenditures for hospital care, for instance, increased by 17 percent during fiscal 1969 alone.[22] Only part of these increases could be attributed to expanded or better services.[23]

These general cost trends had specific implications for Medicaid. Inpatient hospital care represented well over a third (37 percent) of all expenditures for medical assistance in fiscal 1969, and nursing home care another third (30 percent). Moreover, these costs were rising rapidly. Amounts spent on hospital care under Medicaid *doubled* between 1967 and 1970, from $900,000 to $1.9 billion.

The 1965 legislation, as we have seen, specified that inpatient hospital care under Medicaid should be reimbursed on a "reasonable cost" basis, rather than, for example, on a statewide fee schedule.[24] For convenience, the Medicare interpretation of reasonable cost, defined in regulations by the Social Security Administration, was adopted for interim payments under Title XIX.[25] The arrangement greatly facilitated accounting procedures for payment for hospital services on behalf of elderly persons who were recipients of both Medicare and Medicaid.[26] But, at the same time, reasonable-cost reimbursement tied states to the rising costs of hospital care. For instance, the total cost of hospital care for the elderly from all sources of payment rose from $4.17 billion in fiscal year 1967 to $6.53 billion in 1969.[27] As hospital costs rose, so, in large part, did Medicaid reimbursement rates. The states were powerless, both practically and legally.

There was, moreover, some irony in the situation of tying Medicaid hospital reimbursement to Medicare payments. Because of the extent and nature of hospital coverage under Medicare, Medicaid paid out relatively little of its hospital budget for care of the elderly. In 1969, for instance, only about a fourth of the bill for inpatient hospital care provided under Medicaid was for those 65 years of age and over; and the majority of this went toward the costs of care in state mental institutions.[28] But while only a fraction of the whole Medicaid hospital inpatient budget went toward general hospital care for the elderly, the hospital rates for all of the Medicaid categories were tied to Medicare's reasonable cost definition. In the event, reasonable cost under Medicare turned out to mean at least whatever the market would bear, and almost whatever the hospitals chose to demand.

Nursing Homes

Nursing homes, too, were an increasing cause for alarm, although for rather different reasons. Congressional interest in nursing homes up to the 1967 Amendments had focused on their general standards; the need for standards for fire protection, for example, and the level of nursing care. Such questions lay in the realm of public safety and in consumer protection. From the point of view of costs and program limitations, there were, however, two other pressing concerns. One was the widespread development of profit-making nursing homes following Medicare and Medicaid;[29] the other, the classification of services allowable under the two programs.[30] The two were connected. If Medicaid were to pay the bills for all bedridden old persons and all who needed some nursing care, the potential for further expansion of nursing homes was awesome. As more beds became available, the greater would be the cost burden to fall on Medicaid programs.

Two other cost factors were also germane to nursing home expansions. Because the legislation specifically removed from welfare departments any legal entitlement to collect contributions for the cost of care of the elderly from their children, there was a greater initiative to institutionalize elderly parents, at no offsetting income. At the same time, the Medicare legislation, as drafted, positively encouraged elderly persons to go to nursing homes after a period in hospital, a move supposed to be cost-saving. In theory, the patients would be removed from a more expensive hospital bed to the less expensive nursing home and then to the least expensive category of home care services, all covered under Medicare. The problem was that many patients, once in the nursing home, remained there. When Medicare benefits stopped, the bill (for those eligible) landed in the lap of Medicaid.

From the nursing home point of view, Medicare and Medicaid together offered a steady and realistic income that allowed for an appropriate amount of profit. But, as we have noted, there was little effort by either program in its early years to see how public money was being spent. The apparent casualness of nursing home administration was an obvious focus of Congressional criticism. A large number of ineligible nursing homes had been allowed to participate in Medicaid.[31] The 1969 Hearings of the Senate Finance Committee also noted the practices of so-called gang visits by doctors to nursing homes. In the words of Senator Russell Long, "They just kind of walk through and say 'hello' to all of the patients and ask them how they are feeling and bill each one for $8 or $10 as the case may be."[32] Abuse was also noted in some cases in which physicians owned nursing homes.[33]

By 1969, the nursing homes were under open attack, although the primary responsibility for mismanagement in many cases lay with the state agencies for lax certification and insufficient supervision. Audits by HEW in 1969 found $380,000 paid to ineligible nursing homes in California during the period July–December 1968.[34] Generally, utilization review under Medicaid was poor or nonexistent. The HEW audits of 16 states found only four that made systematic reviews,[35] although review was required by the 1967 Amendments and, indeed, a regulation to this effect had been issued in March 1969.[36] Such review was particularly important, because the majority of patients were Medicaid recipients.

In terms of cost, although there was no provision in the 1965 legislation that nursing home costs be reimbursed by Medicaid on the reasonable-cost basis required for hospitals, there was considerable pressure on states to do so. According to the law, suppliers of services (other than hospitals) were to be reimbursed according to state policies, which were to "provide such safeguards as may be necessary to assure that . . . such care and services will be provided, in a manner consistent with simplicity of administration and the best interests of the recipients."[37] This principle was elaborated in the requirements for a state plan of medical assistance in terms which defined the "best interests of the recipients" as receipt of medical care and services included in the plan "at least to the extent these are available to the general population."[38]

What did this mean? California was one state which interpreted the intent of Medicaid as being to provide services to the poor on the same basis as services were provided to the middle-class population through the private sector, a stand that argued for payment of Medicaid services under arrangements similar to those made by private insurance schemes or Medicare. This interpretation appeared to be also the original policy of the Social and Rehabilitation Service of HEW. For institutions other than hospitals, states were advised that fee structures should focus on payment on a reasonable-cost basis, equivalent to the reimbursement methods under Part A of Title XVIII.

The situation was, however, extremely confused, and there was some apparent backtracking. Thus a letter dated March 13, 1969, from the Social and Rehabilitation Service, when nursing home costs were causing considerable alarm in Congress, stated that the policy of reasonable costs was not to apply to skilled nursing home care. Provisions for the application of upper standards of reimbursement for skilled nursing home care would, it was promised, be "clarified" when regulations governing the standards for payment for such care were issued. These clarifications, however, were not issued until 1970.[39] Thus, whereas prior to Title XIX the usual method of vendor payment for skilled nursing home care by state welfare departments was on the basis of negotiated fees, per diem or monthly flat rates in many cases below the institutions' operating costs, with the passage of Medicare and Medicaid both costs and expectations began to move upward. In states which shifted to reimbursement methods more nearly reflecting the costs incurred, immediate increases in expenditures were observed.[40] As at the same time the number of nursing homes was also rising, largely through private investment, the states were faced with a second series of cost increases over which they had relatively little jurisdiction.

The nursing home question was of particular importance for states that had previously had relatively generous nursing home benefits. In Vermont, for example, nursing home costs under Medicaid in the period June 1968–June 1970 outstripped general hospital costs, with payments of $9.5 million and $7.1 million, respectively, and represented 37 percent of the Medicaid budget.[41] Well over 90 percent of these nursing home costs were for elderly recipients. In Connecticut, nursing home costs had dominated medical vendor payments since the Kerr-Mills era. Approximately half of the Connecticut Medicaid budget had been spent on nursing homes from the beginning, but as over-all costs rose, so did the state's nursing home costs, from $14 million in fiscal 1965 to $36 million in fiscal 1970 (and on to an estimated $58 million in fiscal 1973).[42]

The nursing home question was vexing because, in all the states, the bulk of nursing home expenditures went for care of the elderly: the national figure was 80 percent. Throwing old people out of nursing homes was scarcely politically acceptable, unless organized alternatives were available —and they were not. Keeping the elderly from entering at all was a more realistic solution, but this was difficult to do when new nursing homes were being built and when Medicare encouraged the elderly to enter into extended care facilities. Intermediate care facilities, which qualified for federal subsidies under the 1967 Amendments, offered a supposedly less expensive alternative to skilled nursing care; but these were still "nursing homes." Although they were not directly reimbursed as part of Medicaid until 1972, they still came under the state welfare umbrella. The states were caught in the middle of the whole cycle.

Physicians

Where, then, were the villains of rising costs whom the states could most readily attack? There was one obvious answer: the health care professionals, especially physicians. They were not only responsive to fee controls at the state level; it was they who certified which patients went to expensive health care facilities and decided how long they remained, once there. And they, too, had benefitted from rapidly rising reimbursement levels, even though they were already among the best paid members of society.

It was perhaps unfortunate that the notion of "mainstream" medicine was equated with the exchange and receipt of private fees. But the very structure of fee-based practice, the effect of the passage of Medicare and Medicaid in the same legislation, and a prevailing mood in Secretary John Gardner's Department of Health, Education, and Welfare that medical care for the poor should be provided with equal dignity and through similar channels as the medical care for other members of the population[43] made this approximation inevitable. But although, to some physicians at least, the private fee was a symbol of professional independence, for state welfare departments fee levels were a matter of strategy. HEW was urging them on. Fee structures, it was emphasized in 1966, should be "realistic to assure eligible persons medical care and services in sufficient quantities."[44] The goal was to include two thirds of the practitioners in each state.[45] Not surprisingly, there was a movement led by state medical societies to establish payment of physicians on the basis of their "usual and customary fees" in the developing Medicaid programs. A review in 1967 found that 15 Title XIX programs had established payment of physicians through their usual and customary charging structure; only one of these states (Idaho) had previously paid on this basis.[46]

The success of this policy of encouraging physician participation was universally commended by physician organizations. The president of the Illinois State Medical Society, for example, ascribed the jump in physician involvement in Medicaid in that state, from 3,228 MDs in 1967 to over 6,000 in 1969, to the abandonment of the previous pattern of closed-panel "welfare physicians" to one which allowed all physicians to participate.[47] Participation appeared directly tied to fees. Indeed, 14 states reporting unwillingness of physicians or other providers to participate in 1968 cited inadequate fees as a major reason.[48] But participation was gained at a high price. Under the combined impact of extended services and rising fees, the amount paid to physicians under medical assistance programs increased almost fivefold between 1965 and 1969, from \$121.6 million to \$523.3 million.[49] While many of the additional expenditures represented extra services and possibly extra time spent with medical assistance patients (and perhaps even less tangible elements such as greater personal attention to welfare recipients), at least some of this was pure profit.

Physicians found themselves hoisted on their own petard. The American Medical Association had opposed health insurance for the aged in 1960 because, it was claimed, care was given to the needy by physicians on a charitable basis.[50] Similar claims were made in 1965; at the same time, the relatively modest level of previous increases in medical fees had been emphasized.[51] Yet once Medicaid was enacted, it seemed to be the physicians who gained the most. (Hospitals always had the excuse of union demands and technological breakthroughs to explain their rising expenses.) Thus, while the states looked to the medical societies to help them develop their Medicaid programs,[52] the politics of fees soon jaundiced these co-operative relationships. In some instances, the physicians proved tough barterers. In Virginia, for example, the Medical Society urged the Governor to begin a Medicaid program, provided the state reimbursed physicians in the same way as they were paid under Medicare.[53] As medical societies pressed for the elimination of payment by the old welfare method of fixed fees, they dropped the aura of benevolent contributors to the general welfare and became much more like union negotiators.

As has been seen, in the early stages of Medicaid HEW urged the payment of physicians according to their usual or customary fees on the grounds both of encouraging their participation and of tying Medicaid to Medicare. Dr. Francis Land, MSA Commissioner, said in the July 1969 Hearings before the Senate Finance Committee that there had been "an urging on my part that we try to approach as closely as possible those fees that were being paid under the Title 18 provision, but not above it"[54] But this line was fraught with difficulties. It was in the end to lead to intervention at the White House level: In 1969 the signals were changed, and a Republican President called for the curbing of fees of private physicians.

In the meantime, the change soured relations in many states. A large state with a powerful governor was able to resist pressure from physicians. For instance, California, while providing for reasonable charges in the light of usual and customary fees, put ceilings on the amounts the fiscal agents could in fact pay.[55] New York, too—and New York City especially—was able to battle the providers on an almost equal basis. But in the smaller states the fight was often uneven. In some states too, for example in Massachusetts, physicians lobbied for the appointment of Blue Shield, a physician-dominated organization, as Medicaid's fiscal agent, and the state then found it difficult to control fees.[56]

Elsewhere, too, physicians' monetary concerns were much in evidence. In Pennsylvania, the state medical society organized an elaborate lobbying program to show how much physicians were subsidizing Title XIX because they were being paid on a fee scale rather than their usual and customary fee. Each physician was asked to send statements to patients and to the state welfare department showing the degree of "subsidization" in each case. The bills were to be marked: "The difference between the state payment and customary fee represents the service gratuitously provided by the physician."[57] Yet, this was a state whose medical society had claimed proudly only eight years before:

> *. . . Pennsylvania physicians provided $41,969,000 worth of free care during 1960. This free care was apportioned on the following basis: 28.4 percent resulted from treating private patients without charge;*

> *37.3 percent resulted from hospital ward service; 24.2 percent was provided in outpatient clinic service; 10 percent resulted from free care to all other persons . . . .*[58]

It was scarcely surprising that physician earnings began to soar, especially after the passage of Title XIX, when these services suddenly became reimbursable.

Connecticut's experiences were similar. While the physicians in general had opposed federal involvement in medical care because, among other things, they alleged that "charity" patients were already treated gratuitously, Connecticut physicians were no different from those in other parts of the country in demanding usual (private) fees, if any fees were to be paid at all. Even before the program came into existence, the State Medical Society expressed concern about the fee scale the Connecticut General Life Insurance Company, the fiscal agent, would pay. The Society refused to accept the word "reasonable" in the documents relating to the determination of fees.[59] Nor did organized medicine restrain itself politically, and the 1967 Connecticut Legislature passed Public Act 548, which gave the providers many of the things they asked. Although the Act established a Professional Policy Committee on which the administration was predominant, that committee was to be advised by a Professional Advisory Committee dominated by the providers' associations and a Medical Advisory Committee whose members were nominated by the State Medical Society; a resulting configuration which helped to confuse even federal officials.[60] Additionally, the Act increased the fees of dentists and other practitioners effective October 1, 1967, while decreeing that from April 1968 to March 1969 physicians should experimentally be paid on a "usual and customary" fee basis.

The Connecticut experiment was interesting both in its results and in its implications. Physicians participated more readily, but costs skyrocketed. For April 1968, physician services had cost Connecticut Medicaid $66,718. By December, the monthly sum was $518,347.[61] After hearings in February 1969 and the listing in local Connecticut newspapers of the names and amounts of payments to physicians for Medicaid services, the state returned to a fee schedule. But all was not as it was before. Physicians had been publicized as apparent exploiters of the state taxpayers; the medical profession was displeased; but in the end it was the recipients who suffered. It became much more difficult to persuade a physician to take a Title XIX patient.[62] Compared with the physicians, the other Connecticut providers had low visibility, but they too were engaged in fiscal skirmishes with the state. The worst problem came from the dentists, whose leadership boycotted the program from time to time; while roughly half the dentists in the state actually participated.[63]

By the summer of 1969, then, the idea of "usual and customary" fees was almost a dead issue in the Title XIX program as a whole, for the federal government had moved to freeze physician fees.[64] The rather rapid change of heart was generated not only by the general rise in costs, but by increasing publicity, as in Connecticut, of the extent of provider gains. A pattern of excessive payments to physicians and dentists had emerged throughout the participating states. With these disclosures came growing evidence of fraud on the part of various groups of providers.

The Fine Sport of Fee-Hunting[65]

Besides changes in reimbursement procedures, the fee levels in private practice had been rising. One unforeseen result of Medicare and Medicaid was that in formalizing the system of doctors' charges by developing profiles of the "usual and customary" fees prevailing in each area, some physicians became aware of what others were charging. Quite clearly, there was some "standardizing-up"; that is, a physician charging well below average charges in an area would revise his fees to the average level, sometimes apparently encouraged by the insurance carriers nominally acting as the government's agent. As fee rises tend to be fairly substantial—an increase in a fee from $8 to $10 is, after all, a 25 percent increase—the cumulative effect was a jump in physician charges. The Social Security Administration noted a rise of 14.4 percent in fees in the first two years of Medicare; a *Medical Economics* survey found a rise of 11.1 percent in the fees of self-employed physicians between 1965 and 1966 alone, with the greatest increase in the East.[66] Physician fees thus became a focus of debate for both Medicare and Medicaid.

The Senate Finance Committee conducted its inquiry into Medicare and Medicaid in May and June 1969 and held hearings in July. These hearings were largely a fleshing-out of what the Committee already knew or suspected. Senator Long set the tone of the hearings with his opening remarks about "these runaway programs." Citing the example of one doctor who had billed Medicare $58,000 in 1968 for house calls to 49 patients, he asked, "Who says you can't get a doctor to make a house call anymore?" He added that there might be as many as 10,000 individual providers each making more than $25,000 annually from Medicare and Medicaid.[67]

As the hearings progressed, the Committee heard testimony from HEW officials that their scrutiny of the programs was intensifying and that some 700 cases of possible fraud were under investigation, although the worst problem was not with fraud but with abuses short of fraud.[68] Like many public Congressional hearings, these seem to have consisted of equal parts of fact-finding and publicity. Senator Byrd (Virginia) compared payments for Medicaid's extended care benefits to cost overruns on the F-111 and C-5A,[69] Senator Curtis incredulously "discovered" from Dr. Francis Land, then Commissioner of MSA, that New York's program was open-ended;[70]

and much of the testimony consisted of questions on the specific abuses that had been uncovered, with most of the committee members getting their chance to be outraged.

By this time, however, HEW was also deeply concerned about physician fees. Indeed, the Nixon administration inherited accumulated evidence of fraud on taking office in 1969. The Undersecretary of HEW, John Veneman, announced, "We have to move toward eliminating greed in Medicare and Medicaid whether on the part of the recipients or the vendors."[71] The press was increasingly reporting incidents of fraud; and the position was not helped when HEW announced that 47 doctors had been paid more than $50,000 each under Title XVIII during 1968. The collapse of the Medicaid program in New Mexico was attributed by some to the greed of the providers;[72] in May, in reporting the Senate's investigation, the Associated Press report carried the theme that "Medicaid Reported Bilked Out of Hundreds of Millions of Dollars."[73] Even the *Chicago Tribune,* normally more harsh on recipients than providers, was forced to admit that "in the health programs the cheating is being done mainly by unscrupulous doctors and sticky-fingered functionaries."[74]

There was inevitably a demand for the publishing of the names of high-paid physicians. As Senator Williams put it, "The only way to end this sort of thing is to name names and sums of money and put it on the front pages all over the country.[75] The states complied. For instance, in Maryland it turned out that one fifth of the $4 million paid to 2,470 physicians under Medicaid had gone to 28 of them. One physician received almost $50,000 while 13 others got more than $30,000. Thirty-nine dentists were paid more than $10,000, and one drug store received $245,497.[76] By April 1969 the Senate Finance Committee was notifying states that it wanted data on all physicians paid more than $25,000 under Title XIX in 1968.[77] The AMA expressed concern about abuse by physicians,[78] but many local medical societies were protective about their members. Meanwhile the California legislature introduced special legislation to punish defrauding providers[79] and Senator Long pressed for sending the data to the Internal Revenue Service.[80] Changes were in fact made in the IRS reporting requirements in November 1969, but the 1970 *Staff Report* still considered the arrangements open to abuse.[81]

Although some doctors no doubt were paid large sums under Title XIX because they chose to work in low-income areas, some of the data which gradually emerged was remarkable.[82] The figures, as originally issued, had shown 68 physicians collecting more than $200,000 per annum from Medicaid. In Maryland, after a "nolo" plea, six physicians and a dental intern were put on probation and returned $68,000 to the state, a sum that had been illegally billed to Medicaid. In the recorded figures, the highest payment to a physician in Michigan proved to be $169,000, while three osteopathic physicians were alleged to have filed over $800,000 in claims.

In Kentucky, ten physicians received more than $50,000 each; the highest payment to a physician in Illinois was $110,806; and Kansas reported cases of revoking licenses and banning participation for fraud.[83] It emerged that, in 1968, at least 1329 MDs received more than $25,000 and 290 received more than $50,000 from Title XIX, while over 7000 received more than $25,000 from Medicare.[84] Yet even these figures were incomplete and later had to be revised upwards.[85]

There was further agitation when, later in 1970, the Treasury Department claimed that one third of the physicians with large payments under Medicaid had cheated in their tax returns. The evidence presented by the Treasury Department to the Senate Finance Committee showed that some 4000 of those 11,000 physicians who had earned more than $25,000 from Medicare and Medicaid in 1968 had failed to report all or most of it. In some cases the unreported income exceeded $100,000.[86] It was reported that Bernard Cornfeld's ill-fated I.O.S. Empire was the recipient of much "hot" money paid to physicians under Titles XVIII and XIX.

In the meantime administrative controls on physician fees were developing. On April 15, 1969, Undersecretary Veneman announced that as of July 1, 1969, physician and dentist payment schedules would be set for Medicaid. In June (one week after the announcement by Senator Long that the names of physicians earning $25,000 or more under Medicaid in 1968 would be turned over to the Internal Revenue Service) HEW officials revealed that payment schedules would be based on the lowest Blue Shield payment plans.[87] Fees would thus be deliberately fixed on a lower scale than those for Medicare, which were actually higher than the average Blue Shield fees.[88] This announcement, which came as a shock both to physicians and to those who still hoped to see Medicaid with a reimbursement program tied to full private fees, was followed by a statement from HEW Secretary Robert Finch in June 1969 that payments to physicians would indeed be limited. Also to be eliminated from both Medicaid and Medicare was the 2 percent "cost-plus" beyond identified costs, a payment which had been allowed to nonprofit hospitals and nursing homes, and a similar 1½ percent cost-plus factor which had been granted to proprietary institutions.[89]

Following a series of discussions in HEW and with professional organizations, the interim regulations for physicians and other individual practitioners appeared in July 1969.[90] The link to Blue Shield was dropped. Instead the regulations limited Medicaid fees to 75 percent of physicians' customary charges in January 1969. Subsequent increases would be tied to changes in the Consumer Price Index or in an alternative index developed by the Secretary. Moreover, before increases were to be allowed there had to be evidence that the state and the profession concerned had established an effective utilization and quality-control system, including provision for disqualifying practitioners found to have defrauded, overutilized, or otherwise abused the program. These regulations thus froze physician fees at a given level (although administratively that level was difficult to define), providing for each physician a kind of personalized fee schedule. With the new regulations two levels of payment were recognized, one for Medicare and one for Medicaid, with lower fees for the latter.

For the elderly persons who were entitled to Medicare, but part of whose medical bills were picked up under Medicaid, the situation was anomalous. On the one hand they possessed recognized rights to medical care in the private sector; on the other, they were once more "welfare" patients with physicians donating to them at least one fourth of their normal fee. Physicians themselves responded in different ways. The announcement of the regulations coincided with the withdrawal of the nomination of Dr. John Knowles as Assistant Secretary of HEW, a move widely heralded as a victory for the AMA, but one which cost the Association dearly in terms of further political leverage. Protesting the price-fixing move, the AMA questioned whether HEW had the authority to set up nationally applicable regulations.[91] But meanwhile the AMA itself urged local medical groups to establish effective control mechanisms to review services and fees, a requirement for future fee increases.[92] Peer review was also made the central topic of the AMA Clinical Convention in December 1969 and led to AMA endorsement in 1970 of so-called peer-review organizations as an integral part of national financing schemes.

Although it was increasingly accepted that the freezing of fees and changes in utilization procedures in 1969 had taken care of the worst abuse problem, the physicians' public image had plummeted. The president of the New Haven County Medical Society (Dr. Charles Verstandig) warned members "We've got to quit strangling the goose that can lay those golden eggs. . . . The temptation to get rich while the getting's good is powerful. . . . A lot of our group have payments to make on their apartment house complexes, their shopping centers, their outside business interests. . . . You can't blame the average patient for thinking that we doctors are living much too high on the hog."[93] That the problem has survived is reflected in the frankly mercenary approach to Medicaid on the part of some professionals.[94] But the main action appeared to have shifted to the government's right to police the quality of care in Medicaid and other programs of governmental health care. In July 1969, the AMA had passed a resolution opposing any governmental auditing of quality of care in favor of professional peer review. Significantly it was to be another member of the Senate Finance Committee, Senator Wallace Bennett of Utah, who was to emerge in the summer of 1970 as the champion of stringent procedures for peer review—more stringent, indeed, than the profession was willing to concede.[95] By then, it was clear that federal review of fees, in one form or another, had come to stay.

Recipients

Fraud on Medicaid is not limited to providers. There have been well-documented frauds among recipients ranging through the usual frauds associated with any means-test program to examples of impersonation and "doctor shopping."[96] But a study from the New York City audit program concluded: "In comparison to the abuse emanating from providers of care, we estimate the dollar cost of patient abuse to be relatively negligible." Indeed, the interim McNerney Report, in its effort to provide a method "for determining eligibility" that would "be simple and fast and . . . preserve dignity and self-respect of applicant" came down in favor of the declaration system in place of the formal investigating means test.[97]

If anything, the recipient problem has been not waste, but underutilization. Unfortunately, getting Medicaid has not always been as easy as it might have been. It will be remembered that, in New York, Governor Rockefeller justified the apparently generous eligibility level on the ground that he was expecting only 20 to 25 percent of those eligible to sign up, an expectation which was largely fulfilled. Connecticut claimed to have handled its sign-up program more vigorously. Indeed, State Welfare Commissioner Bernard Shapiro explained the discrepancy between his claim that Title XIX would cost the state no more than existing vendor payment programs and the $15 million deficit at the end of 1967 in terms of the widespread publicity.[98] But the HEW evaluation report made at the end of 1967 still found that the state did not provide adequate arrangements for emergency eligibility services and that "the agency has been taking far too long to determine eligibility."[99]

The difficulty of obtaining Medicaid care became proverbial in New York, but there were other weaknesses in the system. In some states it was never entirely clear who was eligible for Medicaid. And if potential recipients failed to understand whether they might be eligible, this was no more than the reflection of the confusion felt by many welfare departments about the categories of eligibility under Title XIX. As suggested earlier, out of the patchwork of the 1965 and 1967 laws a series of courageous glossators developed categories of persons who might be covered. But decisions made in the state capital do not always filter down to the local welfare departments or individual social workers. For instance, the Title XIX informational pamphlet issued in July 1969 and entitled *Medical Care for People in Connecticut* classified as a category "Parents or other relatives with whom a child under 21 years of age is living with sufficient income or resources to meet their general living expenses but not enough to meet the cost of medical care." But spot checks during 1970 showed that caseworkers in Connecticut (including those working in the hospitals) had advised their clients that this was not a category of "medical indigence" in Connecticut, except for those under 21.[100]

Moreover, as welfare or near-welfare recipients, Medicaid patients were often treated as social dependents rather than "consumers," even in the thick of the consumer movement. Not only did recipients frequently find it humiliating trying to get on Medicaid, they often faced humiliation when they had a complaint about the program, or there was some doubt about their continued eligibility. Grievances come in various shapes, and complaints may be handled in a number of ways, formal or informal. But the refusal or termination of some federally assisted welfare programs (including for this purpose Medicaid) requires the state to hold a quasijudicial "fair hearing" to determine the issue. Thus, in all states the so-called fair-hearing procedures under Title XIX are handled by the Welfare Department. At least until the welfare rights pressures culminated in *Goldberg v. Kelly*,[101] the departments were often lax about ensuring "due process." Moreover, MSA with its inadequate staff was scarcely in a position to press for more affirmative action in the states, even had it been so minded. The result has been that for much of the history of Medicaid there has been relatively little emphasis on "fair hearings."[102] Regulation of recipients has thus largely been repressive rather than protective.

In a detailed study of the Connecticut fair-hearings procedures within Medicaid, a relatively unsympathetic observer conceded that in terms of the existing system the procedure was not working particularly badly.[103] Yet, problems there were; and some sense of these emerged in the Circuit Court case of *Peters v. Shapiro*.[104] In that case, Peters, who was blind, sought to have a tooth removed from his lower jaw and to have a tooth added to his bridge, because, under his existing arrangements, he had to take a painkiller whenever he had a hot or cold drink. His "prior authorization" was denied because the dental consultant decided that the man had enough teeth. On the strength of this advice, and also a social worker's argument that the Welfare Department did not provide partial denture work, in a "fair hearing" procedure his appeal against the decision was denied.

On appeal to the regular courts, Judge Jacobs sent the case back, holding that:

> *The hearing officer accepted the staff report as gospel. His function was nothing more than "signing on the dotted line." The law requires proof by evidence, not by staff memoranda. There must be a responsible finding. There was no such finding here.*[105]

Judge Jacobs did not find that all the rules of evidence had to apply in fair hearings, since one of the functions of such hearings was the exchange of information (by implication a sad reflection on the effects of the adversary procedure), but he did criticize the fact that the dental consultant did not appear at the hearing and had never seen the patient. Some logically probative evidence was necessary.[106]

In a parallel study of fair hearings in New York City,[107] the criticisms were appreciably more extensive. There was an even larger social and psychological gap noted between the complaints officers and the complaining recipients than was the Connecticut pattern, and hearing officers were thought to be more subservient to the welfare establishment. Moreover, delays in holding "fair hearings" were far more extensive. While, in theory, fair hearings were supposed to be held within 30 days, they frequently dragged on for months. Nothing could have underlined more graphically that, at least to the states, Medicaid was but another welfare program.[108]

The social difference between Medicaid's beneficiaries—providers and recipients—was underscored by studies such as these. Mr. Peters continued to swallow painkillers, while physician reimbursements in the thousands of dollars were being publicized in the national press. From the recipients' as well as the providers' points of view, some of the disparity in regulation was, however, about to be recognized. The studies of "fair hearings" mentioned above were undertaken in 1969, before the Supreme Court decision in *Goldberg v. Kelly* in March 1970.[109] In this appeal from New York, the Court held that procedural due process required an evidential hearing before public assistance payments were terminated, and this was held automatically to apply to Medicaid. The decision also gave recipients the right to confront officials who finally determined eligibility, either with or without a lawyer. The decision clearly had a profound impact on the form of the law, and, as far as can be discovered, on its substance also.[110] Less tangibly, some support was given to the position of the recipients as being that of a client in a given social contract, rather than merely a supplicant. It was not entirely fortuitous that redefinition of the recipients' rights coincided with redefinition (limitation) of those of the providers.

Variation or Discrimination

Recipients, however, could scarcely attest to the success of Medicaid as "mainstream" medicine. The potential recipient was faced with a humiliating and complex means test, confusing or inadequate advice, and frequently, problems in resolving grievances. He was also faced with gradually receding eligibility levels, providers disgruntled about reimbursement levels, and marked differences in entitlement and services among the states. In 1968 New York State spent $63.95 per inhabitant while 21 other states spent less than $10 per inhabitant.[111] The year before it had been estimated that potential coverage ranged from 45 percent of the population in New York to 7 percent in Massachusetts, with actual utilization ranging from a high of 11 percent in New York to less than 3 percent in North Dakota.[112]

Recipients might well be thought to be discriminated against by the variation of services available to them in the different states. As we have seen, at least for the "categorically needy," state programs had to provide seven basic services by July 1970 (the original five mandated in the 1965 legislation, plus two added by the 1967 Amendments); but beyond that, states had great latitude.[113] In 1970, 23 states[114] offered no program to the "medically indigent." Mississippi provided no services other than the required ones to the groups compulsorily covered, while Wyoming offered only transportation by way of such additional service. New Mexico, on the other hand, although having no program for the "medically indigent" category, offered to welfare recipients home health services, drugs, dental services, eyeglasses, hearing aids, prosthetic devices, physical therapy, private duty nursing, optometrists' services, podiatrists' services, chiropractic services, clinic services, transportation, and other diagnostic services. At the other end of the scale, California, Connecticut, Minnesota, New York, and North Dakota offered every additional service for which a federal contribution was available to those covered by the categorically related programs.[115] For the "medically indigent" as a whole, the differences were even greater and more erratic. The views of one aging Vermont recipient could be echoed in many states: "Your program isn't much good if you can't help me when my eyes get so bad I can't see and my teeth get so bad I can't chew."[116] It was arguable that the level of medical care in the United States had become more uneven rather than less so in the years after 1965.

Even excluding the issue of different services in different states, there was still the problem recipients might find in attempting to obtain the services to which they were entitled. The professional press was full of examples of appeals to providers to cut back on Title XIX services. For instance, the AMA News for April 21, 1969, reported an appeal by the Kansas authorities to physicians to use restraint in hospitalizing Medicaid patients and a warning by the Governor of Virginia on the dangers of the overuse of Medicaid services. This virtually insured that a Medicaid recipient would be in a different position from a private patient the moment he entered a physician's office.

But recipients sometimes just found that providers refused to join the Medicaid program at all. New York City's problems in encouraging providers to participate and the latter's resort to boycotts have already been chronicled, as have the boycotts by dentists in Connecticut;[117] in October 1970, there was a boycott by skilled nursing homes in Massachusetts. But perhaps the most sordid boycott of all was in the nation's capital—the hospitals' boycott of the D.C. Medicaid program. As the result of a dispute about payment of outpatient services, only two of the city's ten hospitals agreed to cooperate with the program because the D.C. administration proposed paying only 80 percent of the face value of bills.[118] For a year the burden on the few hospitals which were cooperating was virtually intolerable.[119] Although the program had begun in the summer of 1968, it was not until the summer of 1969 that a compromise was finally worked out,[120] and

Medicaid became generally available in Washington hospitals.[121] Reimbursement levels had become the nexus of the whole program.

Perhaps more frequent were the situations where providers were evasive. This appears to have been the situation after Connecticut reverted to a fee schedule for physicians, following the 12-month experiment with usual and customary fees, in March 1969. The medical profession was not well pleased with the change. The *AMA News* finally announced: "Medicaid Killed in Connecticut."[122] Apparently during the year when customary fees applied, 3000 out of a possible 4500 physicians took part in the program. After the fee schedule was reintroduced, these reports suggested that only about 1000 doctors took part. And the reports would seem to be borne out by studies made in the New Haven area early in 1970. A spot check of 15 physicians who were paid more than $2500 in 1968 from Medicaid funds resulted in 8 responses (3 specialists, 5 general practitioners), all of whom had become more restrictive in accepting Medicaid patients after March 1969. In a more general (although not statistically reliable) survey, it was estimated that 58 percent of practitioners in the New Haven area were willing to take some Medicaid patients.[123] Thus, to the geographical and social problems[124] involved in reaching some physicians had been added a noticeable reluctance to treat Medicaid patients on the part of many providers.

It would be wrong, however, not to emphasize the many successes of Medicaid from the recipients' point of view. It was during this period that the Columbia University study on the "Effect of Medicaid on Health Care of Low-Income Persons" was conducted. On the one hand, the study confirmed many of the failings of the program. That many of the eligible were ignorant of Medicaid was also more than confirmed by the study. While 55.9 percent of persons on public assistance knew they were entitled to Medicaid, or at least that they were entitled to free medical services, only 29 percent of those persons who were entitled to Medicaid as "medically indigent" in their particular states knew of the Medicaid program.[125] Much more important, however, in terms of the findings, was that those who were on Medicaid showed a somewhat greater willingness to use preventive services and to seek medical help when they were ill than the low-income population at large. Perhaps most important of all, those who were eligible for Medicaid were likely to have better health than similar groups who were not.

Unfortunately, as we have seen, the economic cost of all of this had been high largely because Medicaid was provided through an unreconstructed, predominantly private system of medical care delivery. By the summer of 1969, Dr. Roger Egeberg, the Undersecretary of Health, was reported as saying that it had been a mistake even to talk of providing "mainstream" medicine for the poor.[126] At least some of the providers might have agreed, as the end result of the "mainstream" approach appeared to be public criticism and the increasing threat of governmental regulation.

NOTES

1. U.S., Congress, Senate, Staff of Senate Committee on Finance, *Staff Data Relating to Medicaid-Medicare Study*, Committee Print, U.S. Congress, Committee on Finance, 91st Cong., 1st Sess., 1969.

2. In 1965 vendor payments represented 32 percent of state and local welfare costs and 25 percent of federal welfare costs. By 1968 these proportions had risen to 46 percent and 41 percent, respectively. *Ibid.*, p. 9.

3. U.S., Department of Health, Education, and Welfare, *National Health Expenditures Data* (Washington, 1973), p. 57.

4. *Staff Data Relating to Medicaid-Medicare Study, supra*, note 1, p. 34.

5. Robert Myers, *Medicare* (Bryn Mawr, 1970), pp. 282–285.

6. U.S. Department of Health, Education, and Welfare, Social and Rehabilitation Service, *Public Assistance Statistics December 1969*, Table 13 (NCSS Report A-2, 1969).

7. *1967 Hearings*, at 275–76.

8. U.S., Congress, Senate, Committee on Finance, *Medicare and Medicaid, Hearings*, before the Committee on Finance, 91st Cong., 1st Sess., 1969, pp. 6–7.

9. The actuarial estimate of 1970 costs for Medicare Part A made in 1965 was $3.1 billion; the 1970 estimate was $5.8 billion. The federal share of Part B costs rose from $623 million in fiscal year 1967 to an estimated $1245 million in fiscal year 1971, with equal matching from the personal contributions of the elderly. *1970 Staff Report Relating to Medicaid-Medicare Study, supra*, note 1, pp. 3–4.

10. U.S. Department of Health, Education, and Welfare, Social Security Administration, *Research and Statistics Note* (Nov. 7, 1969).

11. U.S., Senate, Finance Committee, *Medicare and Medicaid: Problems, Issues and Alternatives*, Staff Report, 1970, p. vii.

12. On the general role of insurance in stimulating demand, see Martin Feldstein, *The Rising Costs of Hospital Care* (New York, 1971).

13. *Medicare and Medicaid: Problems, Issues and Alternatives, supra*, note 11, pp. 3–4.

14. See Rosemary Stevens, *American Medicine and the Public Interest*, New Haven, 1971, Chapter 19.

15. *Medicare and Medicaid: Problems, Issues and Alternatives, supra*, note 11, p. 294.

16. The initial results of a study undertaken during this period by the University of Pittsburgh School of Public Health suggested that hospital administrators were happy with Medicaid. University of Pittsburgh, *Progress Report: A Study of Health Care for the Poor*, mimeograph, July 1970.

17. *National Health Expenditures Data, supra*, note 3, p. 46.

18. *Ibid.*, p. 73. $4.9 billion was accounted for by Medicare, $2.4 billion by Medicaid.

19. See, e.g., U.S. Senate, Committee on Finance, *Social Security Administration, 1967,* Report No. 404, to accompany H.R. 12080, 90th Cong., 1st Sess., 1967, p. 47.

20. Social Security Act, as amended, Sec. 1861 (e) (b).

21. Connecticut was unusual in its use of a State Hospital Cost Commission (HCC) to establish rates for reimbursing the hospitals. The Commission has had a long history in Connecticut, having been established in 1949. N. Gellman, *Hospital Reimbursement Under Medicaid in Connecticut,* 1970 (paper presented at the Yale Law School), 12 *et seq.* Its tradition was so strong that for the first few years of Medicaid it refused to apply the Title XIX formula for reimbursement and actually paid hospitals at a lower rate, a fact which clearly surprised federal officials when Connecticut was given its first PREP at the end of 1967. HEW, *Connecticut Title XIX Medicaid PREP Review,* November–December, 1967. The 1967 Connecticut Legislature passed an act to allow appeals from the HCC to the regular courts and under that legislation a number of hospitals brought a successful action against the HCC, the Commission being found to have abused its discretion. The Commission was ordered by the Superior Court to reconsider its rates in accordance with the mandate of the statute. It refused! The 1969 legislature abolished appeals from the HCC to the courts, substituting binding arbitration. On this and related matters, see Gellman, *supra,* pp. 16–19. Eventually HEW had to threaten to cut off federal money to Connecticut unless it conformed to federal law. Connecticut then resorted to litigation, arguing that 45 C.F.R. §250.30, implementing this Medicaid provision, was "unreasonable." *Connecticut State Department of Public Welfare v. HEW,* 448 F.2d 209 (2d Cir., 1971). The court summarily upheld HEW's position without answering the "unreasonableness" argument.

22. The total cost of hospital care was reported in 1966–67 as $16.8 billion and nursing home care as $1.7 billion. Hospital care rose to $22.5 billion and nursing home expenditures rose to $2.4 billion in 1968–69. These figures refer to expenditures in all institutions, paid from both private and public funds. *National Health Expenditures Data, supra,* note 3, p. 46.

23. A study by the Social Security Administration of the $2.1 billion increase in hospital expenditures for the elderly between fiscal years 1966 and 1968 estimated that 61% of the increase was the result of price changes and another 7% could be attributed to population increases. This left only 32% of the increases for changes in the provision of services. Similar cost rises could be observed for the non-elderly population. *Ibid.*

24. Pub. L. No. 86–97 §1902(a)(13)(B), 79 Stat. 345 (1965).

25. The reasonable cost regulations were introduced in May 1966 as Principles of Reimbursement for Provider Costs. These were adopted by the Social and Rehabilitation Service (SRS) in January 1969 as the standard for hospital reimbursement under Title XIX. The object of the principles was that the public program would pay all allowable costs with respect to an individual patient, while no part of the individual's allowable cost was subsidized by or was subsidizing others.

Methods of apportioning allowable costs under the Medicare regulations included (1) Departmental Method—Ratio of Charges to Costs (e.g., if some percent of a hospital's x-ray charges was for services used by Medicare patients, Medicare paid that percentage of the total allowable costs of the department); and (2) Combination Method, which included the hospital's average daily charge for routine inpatient services, together with appropriate apportionment of charges for special services such as x-ray, laboratory, and operating room.

Besides these two methods, a third and simpler formula was developed by SRS for Medicaid—Gross Ratio of Hospital Cost to Hospital Charges. Under this, the total allowable annual inpatient cost of operating a hospital was divided by the total annual charges for inpatients. The resultant percentage was applied to the bill of each inpatient covered by Medicaid. Following discussions between SRS and SSA (the administrator of Medicare), it was agreed to limit the third method to hospitals not participating in Title XVIII. All formulas were for the determination of interim payments, with final settlement subject to audit. Hospitals were also reimbursed an additional 2 percent of allowable costs for depreciation and other overhead; this was abolished in 1969. See "Reasonable Cost of Inpatient Hospital Services," *CCH Medicare & Medicaid Guide,* par. 14,725; Tierney, *Incentives and Hospital Cost Reimbursement,* Titles XVIII and XIX, Nov. 2, 1967 (paper presented to the Secretary's Advisory Committee on Hospital Effectiveness, Washington, D.C.).

26. Because of the administrative division of Medicare and Medicaid exact figures are hard to obtain. An estimated 2.9 million persons 65 years of age and over received medical assistance (but not all in hospitals) through federally aided programs in fiscal year 1969. *Social Security Bulletin,* Dec. 1969, p. 77.

27. U.S. Department of Health, Education, and Welfare, Social Security Administration, *Research and Statistics Note* (June 18, 1970).

28. In 1969, according to HEW figures, care for those 65 years and over in hospitals accounted for 27 percent of Medicaid vendor payments; and 60 percent of this went to state mental institutions.

29. Of the total of 18,910 nursing care and related homes in the United States in 1969, 14,470 were so-called proprietary institutions. National Center for Health Statistics, *Health Resources Statistics,* 1971, p. 327. Connecticut provides an example of the building expansion: the number of beds in nursing homes rose from 7,725 in 1961 to 11,284 in 1966 and to 14,305 in 1970; and applications for another 900 beds had been approved by the state Hill-Burton agency. This expansion caused the Connecticut legislature to put controls on further construction. Effective July 1, 1970, nursing home construction in the state became conditional upon the issuance of a "certificate of need" by the State Department of Health. The rapid expansion, however, was probably already over. B. Sullivan, *A Patient Origin Study of Connecticut Nursing Home Residents,* 1970 (essay presented to the Yale University Medical School, in candidacy for the degree of Master of Public Health).

30. Federal matching funds were available for skilled nursing home care under Medicaid. In addition the 1967 Amendments had added a new classification of "Intermediate Care Facility" to provide a lower-cost alternative to skilled care, under the same federal matching formula as for Medicaid. The aim was to remove appropriate patients out of the more expensive bed into the cheaper, thus leading to reduced over-all costs.

31. *Medicare and Medicaid, Hearings, supra,* note 8, p. 161.

32. *Medicare and Medicaid: Problems, Issues and Alternatives, supra,* note 11, p. 146.

33. *Ibid.,* p. 136.

34. *Ibid.,* p. 209.

35. *Ibid.,* p. 216.

36. The new regulations were issued in 14 *Federal Register* 3745 (1969).

37. Pub. L. 89–97 :1902 (a) (19), 79 Stat. 347 (1956).

38. U.S. Department of Health, Education, and Welfare, Welfare Administration, Bureau of Family Services, *Medical Assistance Program and Title XIX of the Social Security Act, Supplement D.*, par. D–5320.

39. Effective July 1, 1970, the upper limits for payment for skilled nursing home services, outpatient hospital services, and clinic services are "customary charges which are reasonable." Fee schedules are acceptable provided they fall within the reasonable charges established by Medicare. CCH *Medicare & Medicaid Guide,* par. 14,723. For later developments see "Nursing Home Guidelines for Reimbursement," *ibid,* par. 14,723.82.

40. In Connecticut, skilled nursing homes were reimbursed a maximum of $10.50 a day under Title XIX in fiscal year 1967, and between $15.00 and $16.00 a day in fiscal year 1970—a 50 percent increase. Personal communication from Connecticut State Department of Welfare.

41. State of Vermont Department of Social Welfare, *Social Welfare in Vermont,* Biennial Report, 1968–1970, pp. 16–17.

42. Connecticut State Department of Welfare, personal communication.

43. Cf. John Gardner, *No Easy Victories,* New York (1968), Chapter 10.

44. *Supplement D., supra,* note 38, par. D-5340.

45. The two thirds participation ratio was to be separately determined for each profession and for specialties within a profession. *Ibid.,* par. D–5330.

46. The common pattern prior to Title XIX was payment of welfare patients' physicians according to negotiated fee schedules. Personal communication, Social and Rehabilitation Service.

47. *AMA News,* Jan. 13, 1969.

48. Tax Foundation, Inc., *Medicaid: State Programs After Two Years* (New York, 1968), p. 42.

49. U.S. Department of Health, Education, and Welfare, Social and Rehabilitation Services, *Medicaid, Fiscal Year 1969,* 1970, Table 1.

50. U.S., Congress, Senate, Committee on Finance, *Hearings on H.R. 12580* before the Senate Comm. on Finance, 86th Cong., 2d Sess., (1960), pp. 203, 206.

51. "Physicians have a far better record than hospitals in keeping the price of their services within bounds. In the past 25 years, physicians' fees have risen only 100 percent while the over-all cost of living has increased 115 percent." Quote from Dr. Donovan F. Ward, President, American Medical Association, U.S., Congress, Senate, Committee on Finance, *Social Security, Hearings,* before the Committee on Finance, Senate, on H.R. 6675, 89th Cong., 1st Sess., 1965, pp. 602–612.

52. In Alabama, for instance, the *AMA News* announced in July 1967 that, "The medical profession in Alabama has been given control of the state's future Title 19 (Medicaid) program by an executive order by Governor Lurlene B. Wallace." This claim was justified, it was reported, because administration of Title XIX was to be given to the state health department, which is governed by the State Board of Public Health, "which has the same composition in Alabama as the state medical association's board of censors." The *AMA News* noted, with its customary concept of political objectivity, that "by making the Alabama Title 19 program a responsibility of the health department, the program will be completely removed from politics." The Medical Association of Alabama also noted: "The physicians of Alabama respectfully remind you that we have always given freely of our time and talents for the needy. We desire and expect to continue

to contribute our time and efforts, and we believe that we can best serve our patients without third-party interference." *AMA News,* July 10. 1967.

53. *AMA News,* Nov. 13, 1967. This endorsement was crucial. See *Richmond Times-Dispatch,* Sept. 12, 1967.

54. *Medicare and Medicaid Hearings, supra,* note 8, p. 158.

55. Acton W. Barnes, *A Description of the Organization and Administration of the California Medical Assistance Program: Title XIX,* mimeograph, School of Public Health, University of North Carolina, 1968, p. 108 *et seq.*

56. *AMA News,* Dec. 9, 1968.

57. *AMA News,* April 1, 1968.

58. *Hearings . . .* on HR 12580, *supra,* note 69, pp. 203, 206.

59. Orvan Hess, "The President's Page," *Connecticut Medicine,* vol. 30 (1966), p. 503.

60. See Kate Clair Freeland, *Medicaid in Connecticut: The First Year* (paper presented at the Yale Law School), p. 8 and *passim.*

61. *New Haven Register,* Jan. 20, 1969, p. 1, col. 1.

62. T. Mitchell, *Physician Participation in Medicaid in New Haven, Conn.* (paper presented at the Yale Law School), 1970.

63. For a study of the politics of this, see R. Gomes, *The American Dental Association and the Connecticut State Dental Association Policies Regarding Participation in the Medicaid Program, 1970* (paper presented at the Yale Medical School).

64. For implementation of the 1969 changes see State Letter No. 1063, Medical Services Administration, Social and Rehabilitation Service, March 13, 1969; U.S., Department of Health, Education, and Welfare, Medical Services Administration, *Some Implications of the Interim Policy Published 1 July 1969 of Reimbursement of Individual Practitioners by State Under Title XIX of the Social Security Act (July 10, 1969).*

65. The sport is not necessarily a new one: "For gold in phisik is a cordial / Therefore be lovede gold in special," Chaucer, *Canterbury Tales, Prolog,* the Doctor of Phisik.

66. U.S., Congress, Senate, Committee on Government Operations, Sub-Committee on Executive Reorganization, *Health Care in America, Hearings before the Sub-Committee on Executive Reorganization,* Committee on Government Operations, 90th Cong., 2d Sess., 1968, pp. 502, 515.

67. *Medicare and Medicaid, Hearings, supra,* note 8, pp. 1–2.

68. *Ibid.,* p. 61.

69. *Ibid.,* p. 92.

70. *Ibid.,* pp. 142–144.

71. *AMA News,* Feb. 17, 1969.

72. *Rocky Mountain News,* Feb. 18, 1969 (Denver).

73. E.g., *Press Herald,* May 16, 1969 (Portland, Me.).

74. *AMA News,* July 21, 1969.

75. *Ibid.,* March 10, 1969.

76. *Ibid.,* March 17, 1969.

77. *Ibid.,* April 7, 1969.

78. *Ibid.,* April 12, 1969.

79. *Ibid.*, April 21, 1969, and May 26, 1969. Similar legislation was also proposed in Massachusetts. *Ibid.*, April 29, 1969.

80. *Ibid.*, June 30, 1969. See also *Medicare and Medicaid Hearings, supra,* note 8, p. 92 *et seq*. Rather colorfully, the Finance Committee observed the assignment of identification numbers under Medicare (one physician sometimes having more than one number) as "comparable to Swiss bank accounts." *Staff Data, supra,* note 1, p. 38. However accurate the analogy, the feeling behind it went directly to the heart of the tax watchers on the committee. The Finance Committee attached an amendment to the Tax Reform Act of 1969 (H.R. 13270) to require disclosure of such payments, but because IRS partially closed this loophole administratively, this provision was dropped by the joint committee conference following passage by the Senate. Insurance companies were thereafter required to report physician payments under Medicare to IRS, and the same requirement was made with regard to states and their fiscal agents under Medicaid.

81. *Medicare and Medicaid: Problems, Issues and Alternatives, supra,* note 11, p. 145.

82. *AMA News,* July 21, 1969.

83. *Ibid.*

84. *Medicare and Medicaid Hearings, supra,* note 8, pp. 161–162.

85. It finally emerged that, under Medicaid, solo practioners had been paid the following sums over $100,000 in 1968: California—$101,986; $121,188; $105,513; $132,975; $152,485; $101,061; $132,921; Illinois—$103,698; $104,872; $102,357; $110,806; Kentucky—$119,768; $103,255; $108,490; Michigan—$100,508; $107,758; $112,464; $112,451; $169,061; $203,402; New York—$155,134; $363,101; $356,978; $110,592; $101,604; $292,304; $113,781; $142,208; $113,146; $121,025; $115,752; $123,774; $106,618; $119,611; $151,932; Oklahoma—$100,623. *Medicare and Medicaid, supra,* note 11, pp. 163–198.

86. *New York Times,* Sept. 22, 1970, p. 1, col. 1.

87. *Washington Report on Medicine & Health,* April 14, 1969.

88. *New York Times,* June 23, 1969; *Ibid.*, April 21, 1969.

89. Congressional Quarterly Service, *Congressional Quarterly Almanac 1970* (1971), p. 204.

90. 34 *Federal Register* 11,098 (1969); CCH *Medicare & Medicaid Guide,* par. 14,723.

91. *AMA News,* August 11, 1969.

92. *AMA News,* June 30, 1969.

93. *New Haven Register,* March 28, 1969, p. 1, col. 1.

94. For example in the "Professional Practices for Sales" section of the *New York Times,* Oct. 11, 1970: "General medical practice. Tremendous Medicaid area. Gold mine. Rent or sale."

95. In an amendment to H.R. 17550 in August, 1970.

96. For an example, see *Medicare and Medicaid, supra,* note 11, p. 128. This kind of problem is avoided in the national health programs of most developed societies by requiring that beneficiaries register with one primary physician or facility. Because of the freedom of choice provision, Medicaid patients sometimes see a number of physicians in connection with the same problem.

97. *McNerney Interim Report,* pp. 1–2.

98. Address by Commissioner Shapiro to Lions Club of Hartford, Conn., in *Public Welfare Trends* (July–Sept. 1967). By that time, some 16,218 out of a possible 50,340 eligible for Medicaid as "medically indigent" had signed up.

99. *PREP Review, supra,* note 21, pp. 2, 13. The Commissioner of Welfare nevertheless reported to the Governor that the federal review of Medicaid had been favorable. State of Connecticut, Department of Welfare, *Annual Report to the Governor* 36 (1968–1969).

100. For a study of the procedures for applying for Medicaid in Connecticut and especially the risk of being refused after services have been performed, see Pinah Lahav, *The Treatment of Title XIX Patients in Health Care Facilities* (paper presented at the Yale Law School), 1970.

101. 397 U.S. 254 (1970).

102. Something is, however, known about the procedures. See, e.g., Ann E. Freedman, *Medicaid Grievance Procedures in New York City* (paper presented at the Yale Law School) 1971; Gail Falk, *Grievance Procedures for Recipients of Title XIX Medical Assistance in Connecticut During the Winter of 1969–70* (paper presented at the Yale Law School), 1971.

While the rise of the Welfare Rights Organization and *Goldberg v. Kelly* have led to a rapid rise in the number of fair hearings with respect to welfare—there was a 200 percent increase in Connecticut in one year (State of Connecticut, *Annual Report of the Commissioner of Welfare 1968–1969*, p. 26)—few fair-hearing complaints relate to Medicaid. There are various reasons. For instance, complaints about the quality of care by vendors are often handled by health rather than welfare departments, although, for rather complex psychological reasons, there seem to be few complaints registered in this category. But most important of all is the fact that the refusal or termination of any categorical assistance program automatically includes a Medicaid determination as well.

In terms of numbers, in Connecticut for instance, there were 375 fair-hearing requests between May and August, 1969 (Falk, pp. 17–19). Of these, some 56 appeared to concern Medicaid. Of the 56, 28 involved denials or discontinuance of eligibility. This figure may strike one as surprising, because, for instance, in August 1969, statewide no less than 630 of the 1336 applications for Medicaid were rejected (Falk, p. 21). Eight of the 56 requests concerned complaints by allegedly legally liable relatives (As noted earlier, Connecticut has never been able to accept fully the Title XIX prohibition against making relatives "legally liable.") More legitimately, Connecticut does investigate carefully transfers of property by potential Medicaid recipients to their children (Falk, pp. 19–20). One fair hearing involved the alleged failure to reimburse for CMS (Blue Shield) payments and one related to the payment of a hospital bill. There were also 17 complaints relating to dental problems, because a system of prior authorization was in effect for dental care. Of these 56 complaint procedures begun, some 17 were sent to a final hearing, 14 being decided in favor of the Agency and three in favor of the recipient.

103. Falk, *op. cit., passim.*

104. 5 Conn. Cir. 603; 260 A 2d 133 (Conn. 7th Cir. Ct. 1969).

105. *Ibid.*, pp. 604 and 134, respectively.

106. Falk, *supra,* note 102, pp. 18–19.

107. Freedman, *supra,* note 102.

108. Freedman, *supra,* note 102, p. 5a. In many respects, however, the statistics were surprisingly similar. While there were, at that time, far more people

receiving Medicaid than cash assistance, complaints about the former were appreciably less common than the latter, for the reasons outlined in note 102. Between October 17 and December 8, 1969, there were only 39 "fair hearings" concerning Medicaid although 793,000 persons were enrolled. This, of course, did not mean that there were not more complaints about Medicaid, but that few of these were dealt with through formal procedures. Of these 39 hearings, 35 were decided in favor of the Agency.

109. 397 U.S. 254.

110. In 1971 a new regulation concerning fair hearings was issued, designed to protect the individual who was a recipient or potential recipient. 45 CFR 205–10; *Federal Register*, vol. 36, February 13, 1971 pp. 3034–3035. In particular, those who were denied some request had to be informed in detail about their rights, including the right to be represented (by a lawyer or another) at the hearing. There was to be a heavy emphasis on speed of the hearing and in case of termination, reduction, or suspension, 15 days advance notice of the action had to be given. Perhaps most important of all, if the recipient requested a hearing during the advance notice period, then, "unless the State agency determines that the issue is not one of fact or judgment," assistance was to be continued until the hearing had been settled. (On what amounts to "fact or judgment" see *Medical Assistance Manual*, 6–30–20 G. At least some federal judges seemed willing to extend this protection. See the report of the decision of Judge Clairie in *Porta v. White*, *New Haven Register*, June 7, 1972.) There were also provisions for a second medical opinion where authorization for some procedure had been denied and an attempt to make the proceedings somewhat more independent of the local bureaucracy.

111. U.S., Department of Health, Education, and Welfare, Social and Rehabilitation Service, National Center for Social Statistics, *Medicaid: Selected Statistics, 1951–1969*, (1970) p. 59.

112. Puerto Rico, which presents special problems, is excluded.

113. The seven basic services required by July 1970 were: inpatient hospital care, outpatient hospital services, other laboratory or x-ray services, skilled nursing home services for those over 21, screening and treatment for those under 21, physician services, and home health services.

114. Alabama, Arkansas, Colorado, Florida, Georgia, Indiana, Iowa, Louisiana, Maine, Mississippi, Missouri, Montana, Nevada, New Jersey, New Mexico, Ohio, Oregon, South Carolina, South Dakota, Tennessee, Texas, West Virginia, and Wyoming.

115. CCH *Medicare & Medicaid Guide*, par. 15,504.

116. *Social Welfare in Vermont, supra*, note 41, pp. 18–19.

117. *PREP Review, supra*, note 21, p. 5.

118. *AMA News*, Oct. 21, 1968; *Ibid.*, Sept. 2, 1968. See also *Ibid.*, Nov. 18, 1968.

119. Neighborhood Legal Services Program, Washington, D.C., *Medicaid in the District of Columbia*, mimeograph, 1969.

120. *AMA News*, April 14, 1969.

121. For a critique of the services of Medicaid in Washington in October 1969, see Testimony of Margaret Ewing of Neighborhood Legal Services Program before the D.C. Council's Committee on Health and Welfare (Oct. 27, 1969). See also U. of Pennsylvania and UCLA, *Materials on Health Law*, vol. 5, *Medicaid*, 1971 edition, p. 228 et seq.

122. *AMA News,* Dec. 14, 1969.

123. Mitchell, *supra,* note 62, p. 10.

124. For a description of some of these psychological barriers, see Lahav, *supra,* note 100, pp. 6–8.

125. Columbia University, School of Public Health and Administrative Medicine. *Effect of Medicaid on Health Care of Low-Income Persons,* mimeograph, no date, Chap. 6. Some of the variation in knowledge of the program may be related to the remarkable differences in the coverage of the programs from state to state. The Columbia study looked at the nine largest states in 1969. Of the four sample groups it surveyed, it found 14.8 percent eligible in New York, 7.4 percent in California, 5.2 percent in Pennsylvania, 5.0 percent in Illinois, 3.4 percent in Michigan, and 2.9 percent in Massachusetts. All these states covered both the categorically needy and the medically needy. In Ohio and Texas, which covered only the categorically needy, the percentages were 4.3 and 7.0 respectively. *Ibid.*, Chapter 11. New Jersey had no Medicaid program at that time.

126. *AMA News,* July 21, 1969.

11
Reassessments

The growing criticism of the providers of medical care was a tacit acceptance of the limitations of the initial concept of vendor payments. By mid-1970, it was only too clear that comprehensive health services to the needy could not be provided under Medicaid without massive costs, a substantial part of which would go to enrich the providers. States were not willing or able to accept such costs; indeed, their budgets were already overstrained. Their resulting activities had been in two directions: limitations on recipients (and, when possible, on services to recipients) and restrictions on vendor reimbursement rates. But this meant, in turn, a return to a much more limited philosophy of "welfare medicine" than had been implicit in the 1965 legislation.

Although the inability of the states to control expenditures had thrust cost questions into the center of concern at the national level, the nature and desired extent of "welfare medicine" was due for reassessment. The 1967 and 1969 Amendments had allowed more flexibility in the states; but at the same time a stronger federal regulatory role was indicated, affecting both providers and the states. By mid-1970, more general national questions were also evident. These ranged from whether Medicaid should be federalized, in terms of both funding and eligibility levels, to proposals to restructure the health and welfare systems.

Role of the Senate Finance Committee

It would be misleading to suggest that the variety of debates on questions affecting Medicaid were coordinated or cohesive: quite the opposite. There was still no organizational focus for debates on health and welfare programs, either in Congress or in HEW. As in earlier debates, different groups and committees tackled different issues, with greater or lesser enthusiasm: the welfare reformers ignoring health services, the health reformers specializing in relatively small areas or issues. Policies were made, but there was no one policy for the provision of health care under which Medicaid's peculiar dilemmas could be assessed. This absence had two immediate results. Proposed solutions tended to deal with parts rather than the whole, and decision-making was disseminated.

The growing importance of the Senate Finance Committee was a direct result of this lacuna in policy-making. In the absence of stated goals for health and welfare in Congress, Medicaid policy continued to be made in response to demands for cost controls. Senator Long articulated the basic goals. Medical care provided under Medicare and Medicaid, he emphasized, should be of high quality, "but we think it should be provided on the basis that is efficient and economical, not on a basis which is wasteful and extravagant."[1]

One result of this emphasis on controls was, however, that the Medicaid program was in constant danger of having the argument of costs used not to provide services more efficiently, but rather to cut down the provision of services to those who needed them the most. The approach protected taxpayers rather than recipients. While the courts were seeking to define basic entitlements under Medicaid, the legislature appeared to be moving away from protection in pursuit of the goals of administrative efficiency and fiscal restraint. Yet, merely to issue a series of requirements for monitoring and reporting fraud or for collecting information evaded the issue of what, indeed, should be Medicaid's goals. It was the implication of quite another message, namely that Medicaid should be federally organized as a health program rather than an economy drive, that formed the primary theme of the report of the HEW (McNerney) Task Force on Medicaid.[2] Indeed, as will be seen, the Task Force went much further, arguing that the very structure of health services needed to be reformed and that Medicaid should, with other federal programs, play a deliberate part in initiating structural change through providing funds for stimulating new local systems of health care delivery. This argument raised very different implications for administration from those raised by the primary pursuit of cost controls.

The situation was further complicated by the lack of a developing set of policies and goals from HEW within the framework of existing legislation. Administration had not been Medicaid's strong point, at least up to the summer of 1970. Medicaid appeared to have no core. With the accelerating costs and the apparent lack of dynamism, courage, power, or authorization in HEW to take firm control of the program—even to the extent of publicizing standards and detailed critiques of the programs in the states—concern about shortcomings in management grew in the Congress. The Senate Finance Committee, in particular, became a powerful substitute for a board of directors for Medicare and Medicaid. Indeed, the staff of that committee did much of the ferreting out of information that was lacking throughout the administrative hierarchy. By default, then, the committee was involved both in policy-making and in operational decision-making.

The cost emphasis of the Finance Committee was both an important and a continuing element in the development of Medicaid. Other committees might ask—as did Senator Ribicoff's Subcommittee on Executive Reorganization in the *Health Care in America* hearings of 1968—"How soon after the Vietnam War would it take to get a real health program swinging?"[3] but this concern for quality was increasingly a minority viewpoint. Senator Ribicoff's subcommittee, indeed, continued to probe the question of how federal money could best be spent to improve the health delivery system, producing a landmark report, *The Federal Role in Health,* in April 1970.[4] But while the message of that report was the need to coordinate federal health expenditures to eliminate waste and to reorganize the total role of federal health expenditures, the message of the Senate Finance Committee (of which Ribicoff was also a member) was much simpler: it was primarily concerned with how Medicaid and Medicare funds were being spent. As discussion over the health care "crisis" progressed, there was no one committee in Congress charged with responsibility for federal health expenditures.

A series of implications flowed from the fact that Medicaid (and Medicare) came under the jurisdiction of the Congressional tax committees, the Finance Committee in the Senate and the Ways and Means Committee in the House. Medicare and Medicaid together represented $9.7 billion of the total of $14.5 billion of federal expenditures on health in fiscal 1970.[5] Yet, while others talked of rationalizing the health system, expanding health care services, and developing national health insurance, the two most powerful committees were committed to cutbacks in services and expenditures to meet what was felt to be Congress's original intent. However appropriate these goals, there was a schism between the fiscal regulators and the health care developers that only major new legislation would bridge. Nowhere was this more clearly seen than in the different approaches to Medicaid taken by the Senate Finance Committee and the McNerney Task Force on Medicaid, which for the most part the Finance Committee largely ignored. One looked at the impact of Medicaid on the health system; the other, at the impact of the system on Medicaid.

In its managerial role, the Finance Committee had extensive power over Medicaid, but it could only hope to pinpoint difficulties, not provide the strong and imaginative management needed for Medicaid administration in HEW. The 1969 hearings stressed the lax auditing of Medicaid programs in the states, the rise in nursing home valuations and physician fees, poor budgeting, and spiralling costs. Individual members of the committee went to town in the questioning of witnesses, Senator Bennett noting, for example, that his state of Utah "had missed their 1969 costs by $2,400,000";[6] Senator Long remarking (after producing high figures of physician fees in his own state) that "You might think that some of us fellows in Louisiana have really found a way to charge high against Medicaid and Medicare, but if you think we are high you ought to take a look at Oklahoma";[7] and Senator Curtis (Nebraska) teasing Dr. Francis Land, then the Medical Services Administration Commissioner, with a cumulative series of questions emphasizing the widespread coverage of New York's Medicaid.[8] Following his exposure to the Senate Finance Committee at the beginning of July, Dr. Land, after announcing on July 16 that he had not even considered resigning, resigned on July 25, 1969, the day the McNerney Task Force was established. Meanwhile, the Finance Committee was pushing through Senator Anderson's amendment to drop comprehensive services back until 1977.

The Staff Report of April 1970 reemphasized the role of the Finance Committee and, implicitly, the lack of activity in MSA. In its publication of original information on Medicare and Medicaid, notably material on physician fees and intermediaries, the report provided invaluable data. But it also hammered home the need for increased federal control and regulation. Recommendations for Medicaid included the required use of fee schedules for practitioners, drugs prescribed by formulary, procedures for prior approval by state agencies of such services as elective surgery and hearing aids, a requirement that each Medicaid patient have one primary physician (to end costly "doctor shopping"), the establishment of federal and state fraud abuse units, the furnishing to recipients of bills paid on their behalf (so that they too could complain when services were inappropriately reimbursed), federal regulation over state claims-control processes, and the imposition of deductibles and other forms of cost-sharing on the medically indigent. The primary call was for federal leadership: "The Medical Services Administration needs dynamic, concerned and qualified leadership and staff if a complex, costly, and important program such as Medicaid is to be soundly administered."[9]

For Medicaid, therefore, if not for Medicare (which was strictly prohibited from exercising controls over the health care system),[10] the message was regulation; it was this message which was to be transmitted into the series of bills that led to the Social Security Amendments of 1972. Meanwhile the federal administration of Medicaid was to undergo important changes, in large part under pressure from the McNerney Task Force on Medicaid, whose final report was made in June 1970. By the spring of 1970, Medicaid was surrounded by the jargon of change.

The Competing Approaches

The rhetoric represented real political considerations. There was an obvious need to assess the impact of federal funding on the health care system as a result of Medicare and Medicaid. Although regulation and cost controls formed one major approach to the reform of Medicaid, proposals for welfare reform and for reorganizing the health delivery system were also developing. Was it appropriate, for example, to continue to build up dollar amounts in Medicaid, rather than to subsidize additional neighborhood health centers? By June 1970, the Office of Economic Opportunity had developed only 49 comprehensive neighborhood health centers in the whole of the United States. Technically begun for demonstration purposes, they represented a federal flirtation with the provision of comprehensive health care, rather than any firm long-term commitment. But although such centers were expensive, they did something which Medicaid did not. Each provided an array of health services, in one place, to defined poverty populations.

The federal role in health thus represented one channel for Medicaid debate. A special study undertaken by Dr. James Shannon (a former head of NIH) for Senator Ribicoff's Subcommittee noted that of $20.6 billion spent on health activities by the federal government in fiscal 1971, only $4.0 billion actually went to improving the nation's health. Most of the remainder (largely Medicare and Medicaid) was still technically devoted to income supplement, rather than attempts to develop health service.[11] A vital question was therefore whether Medicare and Medicaid funds should be used more instrumentally, to stimulate changes in the health care system. This question was to be tackled by the McNerney Task Force with respect to Medicaid and was to become a core issue in the debates over health maintenance organizations in the early months of 1970.

Alongside the creaking structure of Medicaid and the deficiencies in the health care system, the growing pressures for welfare reform threatened the system on which Medicaid was based. By the end of June 1970 a series of alternatives to Medicaid was crystallizing. There were proposals in the McNerney reports both for federalizing Medicaid and for tying it more closely, as a lever for change, to the health care system. Out of the concurrent proposals for welfare reform, represented in President Nixon's Family Assistance Plan, came new proposals for the replacement of a large part of Medicaid by a system of national health insurance for low-income families: the Family Health Insurance Program, or FHIP. Meanwhile, proposals for national health insurance for the whole population were developing from inside and outside Congress; and a new catch phrase, the "health maintenance organization," was offering conservatives and liberals alike the prospect of locally organized health care systems.

The McNerney Reports

The Task Force on Medicaid and Related Programs, chaired by Walter McNerney, president of the Blue Cross Association, had been set up in July 1969 soon after the Senate Finance Committee's critical hearings and in the midst of debates over regulation of physician fees. The Task Force consisted of 27 members (including the chairman), drawn *inter alia* from health services administration, state welfare administration, academia, and industry. The group's primary charge in examining Medicaid was to focus on program management, effectiveness of use, and eligibility; and it was advised to stress cost controls, review procedures, standards, and better working relationships and cooperation among government agencies.[12] It was, however, bound to make its own assumptions about the basic purposes of Medicaid.

The new Task Force had the double advantage of being created at a politically "hot" period and of being allotted relatively generous staff and resources: The two facts were not unconnected. Secretary Finch announced that the Medicaid Task Force was set up "to deal immediately with the crisis in that program."[13] As initially announced the Task Force was headed jointly by McNerney and by Undersecretary of HEW John Veneman. Its Staff Director was Arthur Hess, Deputy Commissioner of Social Security, and it drew freely on staff from other branches of HEW, most notably from the Health Services and Mental Health Administration (the agency which dealt with most HEW health programs outside Medicaid and Medicare and was also responsible for the development of basic medical standards for Medicare, but not for Medicaid). So rapidly did the staff develop in the early weeks of the Task Force, and so enthusiastically did they throw their energies into examining all the warts of Medicaid, that the Task Force activities virtually eclipsed MSA.

This was not entirely surprising. MSA was directorless between July 1969, when Dr. Land resigned, and December of that year, when the new director, Howard Newman, was appointed. While Congress rang with criticism of Medicaid's organization and administration, MSA was continuing to administer a $5 billion program with a staff of 50 professionals and 35 support staff in Washington and minute staffs in HEW's ten regions. Yet criticism of Medicaid management had become a major sport. Not surprisingly, as the 1970 Senate Staff Committee reported, MSA administration was lackluster in many areas: "Responsibilities had not been discharged," manpower was inadequate, too much time was spent "putting out fires," regulations had been delayed and guidelines implementing them had not been issued, and there was no real procedure for reviews.[14]

Medicaid's official group of consultants, the Medical Assistance Advisory Council (established under the Social Security Amendments of 1967), had foundered. The lack of clear responsibility for the Council was a major problem. But this was compounded, in turn, by the lack of available staff in MSA to undertake routine and special reports for general information or to develop responses to the Council's suggestions. Thus, instead of using MAAC as an advocate group, there appears to have been a mutual suspicion between the Council and the senior staff of MSA. The first chairman, Professor Rashi Fein of Harvard, resigned, reportedly "in disgust over non-use of the group."[15] And by the fall of 1969, the Council was moribund. (It was reactivated, under the chairmanship of Dr. Donald C. Smith, with substantial new membership in November 1969.)

Meanwhile, what forcefulness that did appear in Medicaid decision-making came from special or outside efforts. The nursing home regulations, as has been noted, were developed in conjunction with a special consultant from the nursing home field. The regulations for professional fee guidelines that emerged in July 1969 were the work of a special task force headed by another consultant, Dr. James Haughton, Deputy Administrator of the New York City Health Services Administration.[16] Haughton also played an important part in rescuing HEW from its earlier "erroneous" announcement that physician fees were to be tied to Blue Shield fee schedules (a matter of some concern to the medical profession) and in selling the regulation that limited fees to January 1969 levels.[17] Indeed, the success of this special task force provided a useful forerunner for the McNerney Task Force itself.

Dr. Haughton became chairman of the most important of the three panels set up by the McNerney Task Force at its first meeting in July 1969: the Panel on Effectiveness of Use. Its primary emphasis was clear. By "effectiveness of use" it meant not merely getting the most value out of a limited budget (the Senate Finance Committee emphasis), but also the provision of appropriate health services to the needy population. The two other panels were focused on Program Management and Eligibility. All three panels moved into immediate action. By early August 1969, the Panel on Effectiveness alone had a staff of 27.[18] A library of source materials had been assembled. The staff were setting up state files, including DHEW audit reports, PREP reviews, state Medicaid plans, and other documents and were planning a series of special investigative visits to states, including visits on particular topics such as procedures for utilization review. In addition, a number of special consultants had been assembled from the "health" side of HEW. Indeed, the general tenor of the inquiry was that of "health service administrators," taking a patient-centered point of view, investigating programs set up by "welfare administrators," who were supposedly more tax-conscious and restrictive.

Whatever the initial attitudes, however, it was the administration of the program that demanded the most attention. The basic managerial problems of Medicaid were immense. Even before the McNerney Interim Report was issued, the preliminary findings of the Finance Committee staff had appeared:

> *Federal officials have been lax in not seeing to it that States establish and employ effective controls on utilization and costs, and States have been unwilling to assume the responsibility on their own. The Federal Medicaid administrators have not provided states with the expert assistance necessary to implement proper controls. Also, they have not developed mechanisms for coordination and communication among the States about methods of identifying and solving Medicaid problems.*[19]

Belatedly, in 1968, HEW had set up a scheme for standard audit in 16 major Medicaid states, and these reports were released during 1969. Among the findings were that Illinois had drawn nearly $1 million in federal funds improperly,[20] that New York City had wasted as much as $9.7 million in federal funds because of alleged procedural violations and administrative laxity,[21] and that Texas was using procedures that resulted in the loss of interest income to the federal government of $48,750 a month.[22] All told, the audits reportedly revealed weaknesses in management controls, as well as in procedures for processing claims, eligibility, and other areas amounting to a minimal "questionable dollar impact" (that is, waste) of $318 million.[23]

These audits served to emphasize two major features of Medicaid with which the Task Force on Medicaid had to grapple. The first was administrative inefficiency in the states; the second the lack (based on the initial assumption that the states would be efficient) of federal guidelines, methods, and controls. It is illustrative of the low-keyed central role of SRS in Medicaid's early years that not until June 1970 was a federal regulation proposed for Medicaid to require that a state, in discharging its fiscal accountability, "maintain an accounting system and supporting fiscal records adequate to assure that claims for federal funds are in accord with applicable Federal requirements."[24] A layman (or taxpayer) might have supposed that such records were already available, with state accountants acting busily and inventively to increase productivity and save costs under the watchful eye of federal administrators. But, as we have seen, such was not the case.

Exploration by Task Force personnel emphasized the audits and the Senate Finance Committee's findings. Mismanagement by some of the states or their fiscal agents led to "duplicate payments," inadequate utilization review, and waste of resources in determining eligibility.[25] These events were allowed to occur because there were inadequate staffs in the regions, without clear lines of command and without "definitive guidelines relating to policies, procedures and goals."[26] There was inadequate follow-up of site visits (PREP reports) on the operation of the program in the different states, and there was considerable evidence of approval of plans and arrangements that did not conform to the federal law.[27] For example, a PREP review in New Mexico in February 1968 had found a lack of any focal point for administration of the Medicaid program, inadequate staffing at state and local levels, no effective Medical Advisory Committee (the committee had met once since the program had begun in December 1966), and no specific plan for evaluation of the utilization and quality of medical care. The HEW audit report of April 1969 found, however, that no effective follow-up to these findings had been made by the regional office of MSA in Dallas.[28]

The early activities of the Task Force, responding to this situation, focused on selected areas. One problem was a lack of norms against which services could be measured. The Panel on Effectiveness focused on utilization review procedures, i.e., systems for reviewing the use of services, from which assessments of effectiveness of the programs could be made.[29] But from the beginning, this panel raised the question of how far Medicaid could be harnessed to utilize and influence patterns of the organization of medical care, and what standards should be required of the providers of care. Both of these activities assumed increased regulation of providers. The Panel on Management concentrated on recommendations for improvement in the federal administration, again focusing on the need to go beyond the fulfillment of legal requirements to the encouragement of innovation and experiment. MSA, it was noted, should take a more aggressive role, and the responsibility of the regional offices should be substantially increased.[30] The Panel on Eligibility set out, meanwhile, to review methods of determining eligibility, together with their implications.

The activities of the Task Force Staff were important not only in focusing HEW attention on Medicaid's operation but also in investigating new developments in health care organization and regulation that might be relevant in a government program. Utilization review procedures were of special concern, and attention was paid to the organizational controls built into a number of private health organizations—the Kaiser Foundation prepaid group practice plans, the Physicians Association of Clackamas County, Oregon (which acts as a physician-controlled nonprofit health insurance organization and includes 3500 Medicaid recipients in approximately 25,000 subscribers), and a new primary care health system being set up in Massachusetts under the guidance of Dr. Leonard Cronkhite, to be based on neighborhood centers designed to serve 15,000 to 25,000 people. Thus, while the primary charge of the Task Force was to stimulate change within Medicaid's existing legislative mandate, from the beginning the staff were examining Medicaid within a much wider health care framework.

The reports of the three panels, approved by the whole Task Force, formed the substance of the interim report of the Task Force, published in November 1969.[31] The result was an important smorgasbord of recommendations, ranging from strictly managerial issues to wider questions of the federal role in health. Among the recommendations were proposals for simplified eligibility procedures, better public relations to make information about Medicaid more readily available, broadening the availability of services by sponsoring demonstration projects in comprehensive health care, encouraging consumer participation in decision-making, establishing standard program effectiveness systems in the states, encouraging health care planning, and developing methods of "incentive reimbursement," i.e., new methods of payment to encourage better standards and use of services. Generally, then, the tone was of expansion and improvement of services to recipients.

The most interesting recommendations were, however, the most far-reaching: Medicaid should be federalized and should be used instrumentally.

The Task Force stated bluntly that Medicaid (and related programs such as Medicare) "should not be merely conduits for funds which reinforce the inadequacies of the existing health care system, but should be used as instruments to improve the system."[32] For Medicaid, it was suggested, 5 percent of federal appropriations should be set aside each year for the general development and improvement of health care services and resources, with the primary focus on organized primary care, prepayment schemes, and comprehensive health care systems. It was also recommended that the activities of planning agencies should be tied into Medicaid reimbursement methods, e.g., that corporate planning by institutions should be required as a condition of participation. The need for national standards for Medicaid was stressed. Finally, a series of recommendations were designed to improve federal management capability, with respect to "dynamic leadership" and adequate staffing of MSA and—more generally—to mechanisms for effective policy coordination for all health programs in HEW. As far as MSA was concerned the Task Force called for administrators experienced in health care administration "with a solid management perspective."[33]

The interim report was in some ways more important than the Task Force's final report, published in June 1970, although the final report was both more detailed and more carefully conceived.[34] The interim report was, in effect, a design to develop Medicaid as a federally run basic health program for the poor, with the goal of providing recipients with good medical care in a well-run health system; the underlying philosophy was little different from that of the 1965 Amendments as initially interpreted by HEW. But, after the frenetic activity of its first months, the Task Force staff appears to have lost some of its steam. Secretary Finch had requested the group to look at national health insurance, a subject of increasing general interest and one which would naturally flow from the Task Force's thinking, but this question was dropped in January 1970.[35] The Task Force, whose debates were becoming increasingly diffuse, was rapidly being overtaken by events—some of which the interim report had had a hand in shaping.

The Story of FHIP

While the Task Force on Medicaid was stressing the role of Medicaid in the context of health, welfare reform proposals were reinventing the need which had stimulated Medicaid in the first place. At least some of the poor were poor because they were sick. The structure of welfare was thus interlocked with that of health care delivery. President Nixon announced his proposals for a Family Assistance Plan in a national television address on August 8, 1969, and developed them in his welfare reform message to

Congress three days later.[86] Both messages stressed the "blatant unfairness of the welfare system." One major assistance program, Aid to Families with Dependent Children, would be abolished, to be replaced by a new federal program that would guarantee a family of four a basic payment of $1,600 a year. The others—Aid to the Aged, Blind, and Disabled—would be continued as state programs. However, a national minimal standard for benefits would also be set, with the federal government contributing to its cost and also subsidizing additional state payments above that level.

These proposals were buttressed with proposals for "workfare," designed to get people off the welfare rolls. But the basic program was expansionary in terms of cash assistance, at least for the poorer states. In 20 states the suggested federal floor for family assistance was above the existing welfare levels. For the richer states the proposals also offered some advantage in federal payments for AFDC up to the national level, with the option of state payments above that level. As 6.5 million of the 9.3 million recipients of welfare in March 1969 were in the AFDC program, the impact of the proposals would be considerable. At the same time, the proposals offered an opportunity for cash assistance payments to the working poor, through income supplements to those earning low wages. This program brought up considerably the level of assistance. "Working poor" families could be headed by a worker whose earnings were below $3920 for a family of four. This latter amount was above most states' Medicaid eligibility levels.

One extraordinary feature of the original FAP proposals—a result of the piecemeal approach to decision-making in domestic social areas—was the exclusion of any consideration of Medicaid. An odd situation had been reached. While the "health" critics regarded Medicaid as a failure because it was designed as a program of income supplement, not of health services development, the welfare reformers apparently neglected Medicaid because it was a health program, not a program of income maintenance. Alice could not have done better in Wonderland.

In part, of course, the dilemma was rooted in Medicaid itself, hovering uncertainly as it did between the two classifications. But the exclusion of Medicaid considerations from FAP, at least in its early phases, must also be blamed on the lack of any social-planning agency. FAP itself was not developed by the welfare arm of HEW (SRS) but by the Office of Management and Budget, then known as the Bureau of the Budget. The economists at the Office of Management and Budget were searching for rational fiscal solutions to an apparently straightforward question of cash assistance. Although the solutions might be complex, the problem was basically one of the appropriate transfer of dollar income.

HEW, meanwhile, was not only a sprawling and disorganized agency whose sections tended to work independently; there was, in addition, a rift in views between the relatively "liberal" staff of HEW who were running the health programs of the 1960s and the new management line at OMB, a rift which made communication difficult in both directions. Insofar as one can ever characterize institutional roles or attitudes, from the Executive Office Building the fat, unwieldy, and perhaps ungovernable structure of HEW must have seemed a classical economist's nightmare. It was, indeed, to defeat President Nixon's first appointee, Robert Finch, who resigned as Secretary in June 1970. But while from one direction, HEW might seem filled with "social workers" (a term which implied soft-headedness), from the point of view of HEW staff struggling with often ill-formed and patchwork programs, the apparent attempts to cut costs for cost-cutting's sake were equally unacceptable. While the underlying problem on both sides was the same—the lack of clear Congressional commitment to provide a minimum income to the poor, with basic supporting services—the rift between the body of HEW and the Nixon Administration in 1969–70 added to existing problems of program development and coordination.

Over and above the backstairs bickerings, there remained, however, the stepchild status of Medicaid in the light of welfare reform debates. President Nixon stated flatly in a message in March 1970 that Medicaid was supposed to be a medical program (rather than an integral part of the welfare system). This, it turned out, was a plea for retrenchment: He proposed that long-term nursing-home and mental-hospital care be cut from Medicaid plans, on the grounds that "we direct federal matching funds toward medical treatment rather than custodial care and provide new incentives to the states to emphasize more efficient forms of extended care."[37] This was all very well in terms of health priorities. The removal of such benefits would, however, clearly put stress on other aspects of the welfare system. Otherwise, what would happen to these patients? Cash assistance levels would buy scant service for a bedridden or otherwise dependent person in a private institution. Were persons in nursing homes suddenly to be ejected, and if so, where would they go? If Medicaid were removed, at least some of the costs would have to be picked up by state welfare programs.

In short, for all public beneficiaries, but particularly for the old and the young, Medicaid provided an important buffer; health care was a vital element of income maintenance. This factor was important for all welfare programs, but it became of immediate political importance in the proposals for FAP in 1969 and 1970. If there had been a general health service for the whole population, available to all irrespective of income status (as, for example, in Great Britain), welfare reform could be considered quite separately from medical care. But Medicaid, as it had developed, was an all-or-nothing proposition. The beneficiary was either entitled to it or he was not. It was irrelevant at this stage to point back to the concept of "medical indigence" as a potential gray area in which those not on welfare could be given the support of health services until completely economically independent. The "medically needy" had taken a back seat. Of 6.9 million recipients of medical assistance in the United States in the month of August 1970, only 1.5 million were not also recipients of cash assistance, and these were concentrated in California, New York, Massachusetts, and Puerto Rico.[38] Moreover the concept of medical indigence as it was applied inevitably meant another relatively rigid means test. There were thus no supporting health benefits available to act as a backstop to the FAP welfare reform proposals.[39]

Thus, while the FAP program was designed to provide a graduated national system of welfare from indigence through low-paying or part-time work, important state variations would remain whenever FAP recipients fell sick. Without a national health program, some of the elements of national welfare would be negated. Moreover, Medicaid programs did not taper off by income. In New York, for example, the medically needy eligibility level was still $5000 for a family of four in January 1970; when the family earned more than that, Medicaid would either be discontinued, or the family would be involved in the constant process of "spending-down" to get back on it—scarcely a major work incentive. In other states, of course, the "notch" would be much more evident. At the beginning of 1970, two states (Alaska and Arizona) still had no Medicaid program, 24 offered Medicaid only to those on cash assistance, and 24 (together with D.C., Guam, Puerto Rico, and the Virgin Islands) had programs for the medically indigent.[40] As both eligibility levels and services varied by state, there were considerable differences both in the dollar amounts available for medical care and the cut-off point for eligibility. This deficiency in the FAP proposals was noted by critics at the time. While most of the debate in Congress and in the press centered on the FAP's compulsory job training and work provisions, behind-the-scenes efforts were being made to develop a health benefit system for the poor that would get rid of the unwanted "notch" effect.

As has been seen, the interim report of the McNerney Commission, published in November 1969, recommended the federalization of Medicaid. This proposal would presumably solve the question of differing medical care entitlements in the different states by providing one standard for services and eligibility, but it did not attack the problem of the "notch." If the McNerney provision were adopted, equity would be achieved among the states, but not equity between the poor on FAP and the working poor who were above the FAP assistance levels. The general questions of disincentives to FAP, including Medicaid (as well as public housing and food stamps), were raised with some force by the Senate Finance Committee, which at this time was in the process of examining the welfare reform proposals; and on May 1, 1970 a request was made by that committee to the Administration to develop relevant additional proposals to deal with them.[41]

Thus FHIP (the Family Health Insurance Program) was developed almost by default. In a statement on welfare reform by President Nixon on

June 10, 1970—19 days before the final McNerney Report was submitted to the new HEW Secretary, Elliot Richardson—the revised proposal for FHIP was launched.[42] On the grounds that Medicaid was "inefficient, inequitably excludes the working poor, and often provides an incentive for people to stay on welfare," the President announced that he would propose legislation at the beginning of the 92nd Congress to establish a scheme of family health insurance for "all poor families with children." A major segment of Medicaid would thus be turned into national health insurance, to meet welfare reform's exigencies.

The initial proposal for FHIP suggested a scheme of graduated contributions by eligible families up to a cut-off point. But, because of the high costs of medical care and the goal of graduating FHIP benefits by income, the cut-off point would have to be much higher than the proposed FAP level of $1,600 for a family of four. Indeed, the FHIP proposal suggested a cut-off of $5,620 for a family. At this level the family would have to contribute the sum of $500 a year, but the level was still higher than the Medicaid eligibility level in New York—and it would now be extended across the nation. In effect, therefore, the new proposals represented a new form of Medicaid, nationally applied (although only applicable to AFDC-related categories), with a relatively high eligibility level, with graduated premiums up to that level. The aim, of course, was to slide persons from the public to the private sector, by moving the premium system up to a point where it was not basically different from that of private health insurance. An estimated five million families, or 25 to 30 million people, would be covered.[43] There would thus be a major expansion of coverage, as only about 13 million persons were covered under AFDC-related categories of Medicaid in fiscal 1971.

Although no details of FHIP's administration and structure were described—indeed, they had not been developed—the announcement of the new proposals was important in several respects. First, there was the inherent logic of the situation. The FHIP proposals had arisen out of FAP. Daniel Moynihan, Counsellor to the President, remarked at the time:

> *What we are proposing here is to link up a historic system of income guarantees . . . with a system of family health insurance, based upon the same principles of non-dependency, of work incentives and the elimination of the notch effects and national standards: the three principles being that of not requiring people to be dependent, urging and giving them an incentive to be independent, the principle of national standards and the principle of continued work incentive.*[44]

But in relying on such principles, once again welfare medical care was to be dependent on the social necessity of other programs. In terms of Medicaid itself, the acceptance of FHIP would turn back the clock to different standards of medical assistance for different welfare categories: FHIP would cover only families with young children. The old, blind, and disabled, who represented 5 million out of the 18 million Medicaid recipients in fiscal 1971 would presumably remain under Medicaid.

A second important point in the proposals for FHIP was, however, perhaps of greater long-term significance: the acceptance of the insurance principle for covering the health needs of the poor. By tying the whole structure of FHIP into the logic of private health insurance, the Administration automatically endorsed a form of national health insurance. Here indeed, was a new search for "mainstream" medicine. The next step, which was to form an important part of the Nixon health strategy of the 92nd Congress, was to ensure the provision of appropriate health insurance packages in the private sector. Thus, in the same chain of logic, came other Administration proposals for minimum standards of health insurance for employees and for the regulation of the private health insurance industry.

The Supply and Demand Debate

In FHIP, as well as in the proposals of the Task Force on Medicaid, there arose the important question of how far any reformed system could rely on the operation of the private health care sector. In short, was it enough to ensure that needy persons had an equitable opportunity to obtain medical care (through health insurance or vendor payments), or were more draconic measures necessary to improve the types, availability, and nature of health services? Perhaps both roles were necessary; in this case, the question was where the primary emphasis should be directed. The first assumed that the needy were a minority group whose needs should be met through prevailing mechanisms; the second, that the whole population was "medically needy" in some respects because health services were not operating with optimal efficiency. But whatever the ultimate solutions, the two poles for federal influence remained. Programs such as Medicaid (and the proposals for FHIP) stimulated the demand for health services by allowing the poor to be purchasers of care in the (largely) private sector. The Task Force, on the other hand, would also attempt to influence the supply of health services.

In theory, if the market worked, stimulating demand would also improve the services offered. But here was the rub: the providers were organized in a series of licensed medical monopolies. The market was already too distorted to expect classical demand-supply responses. The huge demands of Medicare and Medicaid had demonstrably not improved the availability, organization, and efficiency of health services. Health care was, if anything, more fragmented in 1970 than in 1965, and certainly much more expensive.

If this fact were to be generally recognized, as it was in abundant evidence in continuing Congressional hearings on all aspects of health care in the United States, a stronger federal role would be necessary to improve the way in which health services were provided. In short, it was not enough to stimulate demand without also guaranteeing an appropriate supply and an appropriate structure for providing it. The replacement of state Medicaid programs with a federal service would fully emphasize these points, both because of national standard-setting and through national visibility.

Already, providers of health care were being subject to increased regulation for reasons of costs and waste, a direct result of Medicare and Medicaid. The need to plan services, particularly expensive hospital beds and facilities, to eliminate overlap was a point made clearly in the 1970 report of the Ribicoff committee. Moreover, federal money, directed through narrowly channeled and uncoordinated programs, sometimes contributed directly to such waste.[45] By 1970 the idea of planning and regulation of health facilities was becoming generally accepted, both at the federal and at the state level. (Indeed, many states now have some form of regulation over hospital construction, mostly developed since 1970.) Because a second reason for planning is to guarantee that services to which beneficiaries are entitled are in fact made available, this argument for equity would have been important if FHIP had been implemented; it has become increasingly important under Medicaid.

In any event, Medicaid had graphically illustrated the point that regulation over planning, together with regulation over prices and fees, becomes increasingly necessary where there are two separate systems of demand and supply: one (governmental) for purchasing and one (largely private) for selling medical care. If beneficiaries could buy their care anywhere in the existing health sector, the corollary was tighter controls on the providers. Proposals for national health insurance, of which FHIP was one, would have to meet this point in one form or another.

Of all the Medicaid critiques, the final report of the Task Force on Medicaid saw these points most clearly and fleshed out some of the implications of a national scheme of welfare medicine. Under the proposals, Medicaid would become a federal program, with a uniform minimum level of health benefits financed 100 percent from federal funds; and although the proposal would start with those covered under the Family Assistance Plan, it would eventually include all those eligible for Medicaid. This expansion would be coupled with much bolder federal intervention in the health care system:

> *The Task Force is convinced that it no longer makes sense to keep pouring new wine in old casks—some of which are leaking. Additional financing must be accomplished now with opportunities and encouragement to physicians, hospitals and others to provide service in ways*

that permit a logical response to sound economic and patient-care incentives, and to engage in a competition of organization and method.[46]

The Task Force thus developed its recommendations in terms of the need for a strong federal policy for health services (including the establishment of a National Council of Health Advisors), stimulation through federal money of changes in the health delivery system (including stimulation of primary care and prepayment plans), a stronger MSA (including 125 additional staff positions), the clarification of roles and strengthening of planning agencies at all levels, and better management techniques (including information systems and other forms of review). In general, it recommended that Medicaid's purchasing power should be used to "increase accessibility of care to the needy and to improve the effectiveness of the care."[47] Medicaid, in short, would mold the "mainstream," in concert with other federal programs.

Such considerations were not, of course, limited to Medicaid. By June 1970, proposals for national health insurance for the whole population were blossoming. The American Medical Association had endorsed national health insurance through a system of tax credits—Medicredit—as early as 1968.[48] Representative Martha Griffiths introduced a far-reaching, labor-sponsored health insurance bill for comprehensive health insurance organized through Social Security contributions—the Health Security proposals—in February 1970.[49] In April 1970, Senator Javits introduced a set of proposals that would in effect have extended Medicare to the whole population.[50] In May, Governor Rockefeller, by then a veteran advocate of national health insurance, formed his own Conference on Health and Hospital Services and Costs, chaired by Joseph Wilson, Chairman of Xerox.[51] This committee, too, was charged to develop plans for national health insurance. Indeed there was already a very strong expression of interest in national health insurance from all potential interest groups, from the health insurance industry to the American Hospital Association. No longer, so it seemed, would it be possible to consider Medicaid outside the context of one or another form of national health insurance: the framework was set for the current debates.

Health Maintenance Organizations

Even if Medicaid had become a stimulator of proposals for national health insurance, rather than (as originally designed) an alternative to more sweeping proposals, Medicaid's immediate philosophical, practical, and managerial difficulties remained. Already the proponents of national health insurance were offering more compelling proposals than had been produced at other times in history when national health insurance had been in vogue. All of the proposals (including FHIP) were vague in administrative details and implications. At this time in the history of welfare medicine, there was no straightforward incremental approach to take. Revision of Medicaid would rest upon large-scale changes either in welfare or in health care provision, and there was as yet no general agreement on which would predominate.

In the meantime, however, there remained a relatively uncontroversial middle ground for influencing the health care system, using accepted payment mechanisms without going massively into federally-organized insurance schemes or developing wholesale federal regulation of the health care industry. It was this ground the Task Force on Medicaid explored in looking at programs such as prepaid group practice, particularly in its early meetings. And it was this middle ground that was in the long run to prove so appealing in the developing proposals for health maintenance organizations.

The idea of a health maintenance organization surfaced in February 1970.[52] As initially devised, the health care system would be reformed at the local level into a series of competing private health service organizations, each of which would offer patients a "health maintenance contract," i.e., a contract specifying services designed to protect the patient's health. Programs such as Medicaid would buy such contracts for recipients, instead of purchasing insurance or making vendor payments. At first glance this proposal might seem as wide-eyed as the concurrent proposals for national health insurance. The "health maintenance organization" (HMO) was, however, perhaps the most politically realistic and shrewd of all proposals offered to the 91st Congress. First—and not to be scorned—it provided a new rhetoric. The prepaid group practice, of which the Kaiser Foundation plans were a major example, had long been associated with the liberal left. The HMO was presented, in contrast, as the reasonable businessman's approach to offering medical care. The terms "group practice" and even "insurance" were avoided. Primary emphasis was given to the reinvention of a market system in medicine. The consumer would buy a contract at the HMO of his choice and certain services would thus automatically be available to him. One HMO would compete with others for clients, and there would in theory thus be automatic incentives to efficiency, advertising, and good public relations.

Beyond this, the HMO capitalized on other political themes of the New Federalism. National health insurance, by its very nature, requires centralized authority and regulation. Whichever form was eventually chosen, the federal government would have increasing control over health care, rather than less. The HMO, on the other hand, was presented as a direct antithesis to this proposition. By offering self-contained organizations at the local level, HMOs would stimulate decentralized government decision-making. In terms of Medicaid, for example, the state (or federal government if Medicaid were federalized) would buy into HMOs for a fixed fee and would rely on the built-in efficiency of the HMOs rather than impose widespread regulation on the whole health industry. Besides decentralization there would thus also be flexibility—a premise central to the ideas of creative federalism generally mooted within the Nixon Administration.

Finally, the HMO offered two other important elements, which were apparent in its title. Health maintenance implied a commitment to preventive medical care, as well as to crisis medicine: it would go beyond then-current conceptions of Medicare, at least, and in some respects of Medicaid. Even the phrase *health maintenance* provided an obvious balance to the parallel proposals for income maintenance.

The term "HMO" came to be applied to prepaid group practice plans (which range in size from under 10,000 to more than 1 million persons) and also to other organizations, including medical-society foundations. But, in the classic tradition of social change in America, the details were less important than the rhetoric. The HMO offered a new, potentially acceptable, prospect to both the political right and the political left. As with similar programs for the use of "vouchers" in education, the old liberals appeared to have been overtaken in radicalism by the new conservatives. HMOs joined FHIP to become an intrinsic part of the Nixon Administration's "Health Strategy."

In the meantime, HMOs had an obvious appeal for the potential development of Medicaid. If states could buy contracts for specified services from private organizations on behalf of their Medicaid beneficiaries, in one fell swoop there would be cost containment (as a system of fee-for-service bills would be replaced by a flat prepayment fee), guarantees of organized medical services, and acceptance of Medicaid patients within a one-class medical service system (as, presumably, the HMOs would serve the whole population, not merely poverty groups).[53] The Task Force on Medicaid therefore readily endorsed the concept of HMOs in its final report of June 1970.

But by this time the HMO movement was gathering support from other directions. The critical Senate Finance Committee report on Medicare and Medicaid appeared in February 1970. In May, the House Ways and Means Committee reported out new Social Security Amendments proposing important changes in Medicaid, together with Medicare and maternal and child health programs, "with emphasis upon improvements in the operating effectiveness of such programs."[54] The Amendments also introduced into Congress the concept of a "health maintenance organization" as an option for Medicare and Medicaid, which was to form a further strand in debates over medical care.

The only problem with HMOs was that, while they were politically subtle and able to take on the hues of right and left, there was no hard evidence that they were any more than yet another gimmick. Even assuming that private prepayment plans were in fact an economical way of providing medical care—and the evidence was not conclusive—could the principle be applied to poorer groups that might have different medical needs and different social outlooks? HMOs had the aura of yet another demonstration project. They might be the wave of the future; they might also be primarily a subsidy to protect providers in their existing professional structures and yet another hoax as far as the recipients of Medicaid were concerned.[55] Once again, a clear definition of welfare medicine had been delayed, in favor of piecemeal "solutions."

But, by 1970, at least new patterns, or suggested patterns, were emerging. The Social Security Amendments, which were to become H.R. 1 in the 92nd Congress, marked the beginning of a new period. By the end of June 1970, Medicaid was at the vortex of proposals for change. In Congress in 1970 were more than 200 proposals for change in Medicare and Medicaid, ranging from relatively simple suggestions for managerial change to proposals that would abolish Medicaid altogether. In the two and a half years since the 1967 Amendments, the context of Medicaid had changed radically. Although there were increasing criticisms of Medicaid's waste and continuing pressures for stronger management and regulation, from the Senate Finance Committee, from the Task Force on Medicaid, and in the new Social Security proposals, the future of Medicaid was inexorably linked to the wider scene, whether through FHIP, through HMOs, through national health insurance, or through other proposals for federal policy-making.

NOTES

1. Senate Committee on Finance, press release, June 26, 1969.

2. U.S., Department of Health, Education, and Welfare, *Report on the Task Force on Medicaid and Related Programs,* 1970, pp. 2–3 and *passim.*

3. U.S., Congress, Senate, Committee on Government Operations, Sub-Committee on Executive Reorganization, *Health Care in America, Hearings* before the Sub-Committee on Executive Reorganization, Committee on Government Operations, U.S. Senate, 90th Cong., 2nd Sess., 1968, p. 511.

4. U.S., Congress, Senate, *Federal Role in Health,* Report of the Committee on Government Operations, U.S. Senate, Made by its Sub-Committee on Executive Reorganization, Pursuant to S. Res. 320, 91st Cong., Report No. 91–809, 1970.

5. Medicare $7.1 billion; Medicaid (federal share) $2.6 billion. U.S., Department of Health, Education, and Welfare, Office of Research and Statistics, *Compendium of National Health Expenditures Data* (Washington, 1973), p. 56.

6. U.S., Congress, Senate, Committee on Finance, *Medicare and Medicaid, Hearings* before the Committee on Finance, 91st Cong., 1st Sess., 1969, p. 138.

7. *Ibid.,* p. 161.

8. *Ibid.,* pp. 142–144.

9. U.S., Senate, Finance Committee, *Medicare and Medicaid: Problems, Issues and Alternatives,* Staff Report, 1970, p. 127 and *passim.*

10. P.L. 89–97, Sect. 1801; 79 Stat. 291 (1965).

11. U.S., Congress, Senate, Committee on Finance, *Health Activities, Federal Activities and Public Purpose,* Committee Print, June 1970, Pursuant to S. Res. 320, 81st Cong.

12. Memorandum Draft of Secretary's Task Force on Medicaid—Charge, July 9, 1969 (Papers of the Task Force on Medicaid, Departmental Archives, HEW).

13. A Report on the Health of the Nation's Health Care System, July 10, 1969, mimeograph (Papers of the Task Force on Medicaid, Departmental Archives, HEW).

14. *Medicare and Medicaid: Problems, Issues and Alternatives, supra,* note 9, pp. 239–242.

15. *Washington Report,* Nov. 3, 1969.

16. *Washington Report,* June 16, 1969.

17. If the payments for January were below the 75th percentile of customary charges, they might be raised to the 75th percentile upon approval of the Secretary of HEW. 34 *Federal Register,* 11098 (1969).

18. Progress Report, Panel on Effectiveness, Aug. 4, 1969 (Papers of the Task Force on Medicaid; Departmental Archives, HEW).

19. U.S., Congress, Senate, Staff of Senate Committee on Finance, *Staff Data Relating to Medicaid-Medicare Study,* Committee Print, Committee on Finance, 91st Cong., 1st Sess., 1969.

20. *AMA News,* July 21, 1969.

21. *Ibid.,* Sept. 8, 1969.

22. See Medicare and Medicaid Hearings, *supra,* note 6, pp. 72–73; U.S., Congress, Senate, Committee on Finance, *Medicare and Medicaid, Hearing* before the Committee on Finance, 91st Cong., 2nd Sess., 1970, *passim.* The Texas case is particularly interesting as an example of the type of situation that occurred. The State Department of Public Welfare had made an agreement with Group Hospital Service, Inc. (Blue Cross–Blue Shield of Texas) to "insure" Medicaid recipients; the audit found that in fact GHS was acting under a "fiscal agent" agreement of the state, merely administering the state program rather than providing full insurance coverage. Between September 1, 1967, and June 20, 1968, it was noted that GHS had accumulated more than $14 million of state money as premiums for medical services in excess of actual disbursements. The state held that this was in accordance with the state interpretation of the agent function and that such accumulations were a hedge to offset future claims. Experience bore this out; by June 30, 1969, GHS expenditures exceeded receipts by almost one-half million dollars. The state claimed that this method resulted in a reduction in premium rates and better administration of services. The HEW Audit Agency ruled that the arrangement with GHS was not insurance because no element of risk for GHS existed, and it therefore did not comply with the requirements of *Supplement D* (paragraphs 5520A and 5830). This ruling was upheld by the administrator of SRS. Also at issue was nearly $888,000, the difference between federal matching at the 50 percent rate for administrative costs and the higher matching at the medical assistance rate. This sum was still in dispute in 1970 in appeals and decisions involving the state, SRS, and the HEW Regional Office.

23. The greatest single cost ($126 million) lay in determining eligibility. *Medicare and Medicaid: Problems, Issues and Alternatives, supra,* note 14, p. 245.

24. *Federal Register* 8780 (1970). This regulation also applied to Titles I, IV-A, X, XIV, and XVI of the Social Security Act. Agencies would be required to maintain accounting records for each title for a period of a minimum of 3 and a maximum of 5 years after the end of each fiscal year, subject to the timing of federal audit.

25. *Medicare and Medicaid: Problems, Issues and Alternatives, supra,* note 14, p. 204.

26. *Ibid.*, p. 236.

27. *Ibid.*, pp. 238–239.

28. Audit of the Regional Administration of Title XIX of the Social Security Act by the Regional Medical Service Staff, Region VII, April 1, 1969, Audit Control No. 07-90202 (Papers of the Task Force on Medicaid; Departmental Archives, HEW). The general pervasiveness of the laissez-faire attitude during the early years of Medicaid was reflected in the reports of the Task Force staff. The State of Washington, for example, with Medicaid expenditures of over $51 million in fiscal 1968, was reported to lack qualified personnel in the areas of data processing and analysis and the implementation of utilization-review procedures. The Kentucky Medicaid program, while commended for its use of advisory committees and development of computer capability, was six months behind in paying physicians' claims.

29. Existing procedures for utilization review ranged from relatively sophisticated systems in Rhode Island and Connecticut to an "unacceptable" situation in Massachusetts (Papers of the Task Force on Medicaid; Departmental Archives, HEW).

30. Memorandum, Task Force on Medicaid, 28 Aug. 1969 (Papers of the Task Force on Medicaid, Departmental Archives, HEW).

31. Task Force on Medicaid and Related Programs, Interim Report, Nov. 12, 1969.

32. *Ibid.*, p. 9.

33. *Ibid.*, p. 37 and *passim.*

34. *Report of the Task Force on Medicaid and Related Programs, supra,* note 2.

35. *Washington Report,* Jan. 5, 1970.

36. U.S., Public Papers of the President, *Public Papers of President Richard Nixon,* 1969, p. 647. "Special Message to the Congress on Reform of the Nation's Welfare Program."

37. Reported in *Washington Report on Medicine and Health,* March 2, 1970.

38. U.S., Department of Health, Education, and Welfare, Social and Rehabilitation Service, National Center for Social Statistics, Report B-1, August 1970.

39. An example illustrates the difficulty. In the month of August 1970 in New York there were 507,000 Medicaid recipients eligible as AFDC recipients or in the AFDC categorically related or categorically medically related categories. Of these, 389,000 were also authorized for money payments (i.e., were welfare recipients). In the same month the state of New York spent $23.7 million on medical care for the whole 507,000 AFDC recipients, including $15.1 million

for the 389,000 on cash assistance. Two points in these figures deserve emphasis. The first is that the cash recipients were receiving an additional benefit for medical benefits, to the value of $40 in that month. The second point is that the medical expenditures for those not on cash assistance were higher—in this case about $70 in that month. *Ibid.*, Tables 12, 20.

40. U.S., Department of Health, Education, and Welfare, Social and Rehabilitation Service, *Medicaid Services—State by State*, January 1970.

41. Press Conference, Mr. Ziegler, Office of the White House Secretary, June 10, 1970.

42. Statement by the President on Welfare Reform, Office of the White House Press Secretary, June 10, 1970.

43. Statements made by John G. Veneman, Undersecretary of HEW, White House Press Conference, June 10, 1970.

44. White House Press Conference, June 10, 1970.

45. For example, at Vallejo, California, and Belle Glade, Florida, federal grants to competing hospitals had produced more beds than were actually needed. *Federal Role in Health, supra,* note 4, pp. 23–25.

46. *Report of the Task Force on Medicaid and Related Programs, supra,* note 1, p. 106.

47. *Ibid.*, p. 112.

48. Under its proposals the federal government would provide persons of low income with certificates for the purchase of health insurance policies from approved health insurance carriers; persons with higher incomes would receive federal benefits in the form of scaled credits on their income tax. The proponents of this program, waylaying criticism that it would stimulate demand without affecting health care supply, linked Medicredit with a series of proposals for utilization review, which the AMA was also endorsing. Rosemary Stevens, *American Medicine and the Public Interest* (New Haven, 1971), pp. 492–493.

49. H.R. 15779, 91st Cong., 2d Sess.

50. S. 3711, 91st Cong., 2d Sess.

51. The committee reported in June 1971. State of New York, *Report from the Governor's Steering Committee on Social Problems of Health and Hospital Services and Costs*, 1971.

52. On the development of the HMO concept, see Clark C. Havighurst, "Health Maintenance Organizations and the Market for Health Services," *Health Care* (Duke University, 1971), pp. 246–325; Herbert E. Klarman, "Analysis of the HMO Proposal—Its Assumptions, Implications, and Prospects," in *Health Maintenance Organizations: A Reconfiguration of the Health Services System*, Graduate Program in Hospital Administration and Center for Administrative Studies, Graduate School of Business, Univ. of Chicago, 1971, pp. 24–38.

53. Some Medicaid plans were, indeed, buying into prepaid groups, but as there were few HMOs—group practices for example, served only an estimated 2 percent of the whole population—the proportion of such contracts for Medicaid was insignificant.

54. H.R. 17550, 91st Cong., 2nd Sess.

55. For a bullish view on HMOs see Daniel Schorr, *Don't Get Sick in America* (Nashville, 1970), Chap. VII; for a bearish view, see Harry Schwartz, *The Case for American Medicine: A Realistic Look at our Health Care System* (New York, 1972), Chap. VI.

PART IV
Benign Neglect

JULY 1970–JUNE 1973

INTRODUCTION

The dazzling infusion of new acronyms under the new Republican Administration by now had made Medicaid's problems seem unimportant, unstylish, and uninteresting. When a President of the United States, renowned for a businesslike approach to social issues, was recommending a guaranteed minimum income for all Americans with a form of national health insurance thrown in, and while others were advocating medical care systems that appeared, gift-wrapped, as the logical outcome of the economic marketplace, Medicaid's existing dilemmas appeared both parochial and transitional.

The new ideas were, indeed, both heady and far-reaching. FHIP offered a quite different construction of the term "welfare medicine" from that of Medicaid. Instead of state-operated programs run on a paternalistic basis, FHIP suggested nationwide entitlements to standard health insurance benefits. Structurally, FHIP was remarkably similar to the early European health insurance schemes stimulated by Bismarck, although it included the nonworking as well as the working poor. HMOs, meanwhile, promised the development of local health care corporations or polyclinics, which would offer an array of services for standard annual premiums, a kind of private taxing and service system at the local level.

It should be remarked, however, that the primary emphasis of the debates in the 91st and 92nd Congresses was not on the actual services to be provided, but on the rhetoric of the alleged philosophies underlying services. Once again, as in the debates leading up to the Medicare legislation, rhetoric was an important vehicle for bridging divergent opinions: the rhetoric of FHIP and HMOs allowed conservatives to embrace what were previously labeled liberal views. A consensus for national health insurance was steadily developing. But at the same time, the process of consensus obscured the practicalities of welfare medicine. While there was a spate of hearings on the need for national health insurance in the 92nd Congress, Medicaid programs continued to be attenuated.

No one can observe Medicaid for long without a sense of schizophrenia. While the latest movement for national health insurance began to bloom, through 1971 and into 1972, Medicaid became even more clearly tied into the welfare process; by 1972 it was little more than the medical arm of the categorical public assistance programs. As in the earlier periods, medical costs rose, while relations with providers deteriorated. There were patchwork aid solutions to attempt to remedy both these problems, but the possibility that the long-term solution might lie in restructuring the providers was not seriously canvassed. The conservative mood of the country continued and was probably accentuated. In both Congress and state legislatures there were demands for further economies, but in almost every case economy meant cutting back still further on the level of eligibility for recipients. The courts, having toyed with the idea of policy-making in the medical care field, beat a strategic retreat.

Yet there was progress in one important respect. After the first flush of enthusiasm for new ideas had evaporated, the federal administration of Medicaid under the Medical Services Administration (MSA) was finally strengthened. The federal bureaucracy, and particularly HEW, may be institutionally incapable of dynamic action. But at least in MSA a real effort was made to provide competent leadership and acceptable day-to-day administration. Regulation of nursing homes and the challenge of implementing the legal requirement (under the 1967 Amendments) for the health screening of children also brought MSA an enlarged role as an enforcement agency. If MSA's pace was slowing as the period ended, it could be attributed more to the crisis created by Watergate than to any inherent weakness in HEW.

But, as before, the real development and administration of Medicaid has continued to depend on the combination of institutions, activities, and conflicting expectations. While MSA has been attempting to develop norms for administration, the particular problems of Medicaid have continued to vary in the states; in this, our last look at the states, we review, in particular, recent developments in Illinois, New York, and California. The courts have continued to play a role in defining and enforcing Medicaid's provisions chiefly from the viewpoint of potential recipients. And last, but by no means least, the Congressional tax committees have continued to provide national surveillance of the program on behalf of federal taxpayers; once again Medicaid was to be tightened administratively, with the passage of the Social Security Amendments of 1972. The interweaving of these various institutional processes forms the substance of this section.

12
Federal Administration

The fate of the Medical Services Administration (MSA) up to 1970 has been cataloged in sad detail. It was despised by other arms of HEW and ignored on Capitol Hill. MSA, in the early days, was small, welfare-oriented, and poorly led; and it had little authority over the states. Commissioner Howard Newman, who arrived in Washington in February 1970, was to go some way toward changing that image. Certainly, in the wake of the Senate Finance Report and the McNerney Report, there was a dramatic increase in staff and effectiveness.

In part, however, the real change was the realization, dramatized in Congressional hearings, that if federal costs were to be contained, there had to be stronger federal direction. While there were, indeed, continuing requests from states for more flexibility in state administration, that was primarily to cut costs; there were few advocates of states' rights pressing for returning welfare medicine to the states. The states were, rather, pressing for federalization. All governmental activities were thus in an upward administrative direction. Medicaid was moving slowly from being a state program with federal subsidy to a program more akin to a federal system with administration delegated to the states. In 1970, this process was just beginning. MSA was in the middle.

New Broom Newman

Specific recommendations for the federal management of Medicaid were, in retrospect, perhaps the most important achievement of the McNerney Task Force, for it was these recommendations, set out in the interim report of November 1969 and expanded in the final report the following June, which provided the impetus for the strengthening of MSA. On the one hand were questions of administrative capability: Medicaid was not only "understaffed from the outset, and inadequately organized and supported to perform the management task required." On the other was a redefinition of management goals: MSA itself was operating under a "mistaken conception of the Federal role required."[1] The early role of "passive monitoring" was demonstrably inadequate. The stage was thus set for major reform.

Taking the need for a new mission as given, the Task Force provided a blueprint for a reformed MSA, with much more active managerial responsibilities. These responsibilities were to include concern with the nature and costs of services being provided under Medicaid. And such concern was to be made operational through the use of Medicaid's purchasing power, and by strengthening the federal government's leadership role *vis-à-vis* the states through cost controls, information systems, standard-setting, and evaluation. In addition, MSA was exhorted to help develop the Medicaid program at state and local levels by providing management training, through identifying and initiating the federal subsidy of projects and programs which improved Medicaid effectiveness, by "specific, prompt and active" guidance to the states on key administration and program policy issues, and through assisting the states in other ways to strengthen their management of the Medicaid program.[2] Significantly, MSA was also urged to make health services more accessible to the needy. In short, MSA was urged to abandon its traditional role of a welfare payments agency, a conduit for money to pass to the states, and became a true "Administration."

To effect these various changes, MSA would have to be expanded and restructured. The McNerney Task Force urged that 125 outstanding positions in the revised budget for fiscal 1970 be filled. But besides this, a reorganization was necessary to focus on the various new tasks. Besides the Commissioner there were to be two new Associate Commissioners, one for "Program" and one for "Administration." Beneath them would be units focussing on program planning and evaluation, operations and standards (to develop regulations and standards for federal, state and local agencies), technical assistance and training, and management information and payment systems.

Finally, while the program reorganization concentrated on strengthening the central administration of MSA, in keeping with Republican instincts, suggestions were also made to strengthen MSA's skeleton staff in the regions. The regional staff's role was to focus on transmitting information from the states to the central office and on interpreting federal guidelines and regulations to the states, to enable states to benefit from technical assistance, and to maintain coordination at the regional level with other HEW programs related to Title XIX. For both the regional offices and the central office, priority was to be given to recruiting staff "with a solid management perspective" together with experience in health administration and other relevant management fields. As a carrot, it was recommended that grade levels within the central office should be raised selectively and that additional "super grades" be created. For watchers on the Hill this last recommendation was perhaps the core of the recommendations, in terms of HEW recognition of Medicaid's status. Taken together, the Task Force proposals for MSA recognized the Cinderella status it had enjoyed. The magic wand would not waft change overnight; but at least the pumpkin had appeared. And the directions for MSA seemed set.

The appointment of Howard Newman as Commissioner was in line with the tone of the Task Force's recommendations.[3] He came into MSA, moreover, with the expectation that the Task Force recommendations would be taken seriously, as indeed they were. Secretary Finch announced the reorganization of MSA along the Task Force lines in March 1970,[4] while Congress finally approved a supplemental appropriation for additional staff.

Staffing, however, continued to be minimal. On Commissioner Newman's arrival in February 1970 MSA had a total of 80 on its staff in Washington, including secretaries, with responsibility for disbursing over $2 billion in federal money. While the HEW reorganization and new leadership promised a new lease on life, and the additional appropriations provided for another 80 persons, a doubling of MSA's staff, there were still only 160 people in MSA in Washington, and these henceforth had the heavy duty of monitoring and managing Medicaid. (As a note of comparison, there were about 800 people running Medi-Cal in Sacramento.) Nevertheless, the time was ripe for change. Under Newman's direction, MSA was reorganized in 1970–71 around the two basic themes of better management and health care delivery. A new management and information systems division was established, to make technical assistance more readily available to the states. At the same time, the procedures for developing policy guidelines and regulations were strengthened.[5]

One further element of importance in stimulating the managerial focus of MSA was a simultaneous movement in HEW, as part of President Nixon's decentralization program, to delegate more responsibility to federal offices outside Washington, in HEW's ten regions. As far as Medicaid had been concerned, the role of the tiny MSA staff in the regions had been anomalous. In its early years the Washington staff of MSA had dealt directly with the states and organized the PREP reports. Lines of communication between states and regions and between regions and Washington were—to say the least—not always clear.

The general move toward decentralization of certain HEW functions to the regional offices in one sense came at a fortuitous time for MSA, in that central and regional reorganization could be considered interdependently. Two important tasks were delegated to the regional offices in 1970: the approval of state Medicaid plans (including amendments to the original plans) and responsibility for undertaking selective reviews of state activities (the PREP reports were abandoned). Both were part of a growing emphasis by MSA, spurred on by the Task Force report and Congressional criticism, to ensure that states were complying with federal requirements. Whether the delegation has worked as well as had been hoped may be seriously doubted; certainly the emphasis on compliance has grown rapidly since 1970 and has been facilitated by a more directive view of the role of the regional office. But the chief reason for the tougher approach was probably that MSA's central office had been strengthened; and it is arguable that, as the regional offices grew larger and stronger, they fitted in less easily with the emphasis on efficient administration at the center. By 1973 there was evidence that those at the center had to bypass the regions in certain matters to insure effective administration.

The various activities to improve MSA's general management formed the groundwork for a more forceful federal role for Medicaid. Other aspects of the reorganization focused on the second series of functions described by the Task Force: the use of Medicaid to influence the health care delivery system. The final report of the Task Force had included an appendix delineating the various functions of the new units in MSA[6]; by the fall of 1971, the "health delivery" aspects of MSA were getting underway. MSA had relatively little money to use for direct experiment, as the Task Force's radical proposal that 5 percent of federal money be set aside had died a rapid death. But although the activities were modest, the seeds were sown. MSA's Office of Program Innovation collected information on Medicaid prepaid contracts in the states.[7] All told, by March 1972 about 280,000 Medicaid enrollees (out of the total caseload of 20 million) were covered through some kind of prepaid arrangement.[8] MSA's own "seed money" has been used for selective purposes: to subsidize experimental Medicaid prepayment arrangements and to fund evaluation projects to see how well such arrangements actually worked.

Meanwhile, the Office of Program Planning and Evaluation began to examine Medicaid's wider aspects. For the first time, MSA had a mandate—or accepted responsibility for such a mandate—to review the relative costs of services provided under Medicaid and to review and stimulate legislative proposals. In August 1971, MSA published an analysis that was appreciably more sophisticated than earlier MSA publications, which had consisted almost entirely of compilations of statistics gathered from the states. The new publication compared the existing provisions of Medicare and Medicaid with the provisions of the most important legislative proposals then before Congress.[9] These included the provisions incorporated into the new House-passed Social Security bill, H.R. 1 of the 92nd Congress and the Administration's bill for family health insurance (FHIP) for the poor with children and for compulsory health insurance for employees.[10] This publication was important in two respects. Not only did it provide valuable information for all those connected with the various proposals, it acted as a symbol of MSA's new authority and direction.

In any event, by the fall of 1971, the first phase of MSA's reorganization under the "New Broom" was about to be succeeded by a second. The first phase had effectively reorganized the central office around revised functions and strengthened the role of MSA in the regions. Efforts had been concentrated on the development of standards, analysis of legislative proposals, and other activities designed to ensure a more active federal role. These ranged from central information-gathering and dissemination (including a new Medicaid newsletter) to the development, under contract, of a model management information system (to be tested in Ohio). Within MSA morale had risen. There was still no doubt a long way to go—there being limits to how far one can transform administrative units[11]—but a healthy start had obviously been made.

But outside MSA, too, the prevailing attitudes toward Medicaid were changing once again, both in Congress and in HEW. While costs continued to be of primary concern, and better management the sometimes simplistic answer, the FHIP proposals had appeared on the scene, and both cost controls and better management were of limited long-term application if FHIP were to become Medicaid's successor. So long as there was an expectation that FHIP might be enacted, the administration of Medicaid could be viewed merely as a stop-gap measure. As the months rolled by, however, the chances for legislative implementation of FHIP receded, as it became clear that welfare reform would not be a major plank in the President's campaign for re-election in 1972. With FHIP's prospects waning and with no immediate prospect of other forms of national health insurance, Medicaid regained importance.

There was by this time a structure by which Medicaid's renewed importance might be focused, but numbers and organizational charts were not the main Newman achievements. What distinguished his administration was that for the first time administrative effectiveness began to appear. While MSA remained a part of the Social and Rehabilitation Service, it slowly shed its aura of being only a part of the Welfare Administration and developed a relatively strong health component. By the end of 1971 MSA was ready for its next phase: to develop an active program not only to set standards for provider participation but to enforce them. Nursing homes provided the opportunity.

Nursing Homes

In Chapter 8 we saw the slow evolution of nursing home regulations. Enforcement of even such regulations as there were, required, however, a rising swell of public opinion that something was indeed wrong with the nursing home industry. Congressman Pryor's description of serious violations of the requirements for nursing home care by Medicare homes provided one dramatic focus for opinion.[12] Continuing audits by the General Accounting Office provided incontrovertible evidence of noncompliance of nursing homes receiving Medicare and Medicaid funds.[13] The nursing home fire in Marietta, Ohio in 1970, in which 32 patients died in a brand-new, licensed facility, gave a tragic illustration of the laxity in enforcing even basic standards.[14] The Nader report on nursing homes, with its added publicity of having been undertaken by a group of girls from a fashionable preparatory school, provoked general public attention.[15] Nearer at hand, a study by MSA of certification procedures in 15 states found that nursing home standards were not being enforced by the state health departments, to which such responsibility had been delegated in each of the 15 cases. Only five of the states had developed a survey form for Title XIX inspection, survey findings were not followed up effectively, and there was insufficient guidance to the states from HEW's regional offices.[16]

Finally, in the summer of 1971, the White House developed its own plan of action for nursing home care. Announced in a speech the President made at a nursing home in New Hampshire on August 6, 1971, the proposals provided the opportunity for developing an enforcement program and the impetus for a major federal effort in reviewing long-term care. The President called for an additional 2000 nursing home inspectors to be trained within an 18-month period. He also announced his intention of asking Congress to authorize the federal government to pay 100 percent of state nursing home inspection costs and to create 100 additional positions for nursing home enforcement at the federal level. Action on nursing homes in HEW was to be consolidated at a single point; investigative units were to be established in states to deal with complaints from nursing home patients; and in HEW there was to be a comprehensive review of the use, standards, and practices of long-term care facilities; short-term training courses were to be established for health workers involved in nursing homes. Finally—and perhaps, most critically—the President emphasized his intention that Medicare and Medicaid funds be cut off from nursing homes that failed to meet reasonable standards.[17]

By no means all of these activities were within the purview of MSA. Indeed, during the period of confusion after the announcement of the President's program, there was an expectation that nursing home inspections would be organized through SSA's district offices (on behalf of Medicare patients), although the staff of these offices had no experience of or actual contact with health care facilities. But the scenario made rapidly increasing MSA activity inevitable. In September 1971, for instance, MSA released a proposed regulation to prevent state boards responsible for licensing nursing home administrators from being stacked with nursing home representatives; they would in the future have to be in the minority.[18]

In October, Marie Callender—a professional nurse, health administrator, and university teacher with respected credentials—was appointed as HEW's Special Assistant for Nursing Home Affairs, thus offering evidence that HEW as a whole was committed to nursing home upgrading. On November 30, HEW Secretary Elliot Richardson announced that federal support would be cut off from substandard nursing homes, effective July 1, 1972, and that by that time each state would have to have completed certification of all skilled nursing homes providing care to Medicaid patients. Homes failing to meet federal Medicaid standards for patient care and safety would no longer be eligible to participate in the Medicaid program.[19] And, just in case further encouragement were needed, the urgency of HEW inspections of patient care in nursing homes was stressed further by a special White House Conference on Aging in November–December 1971 in which some participants recommended that nursing homes should be regulated as "public utilities."[20]

While the date for final compliance was subsequently delayed one month, to July 31, 1972, MSA moved into action at both federal and regional levels. When the regional offices, fortified with additional staff, had gone back to examine certification in the states, 39 states were found to lack adequate procedures.[21] The "New Broom" MSA moved fast. These states were given until February 1, 1972, to establish adequate procedures and were expected to meet the July deadline for full operation. By July 1972, each of the HEW regions included special units set up to deal with nursing home care, a total of 90 persons altogether, who were provided for through special appropriation. An additional three to five persons were also added in each region for medical assistance, and a special unit for long-term care was established at MSA's central office. Thus the number of staff available for compliance purposes rose rapidly.[22] By July 1972 the total authorized strength of MSA had risen to 206 in Washington, together with 150 in the ten regional offices.[23] Long-term care indeed became the focus of MSA attention, possibly to the detriment of other aspects of Medicaid, as the Administration moved to the role of a much more consumer-oriented enforcement agency.

The announcement of the compliance figures for skilled nursing homes in July 1972 marked the apogee of this period for MSA, committed as it was by then to surveillance over nursing homes and to the potential of the threat of the withdrawal of funds from noncomplying homes. As of July 17, 6235 skilled nursing homes were reported as "properly certified." Another 244 were still in the certification process, and 579 (8 percent) had withdrawn from the Medicaid program, voluntarily or through being decertified.[24] As many as 76 percent of the certified homes had, however, only a provisional 6-month approval, instead of approval on the regular 12-month basis. These homes were thus subject to pressures to improve recognized deficiencies, under the threat of decertification.

In some areas, low-standard nursing homes were legendary. A particularly black spot was New York, where investigation proceeded rapidly.[25] As of July 1972, that state had certified 270 facilities and had moved to decertify another 222, including 189 which thereupon entered a court action to block decertification.[26] A court restraining order was in effect in Ohio, through the Ohio Nursing Home Association[27]; and seven nursing home licenses were revoked in Connecticut.[28]

The abuse of earlier effective enforcement was demonstrated only too clearly in Oklahoma's reaction. In that state there were some 300 nursing homes, of which as many as 220 could not meet the skilled nursing home requirements, including basic life-safety (fire) standards.[29] The old question was raised of what would happen to persons in these homes if federal Medicaid funds were not forthcoming; compliance appeared, in some respects, at odds with service. To deal with this latter aspect, the public welfare director of Oklahoma, Lloyd Rader, sent a message to all the affected homes informing them that they could continue as intermediate care facilities—for which there were as yet no definitions or requirements as to standards—and at the same time upped the reimbursement rates for ICFs to that of skilled nursing homes under Medicaid.[30] As a result of the Oklahoma pressures, exerted through key administration figures, the provisions transferring ICFs to Medicaid were pulled out of H.R. 1 by the Congress and enacted separately, effective January 1972.[31] Thus at one fell swoop, MSA became responsible for approving virtually all homes with nursing care in the United States which accepted any welfare or medically indigent patient. From being an agency traditionally involved with purchasing care, MSA was becoming a potentially powerful enforcement agency.

The addition of ICFs to the Medicaid program—while MSA was still surveying the skilled nursing homes—was important in several respects. Federal standards had not been defined under Title XI, the title under which the ICF was previously incorporated. The transfer to Title XIX was accompanied by specifications that federal standards would be developed. MSA thus had to indicate what kinds and levels of care would be covered. At the same time, on transfer to Title XIX, the ICF program was extended to include eligibility for the medically indigent as well as those on cash assistance; this was thus a potentially huge program. A preliminary survey found 34 states with approved ICF programs as of December 1971, but the program was small: There were only 167,000 patients in ICFs throughout the United States.[32] How—and how quickly—they developed would depend on the provisions developed by MSA.

Quite apart from size and lack of regulations, there was the more fundamental question, which had been shelved while definitions were left to the states, of what, indeed, is "intermediate care," compared with skilled nursing care on the one hand and institutional housing on the other. At the same time, there were other immediate questions arising from MSA responsibility. The Oklahoma case raised the specter of what might happen if MSA insisted on the same safety requirements for ICFs as for skilled nursing homes: Who would foot what might prove to be a considerable construction and renovation bill? Care of the mentally retarded added a new area of responsibility which MSA had not so far handled; again, definitions were required. Reimbursement was also at issue. In some states, ICF reimbursement to some homes was higher than reimbursement to other homes in the skilled nursing home category; should there be a fixed reimbursement differential? Finally, there were administrative questions, such as whether a particular nursing home could be recognized as both a skilled nursing home and an ICF and, if so, whether special ICF units would be required or whether the distinction would be by individual patient.[33] In all of these respects, MSA was acting as a health-planning agency.

These questions, together with those of surveillance of skilled nursing homes, were discussed at a series of meetings within HEW and with representatives of the nursing home industry in the early months of 1972. No regulations had been issued by July 1972. But it appeared that efforts would be made to require standards for ICF facilities to be similar to those for skilled nursing homes, while the requirements for staffing would probably be different.[34] At the end of 1972, indeed, it looked as if there would be some federalized form of certification for all types of nursing homes with any patients for whom the homes received vendor payments, and this was further stimulated by the Social Security Amendments of that year that effectively assimilated the certification and compliance requirements for extended care facilities under Medicare and skilled nursing homes under Medicaid. In terms of services, there was even talk of a federal requirement that all nursing homes have "an organized medical staff."[35]

With the slowing down of government during 1973, however, the Administration interest in nursing homes appeared to wane.[36] Whereas, in 1971, President Nixon had declared that federal funds "should not go into substandard nursing homes," by mid-1973 the Administration appeared reluctant to crack down on Pennsylvania. That state, with many nonconforming state-run and county-run nursing homes, used every loophole to avoid Medicaid regulations. While the HEW Regional Office in Philadelphia urged the cut-off of funds, supported by at least some of the Medicaid establishment in Washington, at Cabinet level it looked as if Pennsylvania's bluff would not be called.[37] The effective control over nursing homes was thus far from firmly established.

Early and Periodic Screening

The nursing home activities involved MSA in two types of regulation: encouraging state health departments to enforce certification requirements for Medicaid in each state and insuring that the states enforce the federal standards, by threatening to withhold federal funds to homes found to be out of compliance. At the same time federal officials were attempting to go beyond the basic standards of safety and staffing in a determined effort to appraise the quality of medical care.[38] In no sense, however, did these procedures attempt to inquire whether the number, types, and services of nursing homes available to the needy in a state were in fact meeting the needs for care.

Such an activity was, however, central to another set of activities in which MSA was involved by 1972. The development and implementation of regulations for early and periodic screening, diagnosis, and treatment (EPSDT) of needy children under the age of 21, as required by the 1967 Social Security Amendments, brought MSA squarely into the arena of the direct provision of health care. For the gist of the requirement, which added a new mandatory category to Medicaid, effective July 1, 1969, was to discover all eligible children who needed care.[39] For eligible children, Medicaid was to "ascertain their physical or mental defects, and such health care, treatment, and other measures to correct or ameliorate defects and chronic conditions discovered thereby, as may be provided for in regulations of the Secretary."[40]

In the fashion which was the norm for the MSA of the late 1960s, the date for implementation of this program came and went with nothing having been done. Legal advice had been taken. Apparently MSA had been advised by HEW's general counsel's office that the wording of the legislation implied that no action would be taken until there were regulations; therefore, as they had issued no regulations, no action was necessary. While this was a piece of legal sophistry that probably few federal courts would have been willing to accept, the fact that the delay in implementing the program was not tested in the courts suggests that behind the scenes there were trade-offs between the welfare rights groups and HEW, although the reason given for heel-dragging by MSA was that HEW was loath to pose additional financial burdens on the states.[41]

"Tentative" regulations for early screening were finally issued by SRS on October 30, 1970, 16 months after the program was supposed to have been implemented. The proposed regulations were approved by Secretary Richardson on December 3, 1970, and were finally published in the *Federal Register* on December 11.[42] Still regarded as tentative, they pinpointed the enormous potential scope of Medicaid in this area of preventive medicine. A moral issue was also at stake: Was it enough to discover disease, or should there be a commitment by the state to treat it? The tentative regulations allowed for both early periodic screening and diagnosis of eligible individuals under 21 by July 1, 1973, as well as treatment of the conditions discovered, regardless of the limits imposed by Medicaid under the appropriate state plan. Although in one respect the requirements were narrow —initial concentration was to be in the age group from birth to 6 years—

treatment was to be available widely. This meant, in effect, that at least some states would be required to enter the business of child health services for the poor on a massive scale. As such seemed to be implied by the 1967 legislation, it was not surprising that this Pandora's box had been opened only slowly. The proposals elicited complaints about costs not only from states but also from the federal Office of Management and Budget.

But as far as MSA was concerned, help was at hand from an impeccable authority. On December 11, 1970, the same day that the controversial regulation was issued, the Senate Finance Committee issued its report on H.R. 17550, the Social Security Amendments of 1970.[43] Mindful of the costs of Medicaid, the Finance Committee proposed an amendment to the bill, which would amend the screening requirements before they were implemented. The bill would give initial priority to the provision of screening, diagnosis, and treatment to young children in states that found it difficult to provide services to the entire eligible population under 21. While H.R. 17550 became bogged down in the 91st Congress, there seemed to be a clear message from Congress that a less sweeping implementation of the screening regulation would be acceptable.[44]

It was in this context—which could be labeled either "dishonest" or "realistic," depending on one's point of view—that the regulations were revised. But, for once, children had less political appeal in the United States than the elderly—or at least, poor children compared with everybody's elderly relatives—and screening took a back seat to nursing home care.[45] It was not until November 1971, almost three years after the legislation was enacted, that the final regulations were issued.[46] But by this time, MSA was gathering steam. Although the regulations were narrower than the earlier proposal in some respects, their administrative implications were immense.

The regulations confirmed that states had to provide early and periodic screening and treatment to all eligible children under six and to develop a plan to include all children under 21 by July 1, 1973. The treatment to be provided was less sweeping than in the "tentative" regulations: it had to include only those services available within the limits of the state Medicaid plan, together with needed eye and ear care (including eyeglasses and hearing aids), and dental care, whether or not these were included in the state plan.[47] But here at least was the go-ahead for a much expanded role for MSA in ensuring the provision of health care to 6 million youthful recipients.[48]

The go-ahead for early and periodic screening, diagnosis and treatment, even though coming rather late, put MSA for the first time into the business of preventive medicine. More than that, it put the administration into the position of affirmatively requiring medical services, instead of policing the margins of minimal service. In effect a federal agency was finally in the business of ensuring the provision of minimal care for a section of the whole population. There have been federal programs for specific segments of the population before—for the armed forces, merchant seamen, Indians, and migrant workers—and demonstration projects, such as OEO-funded health centers, for limited general groups. But early and periodic screening, diagnosis, and treatment was a step altogether different in kind and style. The welfare administration of old would not have recognized the new Medical Services Administration.[49]

Nor did the general guidelines see screening as something perfunctory.[50] States were "actively to seek out eligible individuals," the primary target groups being children in families already receiving, or eligible for, Medicaid. Where necessary, interpreters were to be provided, and help was to be given to families in seeking appropriate medical care; service was to range from helping people overcome fear of doctors to providing necessary transportation to facilities. States were urged to work toward the development of coordinated, integrated evaluation processes and health care systems, drawing on the resources of a variety of private and public programs and agencies (with whom the states were to have written agreements). Procedures for reporting and monitoring were outlined.[51]

It is not yet clear what the actual "clout" of MSA will be in guaranteeing that Medicaid children do in fact receive these services; the program began slowly. By mid-1973 some states had yet to comply effectively with the regulations, although the pressure on them was mounting.[52] Perhaps of most significance, as with nursing home regulation, was the threat of withholding of funds, a threat made potentially more effective for screening through the Social Security Amendments of 1972.[53] At least states could be forced to meet basic compliance standards.[54] The states might now find themselves in the position of having to provide basic health services; and, to the surprise of some, it was the southern states, whose health departments were accustomed to providing services, which greeted the prospect with the most equanimity. It is now, however, open to MSA to insist that the states make EPSDT available. If this line of development is followed, MSA could well find itself in the center of health-planning activities. The long-term directions of the program are still, however, open questions.[55]

And May We All Participate?

These activities, strengthening MSA's authority and opening direct lines between a federal welfare structure and a state health department, stemmed from two sets of developments; nursing home regulation from a spate of concern about safety in Congress and the administration, and child health screening from concern about the care available to children. As with previous movements in welfare medicine, the most effective actions focused on the two extremes of the old and the young. But MSA did not, of course, operate in a vacuum. Despite all the internal and external efforts to make it appear more as a health than a welfare administration, it remained an integral part of and a division of Social and Rehabilitation Service. As such, it was caught up in many of the "target areas" of SRS. One of these target areas of SRS in the early 1970s—in a belated response to the pressures of the late 1960s—was community participation. As this was usually taken to mean community participation by articulate adults of working age, another whole area of concern was opened up simultaneously.

During the 1960s, there was increasing public acceptance of the fact that the United States was not a perfect democracy. The Supreme Court and Congress sought to ensure that the franchise could be exercised by blacks and other minorities. In the field of welfare, there was a movement to ameliorate the worst aspects of paternalism, Part of this movement was the attempt to improve the system of "fair hearings" and thus to protect entitlements under existing legislation. Another facet led to the movement to substitute some form of negative income tax for categorical public assistance, discussed in the following chapter. The third manifestation was in the movement for "community participation."

One does not need data from detailed empirical studies to explain the reasons behind the community participation movement. The sense of despair in the ghettos was so great that it burst forth into riots in the blighted cities during the late 1960s. The idea of harnessing this energy for creative ends was clearly a high priority. And—at a different level in a different area—the element of patronizing paternalism in the outpatient departments of the hospitals and in those other places where the poor received their medical care cried out for eradication. One question that might have arisen was whether these two different problems—the need to revitalize the cities and the need to change the charity aura of medical care—were susceptible to the same solution, as SRS appeared to think. The different facets of community representation and participation were, however, not clearly differentiated.

In the 1960s it was assumed by a number of articulate spokesmen that community participation was the solution to virtually all social problems. Nurtured in its early years by the Ford Foundation, with such programs as CPI in New Haven, community participation expanded when the Economic Opportunity Act of 1964 took up the cudgels (and provided the cash) to fund Community Action programs.[56] Ultimately OEO's Poverty Program developed more than 1,000 Community Action projects,[57] and it was inevitable that at least a few of these would attempt to come to grips with welfare medicine. These community action programs[58] rapidly legitimized the requirement of "maximum feasible participation," as OEO moved to develop other programs, including health centers. But the belief in local control (or community control as it came to be known) went well beyond the confines of poverty programs.[59]

Although the medical establishment and government had often failed in the quality and tenor of medical care provided to the poor, the community participation movement became in some respects a misleading panacea. In the area of health, this was perhaps most clearly illustrated by a group of radical medical students in New York, known as Health-PAC.[60] They took a position which seemed to suggest that a community-medical worker alliance would itself solve America's health problems.[61] Some of the rhetoric assumed that the nationwide professional monopolies would dissolve and cash and manpower shortages would disappear, once community representatives were added to various health committees. Local black communities in New York, for instance, were presumed to be able to evaluate manpower policies by hiring and paying physicians, nurses, and other health personnel—decisions which indirectly affected not only the lives of physicians in Illinois but surburban communities in California and, as health manpower is international (with a rapidly increasing number of physicians and others coming from the less developed countries),[62] rural communities in the Philippines and Tanzania.

To pretend that local community boards could have a serious effect on national health policy was from one point of view a cruel deception; from another, yet one more delaying tactic in the continuing groping for a common definition of the governmental role in medicine. But, worse still, the movement seriously undermined the legitimate role for participation—to make the provision of health care more humane and more responsive to local conditions. There was a need to publicize and ameliorate the often shocking conditions to be found in urban medicine; and where community representatives advised local programs, much was often achieved. The Ghetto Medicine Program in New York made considerable strides in improving the psychological atmosphere in the 22 voluntary hospitals where it existed,[63] although there is little to suggest that (publicity apart) the sit-ins attempted by local community groups to achieve control of community health planning agencies achieved anything more than further disintegration in New York City's Health Services Administration.[64]

Nevertheless, belief in community participation in policy making had its supporters in the Medical Services Administration;[65] and there is evidence that MSA, too, failed to distinguish between the need to involve recipients to improve the atmosphere of "welfare medicine" and the danger of misleading recipient groups into thinking that they would be given ultimate control over taxpayers' money.[66] For instance, during 1971, a Study Group on Consumer Involvement was set up within SRS to write a handbook, it having been determined that consumer participation would be a "priority program" for fiscal 1973.

Ignoring the failures in such programs as the Gray Areas and Mobilization for Youth, the idea of consumer participation in policy-making was pushed by some in SRS and MSA, picking up a comment in the McNerney

Report which had also failed to distinguish between consultation and policy-making. As one observer of the process in SRS put it: "It is so much easier to ramble on about 'the community' and 'consumer involvement' than it is to face thinking about taking on the AMA or about how to convince Congress that this step must be taken if good medical care for everyone is to be a reality."[67]

Eventually MSA considered various possible areas of consumer involvement. In the end all turned out to be of the consultative type, where providers had to account to recipients, rather than the involvement-in-policy-making variety. First, there was a suggestion that all states should follow the example of Virginia and send patients a statement of "their" Medicaid "account," so that they could check the accuracy of the statement and the veracity of providers. Second, there has been some support for a nursing home ombudsman in each state, but failing that, the idea was mooted of establishing patient organizations in nursing homes, or having patient advocates in nursing homes.[68]

The reaction of the SRS Regional Commisioners to the SRS *Handbook* are thought to have been negative perhaps because the objective remained one of implying participation in policy-making. So too, it is believed that MSA's enthusiasm for 51 percent consumer representation on Medical Advisory Committees[69] met with some "sales resistance" in the different states. In March 1971, nationwide, only 4 percent of Medical Advisory Committee members were actual Medicaid recipients;[70] and while public welfare administrators generally seemed to think that having recipients on Advisory Committees was a good thing, the effectiveness of the committees themselves was in some doubt.[71] Far from bringing recipients into the decision-making process, there was still an inability to consult them on needs and problems. The overselling of "consumer participation" seemed to have undermined the far more legitimate goal of "consumer consultation," and thus deferred consideration of actual needs. The message was apparently not lost on those on Capitol Hill, where action on Medicaid was being assessed, yet again, in the Congressional progress of the latest Social Security Amendments.

Most Recent Developments

While MSA was becoming better organized and more powerful, it was still, then, dependent on a variety of shock waves from outside: whether these were the result of powerful Congressional interests or the translation into action of new rhetoric, such as "community participation." There was little doubt that MSA was a more effective body than it had been, with far more effective leadership, but it was still caught up in the broader work of SRS and could still waste energy in developing policies that might be irrelevant to the main thrust of its work. The real problem, though, continued to be that there was no one "main thrust," but rather a series of different activities. Nursing home regulation, child health screening, and consumer involvement were going on all at once.

Furthermore, MSA was not only a bureau within SRS, it was an integral part of HEW. Thus, during the period it was also caught up in all the other movements generated by the Secretary's Office. From 1968 onwards, there was an increasing emphasis on management efficiency. Pressure was exerted to see that there was at least some coordination between Medicare and Medicaid.[72] Development of this emphasis further strengthened MSA's administrative role. Audit findings led to the addition of 420 positions in SRS, supposedly to recoup $400 million of federal funds improperly spent by the states on welfare programs. MSA was supposed to be given 75 of these positions, and by the summer of 1972 it was beginning to gear up for stricter fiscal accountability.

Over-all, then, there was a sense that, at least, MSA had some policies. The fact that at least one of its major thrusts, that of nursing home regulation, developed largely through extramural pressures does not deny this point. Given its history as a relatively timid welfare agency, MSA needed a major outside stimulus to develop a tougher image. The focus on management paid dividends. Regulations, while still tardy, at least appeared. And while PREP Reports were abandoned, a regular system of compliance reports was instituted. Failure to comply with any aspect of the Title XIX Program was noted monthly. Failure to comply on some matter for two consecutive months led to political pressure on the state concerned from the Secretary's office. The change was almost Thurberian: "Man bites dog."

The situation must not be overstated. There are several limitations on what an administration within HEW can actually do to bully a state, which may well have a governor with "clout" at the White House or influential congressmen on the Hill. But Newman and the group of senior officials he had gathered around him in MSA were certainly not lacking in ideas for control. Perhaps the most interesting, and certainly the most important development, was with respect to the selective cut-off of funds. As long as MSA is given the mandate to wield this weapon, as in the case of nursing homes and of screening procedures, its authority should increase.

Again, however, it has to be emphasized that MSA remained a part of HEW and was thus subjected to its changing influences and attitudes. The replacement, for instance, in 1972 of Secretary Elliot Richardson by Secretary Casper Weinberger heralded a further emphasis on efficiency and decreasing concern with the humanitarian aspects of social programs. With the help of Booz, Allen and Hamilton, the health side of HEW was scheduled for reorganization,[73] but the Medical Services Administration remained for all practical purposes on the welfare side. As efficiency became ever more the watchword, the rhetoric also changed. There was increasing evidence that the Weinberger administration was less interested in the fate of nursing homes and less committed to HMOs. Utilization review or "peer review" appeared as "top of the pops" for cost-saving. This changing attitude undoubtedly slowed the initiative of MSA. Further regional devolution was also having its impact in terms of MSA's implementation of its decisions; it was unclear how much muscle the new secretary was prepared to put behind programs like EPSDT.[74]

In late 1972 there was a further slowing-down process. After President Nixon's re-election in November, he called for the resignation of most senior officials in all departments, including, of course, HEW.[75] What the effect of this might have been if these persons had been replaced according to plan is unclear. Unfortunately, before new appointments could be made, the country was plunged into the Watergate crisis, and it was not until mid-1973 that many of these appointments came to be made. Again the effect was to retard momentum. By mid-1973, there was a danger that MSA, among others, might revert to its pre-1970 lethargy.

NOTES

1. *McNerney Interim Report*, p. 27.

2. *Ibid.*, pp. 31–35 and *passim*.

3. Newman's background was in hospital administration, law, and government work as a White House Fellow and in the Budget Bureau.

4. *Federal Register*, vol. 35, 1970, p. 4660.

5. It will be remembered that the early interpretation of P.L. 89–97 by MSA was transmitted to the states through *Supplement D* of the *Handbook of Public Assistance Administration;* see previous chapters. After the 1967 Amendments, MSA began to put proposed and final regulations into the *Federal Register* format. Following the usual federal procedure, a regulation is published initially as interim policy or "proposed rule-making," for comment and critique by interested groups. The regulation takes effect when published in its final form in the *Federal Register*. For a while the *Federal Register* format and Supplement D existed side by side, but the latter was subsequently phased out and now has historic interest only. MSA continues to issue policy interpretations to its regional offices and to the states, as well as informational memoranda and other documentation, but these form a separate administrative process from that of the writing and promulgation of regulations.

6. U.S., Department of Health, Education, and Welfare, *Task Force on Medicaid and Related Programs,* 1970, pp. 119–126. Two units had responsibility for the "health" aspects of Medicaid. The Office of Program Planning and Evaluation was to evaluate and explain the mission, goals, and objectives of Title XIX; to measure program performance against agreed objectives and standards; to develop policies and plans for coordinating the financing aspects of the Medicaid program; and to coordinate its own activities with HEW policy-making organizations and with other government and private agencies. The Office of Program Innovation was given a less global task, but one which was

no less ambitious. Basically, this office was to encourage experiments with incentives designed to improve health delivery systems, to analyze alternative concepts for health care (including health maintenance organizations), and to forward any other schemes which promised to improve health services or reduce the disparity in services provided among the states.

7. The oldest Medicaid prepaid contract was that between New York City and the Health Insurance Plan of Greater New York (HIP). This arrangement had begun in 1966, and by 1972 it included 80,000 Medicaid enrollees.

8. U.S., Department of Health, Education, and Welfare, Medical Services Administration, *Medicaid HMO-Type Contracts,* Mar. 1972.

9. U.S., Department of Health, Education, and Welfare, Medical Services Administration, *Health Care Financing Programs and Proposals,* Aug. 1971.

10. The National Health Insurance Partnership Act of 1971, S 1623, included both the FHIP proposals and a new scheme that would require employers to participate in, and subsidize, a standard employer-employee health insurance plan. This latter proposal, embodied in the National Health Insurance Standards Act, would have established a benefit package of basic and catastrophic insurance coverage for eligible workers and their dependents. It was expected to cover three fourths of all U.S. workers and their families. Beneficiaries would have the option of having care provided through a health maintenance organization, assuming one was available in the area.

11. In connection with the philosophical implications of such developments, see Herbert Kaufman, *The Limits of Organization Change,* Alabama, 1971.

12. *Congressional Record,* Vol. 116, pp. 19268, 25481, 27036 (1970).

13. Between October 1969 and April 1970 alone, GAO surveyed 90 Medicaid skilled nursing homes, of which 33 were also extended care facilities under Medicare. Of the 33, whose standards were presumably higher, 8 were deficient in nursing services, 12 were not providing physician visits every 30 days (required under Medicare), 5 were not providing social services, and there were a number of other violations. U.S., Office of the Comptroller-General, Report to the Congress, *Problems in Providing Proper Care to Medicare and Medicaid Patients in Skilled Nursing Homes,* No. B-164031 (3), May 28, 1971, pp. 9740–42.

14. Actually, fire regulations were one area at the time where the Medicaid requirements were stronger than those for Medicare; the latter were subsequently revised. The circumstances of the fire are dealt with in the Nader report. Claire Townsend *et al., Old Age: The Last Segregation* (New York, 1970), p. 63.

15. *Ibid.*

16. U.S., Department of Health, Education, and Welfare, Medical Services Administration, *Report on the Skilled Nursing Home Certification Project,* August 1971.

17. Reported in MSA *Medicaid* (newsletter), October 1971.

18. *Federal Register,* vol. 36, 1971, p. 18106 (Proposed Regulation).

19. SRS, *HEW News,* June 30, 1972.

20. U.S., White House Conference on Aging, 1971, *Health Care Strategies* (1971), pp. 5–6.

21. Deficiencies were listed under five categories: written agreements between the State Medicaid agencies and the survey agency (11 states not complying); application of federal Medicaid standards (20 states); written agree-

ments between State Medicaid agencies and skilled nursing homes receiving Medicaid payments (13 states); establishment of time requirements, six months for those with "correctable deficiencies" (25 states); and other required procedures, including ascertaining that facilities were actually licensed by the state licensing authority (all 39 of the deficient states). MSA, *Medicaid,* January 1972, p. 2.

22. Concern over nursing homes led Congress to authorize and appropriate funds for 150 new positions for nursing home standards enforcement. Eight of these went to SSA, the remainder to SRS (i.e., MSA). Of the SRS positions, 110 were allocated to the regional offices, and 32 to MSA. *Ibid.*

23. Personal communications, MSA.

24. A total of 28,000 patients were involved in the skilled nursing homes that were decertified (27) or withdrew (252). Of these, 16,000 were transferred to the ICF category (almost all in New York), 3000 sent to other skilled nursing homes, and the remainder were subject to a variety of arrangements. Information from MSA.

25. *New York Times,* Nov. 11, 1972, p. 27.

26. For New York's problems in attempting to decertify these homes, see *Bacon v. Levine,* App. Div., 1973, CCH, *Medicare and Medicaid Guide,* para. 26,626; *Maxwell Nursing Home v. Levine,* App. Div., 1973, *Ibid.,* para. 26,652; *Gables Nursing Home v. Levine,* App. Div., 1973, *Ibid.,* para. 26,653; *Cedar Ridge Nursing Home v. Levine,* App. Div., 1973, *Ibid.,* para. 26,654. In general, the courts were reluctant to allow a waiver, once given, to be cancelled unless it was proved that the health and safety of the patient would suffer.

27. Personal communication, MSA.

28. *New Haven Register,* Nov. 4, 1972, p. 38, col. 8.

29. Personal communication, MSA.

30. A demonstration grant was requested, to demonstrate the feasibility of transforming 90 of the homes to ICFs, but legislative approval for this was still pending as part of H.R. 1.

31. P.L. 92–233, Sec. 4, provides for the inclusion of care in an intermediate care facility as an optional service under Medicaid. The Section repealed Sec. 1121 of the Social Security Act. The Act defines an ICF as an institution offering health-related care and services to individuals who do not require care and treatment in a hospital or skilled nursing home, but who do require institutional care above the level of room and board. To be approved for Medicaid an institution must be licensed by the state, meet standards of care prescribed by the Secretary of HEW, and meet any other prescribed standards of safety and sanitation. ICF services may also include those provided in a public institution for the mentally retarded, subject to certain conditions.

The new proposed regulations for ICFs appeared at 38 *Federal Register* 5974 (1973).

32. MSA, *Medicaid,* Feb. 1972, p. 5.

33. Personal communication, MSA.

34. One "loophole" may be the continuance of some federal subsidy to noncomplying homes through the cash assistance titles. Cash assistance recipients have to live somewhere.

35. *New York Times,* Nov. 12, 1972, p. 61, col. 3.

36. For instance, in July 1972, Undersecretary Veneman opined that "although the President has exercised bold leadership, frontline responsibility for

running homes under the law still rests with the states." CCH, *Medicare & Medicaid Guide*, para. 26,489.

37. *Washington Post*, June 17, 1973, p. F8. On July 10, however, it was announced that any SNF that did not meet federal regulations by September 1 would have its funds cut off. Moreover, it was made clear that if Pennsylvania did not make more diligent efforts with its SNFs, all Medicaid funds would be cut off. HEW, *News Release*, July 10, 1973.

38. By the summer of 1972, staff at the regional offices of the HEW were checking procedures in the states in five basic areas delineated by MSA: medical review (whether in fact physicians were seeing patients once a month), utilization review procedures, home health services (whether these were available as an alternative form of care), the application of Title VI (Civil Rights) legislation, and standards for reimbursement. MSA, personal communication.

39. The origin of the requirement was President Johnson's Message on the Welfare of Children of February 8, 1967. In a series of proposals for improving child care under the Social Security system came the need to identify as yet untreated children who needed help.

40. Sec. 1905 (a) (4) (B), as amended by P.L. 90–248.

41. MSA, personal communication.

42. *Federal Register*, Vol. 35, 1970, p. 18878 (Proposed Regulation).

43. U.S., Congress, Senate, Committee on Finance, *Manganese Ore-Suspension of Duties—Social Security Benefits*, Senate Report No. 91-933 to Accompany H.R. 14720, 91st Cong., 2nd Sess., 1970.

44. Interestingly, H.R. 1, which ultimately became P.L. 92–603 in October 1972, did not provide any definitions as to who was to be covered or for what; although, as we shall see (see note 53, this chapter) it did give MSA "clout" by allowing a reduction of federal AFDC matching funds to states that had failed to inform adults in AFDC families of such services or had failed to provide such services. By this time there appeared to be a tacit understanding that child screening applied only to children in AFDC families rather than to all poor children in the state.

45. See, for instance, Rep. William Ryan (Dem., N.Y.): "It's starkly clear that the more than 6 million children who would fall under the operation of the Department of Health, Education, and Welfare's regulation—if only it were formally promulgated—desperately need medical care. They are the forgotten victims of a society which applauds rhetoric, but is remiss in action." *Congressional Record*, vol. 117, col. H 8564 (1971).

46. CFR, 249.10. The regulations were to become effective 90 days after publication, i.e., on February 7, 1972. *Federal Register*, vol. 36, 1971, p. 21409.

47. The state could, however, impose utilization controls on these services.

48. In all 52 Medicaid jurisdictions, children under 21 were covered under AFDC arrangements, when at least one parent was dead, absent, or incapacitated; 30 states included children in families where the father was unemployed; 37 states included children in foster care; and 17 states included all financially eligible children under 21, irrespective of family characteristics, institutionalization, or foster-care placement. Of the 52 jurisdictions, 27 included the medically indigent, as well as those on or eligible for cash assistance. U.S., Department of Health, Education, and Welfare, *Medicaid Children: Who are They?* MSA-804-71, June 30, 1971. Alaska and Arizona had no Medicaid programs as of this date.

49. As to the significance of this new departure, see The Health Law Project, University of Pennsylvania Law School and the National Health Law

Program, University of California School of Law, *Materials on Health Law,* vol. 5, *Medicaid,* 1972 ed., p. 295.

50. The screening itself has to include a full health history, an analysis of physical growth, developmental assessment, unclothed physical inspection, ear, nose, mouth, and throat inspection, vision testing, hearing testing, anemia testing, sickle cell, TB, urine and lead-poisoning testing, as well as nutritional and immunization status reports.

51. U.S., Department of Health, Education, and Welfare, Medical Services Administration, *Medicaid, Early and Periodic Screening, Diagnosis, Treatment for Individuals under 21, Guidelines,* June 28, 1972. For an idea of the potential in the dental care, see Howard N. Newman, "*Early and Periodic Screening, Diagnosis and Treatment of Medicaid Children: The Dental Health Aspects,*" mimeograph (Speech to American Dental Association, March 26, 1973).

52. New York tried to link implementation with prepaid programs. *New York Times,* July 14, 1972, p. 26. Vermont felt the medical resources of the state were so sparse it would have to hire its own physicians to implement EPSDT. Mississippi, for instance, began experimenting with the program before it became mandatory, with dramatic results: 1300 abnormalities were discerned in the first 1200 children screened. Howard M. Newman, "The Challenge and Potential of EPSDT," speech delivered at Regional Conference on EPSDT, Chicago, March 6, 1973, p. 2, mimeographed.

53. P.L. 92–603, Sec. 299F, provides that the federal share of AFDC matching funds will be reduced by 1 percent, beginning in fiscal 1975, if a state fails to inform adults in AFDC families of the availability of child health screening services, fails to provide such services, or fails to arrange for appropriate corrective treatment.

54. In June 1972, 26 states were out of compliance with the EPSDT requirements. PL 92–603, however, with its provision for a 1 percent decrease in AFDC funds for these states which failed to implement EPSDT, had its effect. By March 1973 only 11 states had not begun EPSDT programs. Newman, "*The Challenge and Potential of EPSDT,*" *supra,* note 52, p. 5.

55. The provisions for effective EPSDT have, however, begun to mount. The National Welfare Rights Organization (NWRO) issued material designed "to see that each state has a good EPSDT plan." Moreover, there were WRO plans for working with providers' groups and, as far as possible, taking control of EPSDT programs. In some states, for instance Pennsylvania, such pressures appeared to be successful, at least in the sense that local welfare groups achieved the right to be consulted and to be represented on appropriate committees. In other states—e.g. Michigan—successful litigation was instituted to insure that state plans were effective. In *Dominguez v. Miliken* (W.D. Mich., 1973), a federal district court had no difficulty in holding that Michigan had to provide EPSDT for all children under 6 and to outline a program for all those under 21 by July 1, 1973. CCH, *Medicare & Medicaid Guide,* par. 26,632.

56. 42 U.S.C. § 2808. See William Benjamin, *Participation of the Poor in the Community Action Program: Another Perspective, 1969* (paper presented at the Yale Law School).

57. Some criticized the programs because they were too readily controlled by existing political forces and did not aid the very people for whose benefit they were created. Note, "Participation of the Poor: Section 202 (a) (3) Organizations under the Economic Opportunity Act of 1964," *Yale Law Journal,* vol. 75 (1966), p. 599; Edgar S. Cahn and Jean C. Cahn, "The War on Poverty: A

Civilian Perspective," *Ibid.*, vol. 73 (1964), p. 1317. Others criticized the program because they perceived it as a mindless response to a serious political problem. Daniel P. Moynihan, *Maximum Feasible Misunderstanding: Community Action in the War on Poverty* (New York, 1969), *passim.*

58. Economic Opportunity Act, 1964, § 202 (a) (3); P.L. 88–492; 78 Stat. 516 (1964).

59. *Op. cit.*, 57, *supra.* In the late 1960s, it became a rallying cry for the alienated upper-middle-class radical students, who, as Moynihan analyzed it, sought to assuage guilt about their paternalistic attitudes by seeking nominal involvement of the poor in their schemes.

60. Their arguments became sufficiently fashionable that they appeared in the *New York Review of Books.*

61. See especially, Barbara Ehrenreich and John Ehrenreich, *The American Health Empire: Power, Profits and Politics* (New York, 1971), Ch. XIX.

62. Rosemary Stevens and Joan Vermeulen, *Foreign Trained Physicians and American Medicine,* DHEW Pub. No. (NIH) 73–325, June 1972.

63. Lowell Bellin, Florence Kavaler, and Al Schwarz, *Phase One of Consumer Participation in Policies of 22 Voluntary Hospitals in New York City: A Non-Polemic Analysis of First Year's Experience of Ambulatory Care Advisory Committee,* mimeograph (1971).

64. *New York Times,* August 31, 1971.

65. M.S.A. also had statutory responsibilities in the area. § 1902 (a) (4), added by Sec. 210 (a) (b) of the Social Security Amendments of 1967 mandated some element of community participation:

> *For the training and effective use of paid subprofessional staff, with particular emphasis on the full and part-time employment of recipients and other persons of low income as community aides, in the administration of the plan, and for the use of non-paid and partially paid volunteers in social service volunteer programs in providing services to applicants and recipients, and in assisting any advisory committees established by the state agency.*

66. Hilary Sue Green, *Consumer Involvement in Medicaid: A Reconsideration,* 1972 (a paper presented at the Yale Law School).

67. *Ibid.*, p. 4. The ideal was set forth in the U.S., Department of Health, Education, and Welfare, Social and Rehabilitation Service, *Consumer Involvement Handbook* (1971): "The major goal of SRS is to aid the individual to return or regain his ability for self-care and self-determination—. . . From the point of view of the consumer-client, therefore, the most decisive and immediately apparent form of significant involvement in the agency's program is his own active participation in the determination of what services he needs and may receive through the community program from which he is seeking help."

68. A report by Otto Reid and others found that 10–15 percent of recipients are misinformed about their rights under Medicaid. 53 percent of these who might be eligible as "medically indigent" did not know about Medicaid programs in their states. Cited, Green, *supra,* note 66, pp. 7–8.

69. *AMA News,* Feb. 21, 1972.

70. In New Jersey, however, recipients accounted for 6 out of the 24 members and in North Carolina for 4 out of 12. More typical were Texas (1 out of 27) and Florida (1 out of 34).

71. Otto Reid and Edward O'Donnell, "Citizen Participation in Public Welfare Boards and Committees," *Welfare in Review,* Sept.–Oct., 1971.

72. See, for example, HEW Memorandum to State Survey Agencies; Health Insurance for the Aged and State Agencies Administering Medical Assistance Plans, BHIL-SA No. 165, May 22, 1972: *Joint Policy for Medicare and Medicaid Programs—Limitations on granting of waivers of Certain Provisions of the Safety Code,* CCH *Medicare & Medicaid Guide,* par. 26,474; Comptroller-General's Report to the Congress, *More Needs to be Done to Assure that Physician Services —Paid for by Medicare and Medicaid—are Necessary,* No. B-169031 (4), August 2, 1972 (and see especially Chapter 5, "Need for Greater Co-ordination and Exchange of Information between Medicare and Medicaid") *ibid.*, par. 26,494.

73. American Public Health Association, *Washington News Letter,* May 30, 1973, p. 3.

74. Much of the energy of the Secretary's Office during this period appeared to be going into the development of a comprehensive approach to program planning—the MEGA proposal. Social Legislation Information Service, *Washington Bulletin,* vol. 23, Issue 11 (June 11, 1973) and Issue 12 (June 25, 1973).

75. Commissioner Howard Newman of MSA was the only Bureau chief within SRS to be reappointed.

13
The States

Although the changes in the Medical Services Administration (MSA) and the strengthened power of its staff in the regions indicated a movement toward increased federal control, this was, as we have indicated, a movement that was translated into activity only in selected target areas. MSA was not transformed overnight into a central planning agency. In most respects, indeed, the basic weaknesses of Medicaid remained: a lack of comprehensive goals, a lack of authority over providers, and different perceptions of the program at different administrative levels.

Medicaid thus remained a staunchly state-administered program even as the need for federal policies became more evident. Medicaid's national advisory group, the revamped Medical Assistance Advisory Council (MAAC), did, it is true, join other groups in recommending the federalization of Medicaid in 1971.[1] But the MAAC itself was evanescent; it did not survive the 1972 Social Security Amendments.[2] Meanwhile, state Medicaid programs struggled on. Apart from the crackdown on nursing homes, together with some question of what would be required in the regulations for early and periodic screening, diagnosis, and treatment, the major cause of additional concern, as H.R. 1 moved through the Congress, was the by now familiar confusion as to how yet another series of federal amendments would be interpreted, with what elements of state loss or gain. Aspirations for medical care continued to be dampened by fiscal constraints. At the state level, as well as in MSA, the focus was increasingly on administrative efficiency. It had become clear that it was not politically feasible to have a good medical program for the poor, when there was none for the nonpoor; but it was equally unacceptable for states to move whole-hog into the universal, comprehensive insurance business. In the states, then, Medicaid administration had become a matter of holding the line. Few governors congratulated their legislatures on saving lives, encouraging individual potential, or alleviating misery. The recipient was part of an ever more expensive "caseload."

Skyrocketing Costs

The costs of Medicaid falling on the states, coupled as they were with spiralling budgets for other welfare programs, made this emphasis virtually inevitable. Expenditures administered through the Connecticut Welfare Department, for example, rose from $90 million in fiscal year 1966 to an estimated $292 million in fiscal 1973,[3] the latter amount representing almost $100 per inhabitant of the state. About a third of this amount was directly attributable to Medicaid. Even in states which had approached Medicaid gingerly, there was no apparent means of cost containment. Virginia, for example, began its Medicaid program in fiscal 1970 at a total cost of $55 million, but expected costs of $142 million by fiscal 1974.[4] Meanwhile, the expenses in the larger states became positively awe-inspiring. In calendar 1971 New York State showed expenditures of $1.8 billion for medical vendor payments, while California spent another $1.0 billion.[5] Taking the nation as a whole, the cost of Medicaid *doubled* between fiscal 1969 and 1973[6] and was expected to double again by 1980.

It is important to note, however, that the number of Medicaid recipients also doubled between 1969 and 1973, from 12 million to 23 million, in large part because of the expanding rolls of cash assistance recipients. This statistic has tended to become lost amid the rhetoric. Indeed, from the state budgetary point of view, the figure was disturbing, rather than a matter of congratulation, because of the vast numbers of persons shown to need state aid for medical bills: Where would it end? Moreover, the primary state concern has been balancing the assistance budget, not counting heads. Cost, rather than value, has been the nexus. Even though in 1973 the average state got over half (55 percent) its Medicaid funds from Washington, as total costs rose so also did the sum which was required to be borne by the states. Despite the variable formula of federal grants to the states, the burden fell heavily on large and small states alike: from New York, with its army of 8500 state employees engaged in administering its vast Medicaid program, to states such as Idaho, South Dakota, Wyoming, and Nevada, whose more modest Medicaid activities require the administrative supervision of fewer than ten state employees.[7]

The rising costs of health care have been a general phenomenon, by no means limited to the dependent population, and have raised questions of what, indeed, is value for money in medicine. The Social Security Administration, for instance, has estimated the rise in the amount spent on all types of health expenditure as going from $342 per capita in 1970 to $509 in 1975, with the expectation of a further rise up to at least $670 by 1980.[8] These figures are average costs, over all age groups, and include the healthy in addition to the sick. Nevertheless, they are indicative of the rises in potential costs falling on a family that has one of its members sick and is not fully covered by any form of health insurance: the average middle-class family in America. Thus, with rising costs, the concept of "medical indigence" has been gathering new meaning, far beyond the concept that led to Kerr-Mills and, later, to Medicaid.[9] It was this concept of middle-class medical indigence that formed the backbone of pressures for some scheme of national health insurance in the Congress.[10]

The problems of middle-class medicine were, however, also increasingly evident at the state and local level. If Medicaid programs had reached the full potential envisaged for them in the 1965 legislation, i.e., comprehensive services for all the needy by 1975, those on Medicaid would have had significantly better health protection than any other members of the population—better even than that available in prepaid groups or health maintenance organizations, which usually have limited coverage for drugs, dentistry, appliances, and psychiatric and nursing home care and frequently have some co-payment arrangements. Even with the limited services and relatively low eligibility levels obtaining in state Medicaid programs in the 1970s, the individual on Medicaid may receive thousands of dollars worth of care he would not be able to receive if insured through the private sector. These concerns formed a backdrop to debates and action in both Congress and the state legislatures between 1970 and 1972. As far as the taxpayers were concerned, here was a vital question of equity. In some cases, the old welfare tradition appeared up-ended, with those on medical assistance being "more eligible" than those striving to keep above it. Thus, linked with the questions of cost control and service limitation have been less tangible pressures to make welfare less attractive and welfare medicine more restrictive. There are complex reasons, therefore, why Medicaid has been regarded more repressively at the state level at the same time that MSA has been attempting to make services more effective. But clearly, by tying Medicaid more firmly to the welfare tradition, the states were protecting the interests of the middle class who were themselves suffering from the high costs of medicine.

But whatever the underlying reasons, state actions toward Medicaid have been consistent. Between July 1970 and June 1973, as in the earlier period, the urge throughout the states was to prune back Medicaid programs. In the fall of 1970, for instance, both Utah and New Mexico urged providers to defer elective procedures and to keep stays in institutions to the minimum.[11] By January 1971, an *American Medical News* survey of 34 states revealed that only five expected to expand their programs. No less than 24 programs were running at a deficit, and 18 expected to have to make cuts or to ask for additional funds. In almost every case the chief reason given for the expanding Medicaid budget was that the AFDC rolls, whose beneficiaries were automatically included in Medicaid, had exploded in 1970. Other factors alleged to be adding to the Medicaid burdens were unemployment and court decisions.

Thus the state of Washington, with a 12 percent unemployment rate, cut Medicaid services but expected nevertheless to have 250,000 persons covered by the program as opposed to 200,000 twelve months earlier. Louisiana also made cuts in Medicaid, but extra appropriations were still needed because AFDC caseloads had gone from 18,000 to 62,000 over an 18-month period. In Minnesota there had been a fivefold increase in unemployment claims, while in New Jersey the number of persons on welfare increased by 25 percent. Generally, as in Ohio, physicians' fees were being cut;[12] other states, such as Missouri, reported cutbacks in nursing home rates. The general situation, however, was reflected in the comment by Medical Assistance Director Jack Guveyan in Massachusetts: "We'll have a deficit, we always have a deficit, just like all the other states."[13]

But costs continued to rise during 1971 and into 1972. By early 1972, with costs of the D.C. Medicaid program running far higher than a year earlier,[14] Peter Coppola, director of the city's program, explained that the number of recipients had increased because "a lot of people in welfare rights groups are out in the community beating the bushes to tell people of their right—and so we have more people on the rolls and they're using Medicaid more."[15] But not all increases in cost were the result of more beneficiaries on the Medicaid rolls. In 1972 Maryland reported that in a three-year period costs had risen by 51 percent while the number of recipients had increased by only 16 percent.[16] It seemed that as patients became more aware of their rights, they used services more extensively.[17] Michigan, too, reported that its 28 percent increase in Medicaid costs in fiscal 1971 were represented chiefly by doctors' fees, hospital rates, and drug prices.[18]

Nationally, the urge to cut welfare programs was pervasive. In August 1971, Alabama caused a stir by cutting 33,000 persons from its welfare rolls;[19] but the same process was occurring with greater or less intensity across the country, and Medicaid was inevitably involved. In October 1971, for instance, the medically indigent in Connecticut lost their entitlement to services such as optometry, podiatry, dental care and hearing aids.[20] Indeed, by the middle of 1971, nine states were reported to be cutting back their Medicaid programs that year—a process fought in the courts in at least five cases.[21] Some states attempted to emphasize better administration, including utilization review, in an effort to halt rising costs.[22] Meanwhile other states experimented with regulation of the medical care industry. Connecticut, in particular, sought to experiment with a Health Care Commission to put a price lid on providers.[23]

Excessive Utilization, Near Fraud, and Fraud

In keeping with the earlier experience, the period under review produced its share of providers well rewarded by Medicaid. No doubt many of them deserved such rewards, but some payments were understandably questioned. In Virginia, for instance, it emerged that one physician earned more than $90,000 from Medicaid in 1971 and six earned more than $60,000. But Dr. Edwin Brown, Director of the State Bureau of Medical Assistance, remarked: "We have determined that some doctors misunderstood the billing procedures and there have been a few cases that came close to the abuse line." With reference to the largest payments he added: "These are men practicing in ghetto areas with practices made up primarily of Medicaid recipients. Out of the payments they receive, they pay nurses' salaries, rents, and other costs of practice."[24]

The problems were highlighted even more obviously in Washington, D.C. It has already been seen that costs rose rapidly in the District program, and such rises were not surprising. The hospitals in D.C. had long held out against joining Medicaid, and when they entered they were paid well for services they had previously often provided gratuitously. For instance, it was reported that in 1971 the hospitals were paid over $13 million for services for which they would previously have received some $2 million. During the same year, the People's Drug Store chain was paid $1,122,102 for filling prescriptions—some $435,000 of it being profit.[25] A few days after this was reported, it was revealed that in 1969 alone—the first year of Medicaid in the District—a half million dollars had been wrongly paid out to providers. As in other programs, there were alleged to be administrative weaknesses and inadequate audits.[26]

Once again it appeared to be the physicians in D.C. who were getting the lion's share of the overpayments, some $306,000 of the half million.[27] The year before, the head of the District Department of Human Resources had called on physicians to raise their standard of care,[28] but his plea had apparently had no effect. Certainly the problems were complex. Physicians in ghetto areas had done particularly well out of the program. Two, interviewed by the *Washington Post*, claimed it was normal to be paid $75,000 a year by the program. But they pointed out that much of this went for expenses and that in the meantime they were performing a vital social service.[29]

The situation in the District, however, turned ugly, after the federal government announced the names of those physicians who had been paid more than $20,000 and after the D.C. Medical Society announced it was investigating four physicians who had earned in excess of $70,000 from Medicaid. As most of the physicians involved in these higher payments were black, there was tension between the Medical Society and the predominantly black Medical-Chirurgical Society. The President of the latter organization declared: "It is character assassination to identify physicians in terms of amount of money paid without giving credit for vastly improved patient care rendered." He also noted that "Black physicians are relating more to the community" and are "involved in developing health care programs therein." But it seemed that the issue of "ghetto medicine" was in many ways being exacerbated by the Medicaid system.[30]

In other states, too, there were problems. In New Jersey, where corruption in public affairs is often the norm, it was perhaps not surprising that the state surveillance unit recovered nearly a million Medicaid dollars in 1971,[31] while a number of providers were suspended.[32] But even in puritan Iowa, there were problems. The federal audit of that state's Medicaid program, completed in 1970, suggested the pharmacists might have unlawfully claimed over a million dollars out of a total drug bill of only $10 million.[33] The problems of Medicaid administration in the states seemed hydra-headed.

Nor was a simple solution available. The payment agencies could presumably appear draconian. Commissioner Ball of the Social Security Administration noted as evidence of a "tough claims review process" under Part B of Medicare that in 1970 about 30 percent of all claims involving physician bills were being reduced in at least one of the services shown on the claim.[34] But Medicaid programs were often at a disadvantage in not having a fiscal agent or, if they had, not having effective control over the agent. Undoubtedly there were many state legislators and administrators who warmed to Congressman Mills' experience: "We fellows have to run for office . . . and the best way is to try to work it out so we fellows running for office do not have to run around telling all these doctors we think they are charging too much—that the fees are outrageous and unreasonable. Somebody else ought to tell them that."[35]

The Providers' View of Administration

While it is easy enough to chronicle the various "rip-offs" perpetrated by providers on Medicaid funds, the providers understandably found many aspects of Medicaid irritating. Not only were recipients being cut back in terms of eligibility and services, but in many states provider fees were cut. The reactions to these cuts—particularly from physicians—were frequently strong. In Kansas, the Sedgwick County (Wichita) physicians threatened to see only emergency patients after a 25 percent cutback in fees.[36] The Florida Medical Association asked Secretary of HEW Elliot Richardson to investigate that state's program when physicians' fees were cut to 60 percent of "usual and customary charges."[37] In Massachusetts, physicians actually went to court in an attempt to force the State Rate Setting Commission to increase physician fees.[38]

When the Governor of Michigan proposed that physician fees be discounted by 3 percent if they were paid within 30 days, the State Medical Society protested that: "Once again 10,000 physicians have been isolated from Michigan's nine million people to bear the cost of a particular state financial hardship."[39] Despite this reaction, later in the year the physicians isolated themselves still further from their fellow citizens when the State Medical Society urged a boycott of Medicaid beginning October 1, because they were to be required to sign a single service agreement rather than a separate reimbursement agreement each time they treated a Medicaid patient. The State Medical Society, however, later reversed this stance, advocating instead a program which would cause such administrative chaos that this step towards "socialized medicine" would be abandoned.[40]

But if cuts in fees did not irritate the doctors, administrative red tape did. Low fees and added paperwork became the preferred explanation of why one out of three MDs did not participate in Mississippi's Medicaid.[41] In Ohio it took, on an average, three months to pay a doctor's bill, which was clearly a source of both concern and irritation.[42] A D.C. Medical Society source confirmed the impression that physicians either did not participate in Medicaid because of the paperwork or used the paperwork as an excuse for not participating. But as one respondent put it: "The whole Medicare-Medicaid program stinks of governmental red tape, vagueness and paperwork," while another exploded: "Get rid of that billing system. It drives my girls nuts."[43] But if physicians were irritated, pharmacists—in Texas at least—were so angry with 6-month delays in payment that they formed an organization known as "Positive Action for Pharmacy," apparently intended to topple that state's Medicaid program.[44]

Finally, lack of information about deficiencies in the Medicaid program plagued professionals as well as Medicaid administrators. Government audit reports, inspections, and even the status of institutional compliance with regulations (e.g., in the case of nursing homes) were not usually routinely made public. As the Senate Finance Committee remarked, in its report on the proposed Social Security Amendments in 1972, "in the absence of public knowledge about the nature and extent of deficiencies of individual facilities, it is difficult for physicians and the public to rationally choose among health care facilities and to bring pressures for improvement to bear on those facilities."[45] Too often, it must have seemed that the professionals were being blamed for factors in Medicaid over which, as individuals, they had little or no control. But finally the professionals, too, were regrouping in order to play a more positive role in Medicaid and other public programs. The vehicle for this was to be the rapid development of medical organizations dedicated to "peer review."

The Administrative Response in the States

Slowly, during the period, the more decisive and imaginative direction in the Medical Services Administration in HEW began to have some effect on those responsible for running state Medicaid programs. And not only was there pressure from MSA. The General Accounting Office increasingly investigated specific Medicaid problems, as when it issued a tough critique of the method of paying pharmacists in Ohio.[46] Congressional interest in peer review also had its impact with voluntary peer review appearing in states as diverse as New Mexico and California,[47] and in September 1971 peer review became statewide in New Mexico.[48]

States, too, moved to tighten their administrative systems before costs became completely unrestrained. Moreover, as coverage in the states was cut and as additional cuts were proposed in H.R. 1, as it moved slowly through the Congress from 1970 to the end of 1972, the needs of the elderly began poignantly to emerge again. It was the elderly who found themselves in skilled nursing homes and ICFs whose funds might be cut off for noncompliance, and it was the elderly who suffered most from combined efforts to limit Medicare and Medicaid.[49] In New York City, whose problems continued to dominate the entire Medicaid program, and in Chicago[50] Medicaid had become a symbol of inefficiency and graft in an almost hopeless system of urban poverty and health care chaos. For most states Medicaid was much more clearly a program for the "deserving" poor: the elderly and impoverished children.

Because Medicaid was heavily geared to providing care in institutions (hospitals and nursing homes),[51] administrative action was largely focused on cost-cutting in these. But cost-cutting alone would be myopic, as there were often no alternatives to institutional care and thus nowhere for the patient to turn. The congressional regional hearings on the elderly in 1971 pressed this point home. In Woonsocket, Rhode Island, the waiting period to get an elderly patient into a chronic disease hospital was two to three months.[52] What was to happen to the patient in the meantime? It was not unusual for patients in hospitals or nursing homes under Medicare to be told summarily that they must leave, but where were they to go?[53] Medicaid did not always effect a smooth transition, and in any event the stigma of pauperization remained.

State Medicaid administrations had to struggle along in this atmosphere. It was one thing for Congress to discuss the need to "mobilize community resources to provide alternatives to nursing home care,"[54] and to find "as a shock" that no community in the United States has a comprehensive network of services for the aging and the aged and that this country was far behind other countries in this respect,[55] but state welfare departments were not in the nursing home or hospital business. Indeed, if states did provide well-organized alternatives to institutional care, the total costs of care would almost certainly go up; for hospitals and nursing homes would be able to concentrate on the more acutely ill or needy and would presumably treat more sick persons than are currently treated. In the process, the hospitals and nursing homes might well gain economic benefits, while the taxpayers would be left with a much larger Medicaid bill.

Whatever, then, the motivations at the federal level to provide a full spectrum of medical care and whatever the views and directions of other state agencies—notably the Comprehensive Health Planning agencies developed, under federal subsidy, after 1966—state Medicaid agencies have had limited goals. Administration has mainly meant budgetary efficiency, which in turn has meant patrolling Medicaid reimbursements to providers, largely with respect to health care institutions.

One primary emphasis was the routine function of claims review. In the smaller states the "Blues" proved to be eminently satisfactory for the administration of Medicaid programs. But, as a very rough rule, in the larger states there was increasing concern about the way these physician and hospital organized groups went about their role as fiscal intermediaries. Thus, in 1971, Michigan took back from Michigan Blue Cross and Blue Shield the administration of the state's Medicaid program, claiming it could save $1 million a year on administrative costs. The President of Michigan Blue Shield said he was "surprised and puzzled"; but the state Social Services Director explained: "in taking over this function, first we hope to save some money. It is a peculiar arrangement to farm out the payment of part of the program. . . . It's simply a matter of public responsibility. We will have better control over the program with total responsibility in one place."[56]

All told, seven states discontinued using Blue Cross and/or Blue Shield as fiscal agents between 1970 and 1972. In the later year, there were 24 states with no fiscal agents, and in several others the use of such agents was for limited purposes: In Massachusetts, for example, only the Commission for the Blind used a fiscal agent, while Alabama was unique in employing several fiscal agents simultaneously. The assumption that had grown up in the mid-1960s that public funds were best channeled into the medical care system through private insurance carriers was being severely questioned.

In terms of innovation, however, the most interesting developments seemed to be in the area of experimentation with the delivery of services through prepayment plans. In 1970, the Group Health Cooperative of Puget Sound took on 1000 Medicaid families in the state of Washington, with the expectation that by receiving $38.60 a month for each family they would be able to provide better care with 25 percent less cost.[57] Washington, D.C., also moved tentatively towards a similar experiment. At a cost of $350 a year, 1000 Medicaid recipients were to be provided with prepaid comprehensive health care. Although the cost of care—to be provided by the

Group Health Association (GHA)—was higher than the average cost of Medicaid services in the District ($264.75), the experiment was to include dental and psychiatric services. The *Washington Post* explained that "because of their strong emphasis on preventative medicine, prepaid group health programs have long been believed by many to provide better health care at a lower price than most traditional medicine practiced in this country"; while a GHA spokesman was reported saying, it should take no longer than a year to see if group medicine will indeed provide better and cheaper medical care."[58] Unfortunately, the enthusiasm for developing such prepayment programs was not matched by reliable evaluations of their success, quality, or cost.[59]

Nevertheless, as the White House, Congress, and HEW all became attracted to the concept of HMOs, the tempo of such arrangements quickened. Typical was the report that the Sedgwick County Medical Society in Kansas was thinking of setting up a medical-care foundation to serve the poor.[60] Medical societies across the country began investigating the possibilities of developing prepaid HMO-type programs. Sometimes efforts were made to build prepayment plans into OEO health care programs and health care centers—as in Kentucky.[61] In Michigan, an experimental prepayment plan to provide health care services to the poor was worked out between the state Department of Social Services and Detroit's Model Neighborhood Agency.[62] This perhaps was taken furthest in Newark, where a model program was to absorb Medicaid, OEO, and Model Cities funding.[63]

In a similar vein Governor George Wallace of Alabama put one of his populist ideas to work in this area. In 1972, Alabama developed a prepaid comprehensive medical care program for low-income groups (up to $6400 for a couple with three children) who were not eligible for Medicare or Medicaid.[64] Meanwhile, in Massachusetts, the Assistant Welfare Commissioner, Dr. James J. Callahan, Jr., conceded that while Medicaid was a bargain for the state "it has been inadequate and is increasingly becoming more inadequate."[65] He therefore argued in favor of setting up community medical centers as part of a statewide compulsory health insurance program. There was perhaps a silver lining—in the future—for recipients.

The States and the Courts

Before examining the fate of recipients during this period, we must briefly glance at one further relationship: that between state administrations and the courts. The state (and occasionally federal) courts dealt with other problems of immediate concern to state administrations. Certainly the woolly language of the initial Medicaid legislation invited clashes in interpretation. But even without the initial fuzziness of Medicaid, the courts would have had a variety of roles to play. The open-textured nature of language insures that even the most apparently definitive rules, doctrines, and statutory language are open to considerable discretion in the hands of the judiciary. More generally, however, someone must make determinations in the disputes that arise in any program. Most disputes—especially if a state is involved—are solved through the political process or through negotiations between the state and federal bureaucracies. But administrative problems, involving individuals, are less susceptible of such solutions and are more likely to find themselves being worked out in the courts. Medicaid, especially during this period, has been no exception.

For instance, in addition to the cutback cases, the courts have had to wrestle with disputes between drug companies and the state administration over inclusions in the Medi-Cal formulary.[66] From time to time states have had to be reminded of their basic obligations to the categorically needy or the medically needy.[67] The inevitable cases have emerged in which the dishonest sought to take refuge in technical points, for instance, the ambulance operator accused of submitting false claims to a state agency, who argued that the claims had been submitted to Blue Shield and that that was not a state agency.[68]

In New York, where cutback cases have generally found their way into the federal courts, different types of problems arose. The state courts held, for instance, that a state statute forbidding the attachment of earnings of persons "in receipt of public assistance or care" did not cover the "medically indigent" receiving Medicaid.[69] Under the state's Medicaid rules, prior authorization was necessary to obtain out-of-state treatment. But because there was an exception for emergency treatment, the courts found themselves deciding which factual situations fell within the competing categories.[70] Typical too was the case in which a hospital successfully sued the New York City Commissioner of Social Service for services rendered to a patient who was belatedly discovered to have been eligible for Medicaid. The New York City Circuit Court found that the Department's attempt to impose a 12-month limitation on claims was inconsistent with federal regulations.[71] The state courts, on this type of issue, seemed unwilling to make life too hard for state civil servants.[72]

Generally, but not always, this pattern was reflected in the cases dealing with recipient eligibility.[73] On the other hand, at times the courts have strained themselves to prevent injustices to those who might be cut off from Medicaid by what seemed chance,[74] and this became especially important with the larger than usual increases in Social Security in 1972.[75] The pattern—of state courts generally supporting state administrations—certainly seemed to be followed in the increasing number of nursing home cases that came up during the period;[76] although during 1972 and 1973 there was some evidence that courts might be taking a rather different tack; and extending to providers the right to "fair hearings," which had previously been developed for recipients.[77] Whether this is so or not, before the federal courts the nursing home industry was somewhat more successful —at least in pleading due process,[78] a constitutional problem to be taken up in greater detail in Chapter 15.

The Recipients' Viewpoint

The interactions and controversies of all of these various groups—federal agencies, departments in the state governments, health care providers, fiscal agents, the courts—seemed sometimes to overwhelm the actual recipients. The Medicare and Medicaid hearings of 1970 and the National Health Insurance hearings of 1971 highlighted the weaknesses in Title XIX as seen by the recipients. It was often a pathetic tale—and sometimes a cruel one. Undoubtedly many Medicaid recipients did not value the medical care they received and abused the system.[79] Yet the system they were presented with was often hostile and intimidating. As fees were cut, providers became more difficult to locate and services were provided in a manner increasingly like that of the assembly-line. At the same time, medically indigent persons found themselves part of the welfare system. Rather than change the definition of "welfare" to include a system of basic rights and entitlements, the welfare system seems to have depressed those entering it.[80]

At the local level, service provision is often a matter of resolving demarcation disputes among various payment agencies and confusion (including both overlaps and deficiencies) as to which health provider offers which services. Access to care is often difficult. In Arkansas, where more than half a million persons were living at or below the poverty level in 1971, a common pattern among physicians was to refer the poor to the University Medical Center at Little Rock for potentially expensive or protracted treatment (because treatment was cheaper to the poor at the Center); but a study showed that patients had trouble getting there, and when they did, they might have to wait six to eight hours or find the appointment cancelled; because of time and distance, they would often not take advantage of returning as an outpatient.[81] Nor were such difficulties by any means limited to rural areas.[82]

Even when the Medicaid beneficiary had signed up for the program, it was not always clear who would pay for the care nor where he should go.[83] Such confusion was compounded by the vicissitudes of changing coverage in the Medicaid program on the one hand and, on the other, the ever-rising health care costs. But bewilderment on the part of recipients had become a general trademark of the Medicaid program—and an essential component of the continuing welfare stigma. If anything, this bewilderment has been encouraged by the complex regulations for Medicaid procedures and reimbursement developed independently in each state, which overlay the federal regulations. State welfare officers usually issue minimal (or no) guidelines for potential Medicaid beneficiaries. Federal publications are necessarily vague and often over-idealistic.[84] The welfare tradition puts the potential beneficiary at the mercy of the social worker who must administer the various forms needed in applying for eligibility. As the first meeting between client and social worker invariably culminates in the completion of a form which includes, even in the most liberal states, detailed questions on family history and income—including such items as "Have you Made Funeral Arrangements?"[85]—the caseworker in a sense becomes the guardian of the recipient.

But the caseworker may also be a barrier to available care. A study published by HEW in 1972, involving a sample of Medicaid caseworkers in three states, found that only 83 percent thought they knew the eligibility requirements and Medicaid provisions "well enough to get by." Few of the workers had received special training to deal with Medicaid. Only 32 percent could identify all the benefits in the state Medicaid plan, and a sizeable 20 percent were not even aware that Title XIX payments were possible after maximum Medicare coverage terminated.[86] Not surprisingly, this confusion was reflected in the confusion felt by recipients. While 44 percent of the 948 recipients interviewed in the same study said that their worker had explained Medicaid to them, one is entitled to wonder how accurately.[87] Even then, the continuing variation in terms of income and services by state made generalization difficult. In fiscal 1972, for instance, the average medical vendor payment per family in one state was less than $100; most states fell between $400 and $549; but six states paid between $850 and $999 per family and three paid over $1000 per family.[88]

Some of these discrepancies can be highlighted by looking at the actual services offered at the beginning of 1973. By this time 27 jurisdictions continued to cover the medically indigent,[89] while the different services offered either for the categorically needy or for the medically indigent continued to vary widely. Arizona still had no program at all. Utah not only provided for the categorically needy and the medically indigent but provided both groups with all the mandatory services (inpatient and outpatient hospital services, other laboratory and x-ray services, skilled nursing home services for persons 21 or older, early and periodic screening diagnosis and treatment of persons under 21, family planning services, and physician services),[90] together with all but one of the voluntary additional services for which federal funding was available (prescribed drugs, dental services, eyeglasses, prosthetic devices, physical therapy and related services, private duty nursing, optometrists' services, podiatrists' services, chiropractors' services, clinic services, skilled nursing home care for those under 21, and intermediate care facility services). The situation was at times bizarre. Alaska did not cover the medically indigent and provided only mandatory services for the categorically needy. Connecticut provided all but one of the possible services to both groups. Patterns were not easy to develop. Wyoming and Mississippi were tight; Nebraska and Kansas generous; the most extensive range of services in the whole country was in the state of Washington.[91]

While the variation in eligibility levels for the medically needy was not as great in 1972 as it had been in 1967—some rich states, such as New York, having reduced their levels, others having pushed them up—the definition of "medical indigence" still varied widely from state to state, as indeed the level of categorical coverage varied from state to state depending on the limits of cash payments under state welfare programs.[92] The limits for a medically indigent family of four in Maryland were $3200, in Kentucky and Kansas $3000, $3456 in Minnesota, and $4500 in New York. The old confusion between cash assistance levels and medical assistance levels also remained. In 1972, the maximum eligibility level for medical indigence in some states was appreciably below the income level where cash assistance phases out under the "earnings disregard" provision[93]—i.e., the provision whereby a person on assistance could earn a certain amount and still retain some cash assistance. It was possible, therefore, for someone to struggle up the economic ladder into a job and off cash assistance but have to drop all the way back down the ladder to the Medicaid level if he fell sick, "spending down" any savings on the way, in order to regain medical benefits. Medicaid was thus still involved in the old cycle of pauperization.

The needs of Medicaid recipients, and others, for health care, despite the billions of dollars already spent by Medicaid, formed the backdrop for the series of health insurance hearings held by the House Ways and Means Committee in 1971 and Senate hearings on health maintenance organizations in 1972. While the working population was agonizing over who would pay for liver transplants, there were quite obviously continuing deficiencies in basic health care.[94]

The states, being nearer to the everyday problems of health care than the federal government, became increasingly concerned with the whys and wherefores of health care after 1970. In some cases the stimulus has been the apparently uncontrollable welfare budget; Governor Rockefeller's championship of national health insurance was at least in part so stimulated.[95] In many states the Comprehensive Health Planning (CHP) agencies, established in state health departments with area subsidiaries, have provided a focus for publicity and debate. In others, groups of legislators or private citizens formed, either around problems in the states, or to provide state-based lobbies for national health insurance.[96] The 1971 House Ways and Means Committee hearings rang with the by-then familiar problems: lack of preventive care, high costs, particular problems of certain poverty groups in urban ghettos or in camps for migrants, disorganization of services, lack of facilities in some areas (e.g., Idaho), and the difficulties in attempting to "solve" health care issues through merely increasing available financing.

It was typical of the evolving division of federal and state responsibilities that these statements were most widely publicized at federal hearings. National health insurance was clearly a federal responsibility, which would have to be funded through federal taxation or otherwise sanctioned through federal decree. In the state capitols the urge, at least with regard to Medicaid, was not primarily service-oriented, and debates were fraught with institutional politics. A review of Medicaid's three largest programs, those in New York, California, and Illinois, makes these points abundantly clear.

NOTES

1. *Washington Report on Medicine and Health,* Feb. 15, 1971.
2. See Chapter 16.
3. Gerald E. Bisbee, *The Growth of the Connecticut State Department of Welfare,* 1973. Paper presented at the Yale Medical School.
4. Of which an estimated 63 percent would be federal. Interviews in Richmond.
5. Personal communication from MSA.
6. From $4.1 billion to $8.8 billion.
7. Figures refer to fiscal year 1970. Information from MSA.
8. U.S., Department of Health, Education, and Welfare, Social Security Administration, *Medical Care Costs and Prices: Background Book,* 72–11908, January 1972, p. 90.
9. Senator Kennedy summarized the new victims of health care costs in 1971, in a series of tragic vignettes drawn from evidence to the Health Subcommittee. No longer were these only the "ghetto mother in Harlem, whose oldest son is severely retarded for life because of lead paint poisoning, but whose younger children have not yet even been tested for symptoms of the disease." They included, too, a Cornell engineering student, paralyzed for life by a football injury, whose father, an insurance salesman, carried "the best health policy his company offered," but who was financially ruined; a paint sprayer filing for bankruptcy because he was unable to pay a hospital bill; a college linguistics professor, "dead of brain cancer at 46 after tens of thousands of dollars in expenses. Now, the lives of his wife and children are mortgaged. . . ." U.S., Congress, Senate, Committee on Finance, *National Health Insurance, Hearings* before the Senate Committee on Finance, 92nd Cong., 1st Sess., 1971, p. 27.
10. See Chapters 15 and 16.
11. *Hospital Week,* vol. 6, Oct. 9, 1970, p. 1.
12. *American Medical News,* January 25, 1971. But in Kentucky and Maryland there were reports of increases in doctors' fees. *Ibid.*
13. *American Medical News,* January 25, 1971.
14. The figure for July 1, 1970, to February 28, 1971, was $14,361,651; for July 1, 1971, to February 29, 1972, it was $21,214,765.
15. *Washington Post,* April 13, 1972, p. 1, col. 2.

16. In fiscal 1967–68 payments of $58.1 million had been made for 256,000 patients. In fiscal 1971, Medicaid paid out $88.5 million in connection with 298,000 patients.

17. *Washington Post,* April 14, 1972, Section B, p. 1, col. 7.

18. *Detroit Free Press,* April 24, 1972, p. 5b.

19. *New York Times,* August 31, 1971, p. 22, col. 2.

20. *New Haven Register,* November 9, 1971, p. 15, col. 7.

21. *Health Law Newsletter,* June 1971.

22. Barbara Isenberg, "Physician Panels Are Used Increasingly to Police Skyrocketing Costs of Treating the Aged, Needy," *Wall Street Journal,* April 7, 1972, p. 28, col. 1. Although we shall examine this in greater detail later in this chapter, the importance of utilization review panels as a possible means of curbing costs must be mentioned.

23. See, for example, *New Haven Register,* May 6, 1971, p. 16, col. 1.

24. *Washington Post,* April 19, 1972, Section C, p. 1, col. 7. Perhaps the most extreme example of the complexity of physician billing was the case of Dr. Sanford Potansky of Benton Harbor, who had billed Michigan Blue Shield, the fiscal intermediary for Medicaid in that state, for $169,000 for fees in fiscal 1968. The dispute was still bubbling in the period under review since, irritated by the attacks on him, Dr. Potansky had written out a check for $169,000 and presented it to Blue Shield. The Auditor General of Michigan noted that "he (Dr. Potansky) over-utilized the program—he had people coming back and back who didn't really need to." There was also evidence of "poor record keeping." *Detroit Free Press,* October 16, 1971, p. 3; *American Medical News,* November 8, 1971.

25. *Washington Post,* April 13, 1972, p. 1, col. 2.

26. *Ibid.*, April 23, 1972, p. 1.

27. *Ibid.*

28. *Ibid.*, May 22, 1971, Section B, p. 1, col. 7.

29. *Ibid.*, June 25, 1971, Section C, p. 1, col. 1.

30. *Ibid.*, April 15, 1972, p. 16, col. 2. The department eventually agreed to a "full scale review" of $36 million in Medicaid payments made in 1971. *Ibid.*, May 5, 1972, p. 95.

31. *New York Times,* August 5, 1972.

32. *Ibid.*, December 5, 1971, p. 1, col. 4.

33. *American Medical News,* August 2, 1971, p. 10.

34. U.S., Congress, Senate, Committee on Finance, *Medicare and Medicaid, Hearings* before the Committee on Finance, 91st Cong., 2nd Sess., 1970, p. 14.

35. *Ibid.*, p. 13.

36. *American Medical News,* Sept. 13, 1971, p. 10.

37. *Ibid.*, August 2, 1971, p. 10.

38. *Ibid.*, Dec. 21, 1970, p. 15.

39. *Ibid.*, Feb. 28, 1972.

40. *Detroit Free Press,* Oct. 5, 1972, p. 4a.

41. *American Medical News,* Jan. 25, 1971, p. 7.

42. *Ibid.*, March 22, 1971.

43. *Washington Post,* June 25, 1971, Section C, p. 1, col. 1.

44. *Drug Topics*, April 24, 1972.

45. U.S., Congress, Senate, Committee on Finance, *Social Security Amendments of 1972*, Report of the Committee on Finance, Senate Report No. 92–1230, 1972, p. 288.

46. *Drug Topics*, January 18, 1971.

47. Barbara Isenberg, *supra*, note 22, p. 24.

48. *Hospital Week*, June 4, 1971, p. 1.

49. Even in a broad and well-organized Medicaid program, such as in Rhode Island, there were tragic gaps in coverage. Of the 104,000 persons 65 years of age or over in that state, 102,000 were beneficiaries of Medicare Part A. Of these, 99,000 were voluntarily contributing to Medicare Part B (at an annual out-of-pocket contribution of $67.20), and 63,000 had Blue Cross 65, a private insurance supplement, at an annual cost of $85.80. Despite this type of coverage, however, none of these plans provided adequate institutional care or such basic services as eyeglasses, dentistry, or hearing aids. As a result, almost one fourth (24,000) of the elderly in Rhode Island were on Medicaid. Senator Claiborne Pell posed the salient question in regional hearings on proposed Medicare and Medicaid cuts in Providence in September 1971. Quoting an HEW estimate that health costs would rise by 50 percent in the next two years, he asked providers of health care "how they plan to control this expected 50 percent rise in health costs," and continued, "If this rise cannot be controlled, the senior citizens will unfortunately have to pay the bill." U.S., Congress, Senate, Special Committee on Aging, Subcommittee on Health of the Elderly, *Cutbacks in Medicare and Medicaid Coverage, Hearings* before the Subcommittee on Health of the Elderly of the Special Committee on Aging, 92 Cong., 1st Sess. (Part 3—Providence, Rhode Island), 1971, pp. 227, 276–277.

50. See Chapter 14.

51. In fiscal 1972 the proportion of Medicaid payments going to care in institutions ranged from a low of 32 percent in Iowa (whose program covered only the categorically needy, limited general hospital care to 10 days ["no circumvention permitted"], excluded mental and tuberculosis hospitalization, and had a relatively small number of nursing homes) to 79 percent in Pennsylvania (which covered the medically indigent and had a relatively wide range of benefits).

52. *Cut-backs in Medicare and Medicaid Coverage, supra,* note 51, Part 2, Woonsocket, Rhode Island, p. 165.

53. A sad but graphic illustration was given in a letter dated May 10, 1971, from a man in Los Angeles whose wife was in a convalescent home. On April 30, he had heard from Travelers Insurance, acting as fiscal intermediary for Medicare, that HEW recognized no liability for his wife's care as of the date of entry to the home (Feb. 2, 1971). From April 30, the convalescent home "has emphatically demanded that I pay their bill or remove the patient," and by the time this letter was written the home's administration, which was clearly losing money on the case, had allegedly resorted to daily threats. Letter from R. M. Sterret, *ibid.*, Part I Los Angeles, California, p. 87.

54. U.S., Congress, Senate, Special Committee on Aging, *Alternatives to Nursing Home Care: A Proposal,* Committee Print Prepared for the use of the Special Committee on Aging, U.S. Senate, 92nd Cong., 1st Sess., Oct. 1971, p. v. *et passim.*

55. U.S., Congress, Senate, Special Committee on Aging, *Making Services for the Elderly Work, Some Lessons from the British Experience,* Report to the

Special Committee on Aging, U.S. Senate, Committee Print, 92nd Cong., 1st Sess., 1971, p. iii.

56. *Ann Arbor News*, October 14, 1971; *American Medical News*, October 25, 1971; *Richmond News Leader*, January 20, 1972.

57. *Los Angeles Times*, June 12, 1970, p. 14.

58. *Washington Post*, May 22, 1971, §B, p. 1, col. 7; *Ibid.*, May 26, 1971, §B, p. 1, col. 7.

A similar program was developed in Maryland for a group of 3500 East Baltimore Medicaid recipients. Under this program, the state paid $14.24 per month for each Medicaid recipient included in the Health Cooperative coverage. *American Medical News*, February 14, 1972. Meanwhile, in the same city, a group of physicians signed a contract to provide comprehensive services to Medicaid recipients for a flat $19.73 a visit. Such care was to include dental care and all lab tests. *Washington Evening Star*, June 1, 1971.

59. For a provisional affirmative evaluation, see Clifton R. Gaus, Norman A. Fuller, and Carol Bohannan, *HMO Evaluation: Utilization Before and After Enrollment* (mimeo). Paper presented at the APHA Meeting, November 1972.

For the program to evaluate "Comprehealth" in Montana, see Helen Martz and John Trauth, "Six Ways to Measure Change," *Human Needs*, February 1973.

60. *American Medical News*, August 16, 1971.

61. Robert J. Bazell, "O.E.O. Ledger on Kentucky Program," *Science*, vol. 174, October 1, 1971, p. 45.

62. *Detroit Free Press*, December 24, 1971, p. 4.

63. *New York Times*, September 19, 1972, p. 60.

64. *American Medical News*, March 20, 1972.

65. *Boston Globe*, June 24, 1971, p. 5, col. 3.

66. *California v. A. H. Robins*, 93 Cal. Rptr. 663, 16 C.A. 3d 87 (Ch. App., 3d Dist. of Calif. 1971).

67. E.g. *Dominguez v. Milliken*, W. S. Mich., 1973, where a federal district court firmly held Michigan to the standard laid down in 45 C.F.R. § 248.21, namely that the income test for the "medically indigent" had to be at least as high as that for the state's most liberal categorical program.

68. *Smith v. Superior Court*, 85 Cal. Rptr. 208, 5 C.A. 3d 260 (Ct. App. 5th Dist. of Calif., 1970).

69. *Izzo v. Kirby*, 287 N.Y.S. 2d 994, 56 Misc. 2d 131 (N.Y. Supr. Ct., Special Term, Suffolk County, Part I, 1968).

70 E.g. *Henegar v. Wyman*, 313 N.Y.S. 2d 318, 63 Misc. 2d 688 (N.Y. Supr. Ct., Special Term, Greene County, 1970).

71. *Society of the New York Hospital v. Mogersen*, 319 N.Y.S. 2d 258, 65 Misc. 2d 515 (N.Y.C., Cir. Ct., Special Term, N.Y. County, Part I, 1971). For another aspect of the limitation problem see *Knickerbocker Hospital v. Downing*, 317 N.Y.S. 2d 688, 65 Misc. 2d 278 (N.Y.C. Cir. Ct., N.Y. County, 1970).

72. See, for instance, *Glass v. Dept. of Health of City of New York*, 316 N.Y.S. 2d 306, 64 Misc. 2d 880 (Supr. Ct., Special Term, Kings County, Part I, 1970), where the court refused to interfere when Medicaid children were sent to hospitals for their school health examinations, while non-Medicaid children were examined in school.

73. In *Loehr v. Wisconsin Department of Health and Social Services*, the Court held that mortgages on the plaintiff's livestock and farm machinery had

to be deducted from the value of this property to determine whether his resources exceeded the $3100 allowed for a family of four under Wisconsin legislation; CCH *Medicaid & Medicare Guide*, par. 26.311 (Wisc. Cir. Ct., 1971). In *Arlasky v. Dimitri*, the plaintiff, a nursing home patient whose Medicare entitlement was about to expire, had transferred her income-producing property in trust to her retarded son and then applied for Medicaid. The Supreme Court of New York affirmed the local social services commissioner's determination that she had made the transfer in order to receive Medicaid and hence was ineligible under the provisions in the New York Social Service Law, which prohibited eligibility in such cases; 327 N.Y.S. 2d 177, 38 A.D. 2d 665 (Sup. Ct., App. Div., 3rd Dept., 1971). *Gillett's Will*, a somewhat less touching case, involved a claim by New York to recover Medicaid payments improperly made to Ms. Gillett during her lifetime. It was proved that she had owned IBM stock worth nearly $10,000 which she had kept hidden in a safe deposit box. As this put her well over the allowable liquid assets, the state was allowed to recover most of what it had paid on her behalf; 310 N.Y.S. 2d 574 (N.Y. Supr. Ct., Broome County, 1971).

74. In *Baca v. New Mexico Health and Social Services Department*, it was held that New Mexico could not terminate the plaintiff's OAA and Medicaid payments because of an increase in Social Security payments that put him slightly above the OAA level. The state had been paying his Medicare premiums while he was eligible for Medicaid and OAA; if his eligibility were terminated, he would have to pay the Medicare premium himself, which would place his resources below his need level again. The court saved him from the horror of this dilemma by interpreting the state law and 45 CFR §233.20(a) (3) (iii) (c) as requiring the defendant department to consider only available resources exclusive of Medicare premiums in determining need level; CCH *Medicare & Medicaid Guide*, par. 15.468 (N.M. Ct. of App., 1971). In *Green v. Wyman*, the New York courts held that the plaintiff was entitled to reimbursement for $72 she had paid for medication for fertility treatments after she had become ineligible due to cutbacks in Medicaid in April 1968. The treatment had started while she was eligible under the former standards, and the New York Attorney General had given an opinion in March of that year opining that such persons should remain eligible for continuing treatment. This did not extend, however, to the point of making her eligible for payments to cover her resultant pregnancy; 162 N.Y.L.J. No. 79, p. 2 (N.Y. Supr. Ct. 1969); 316 N.Y.S. 2d 189 (App. Div., 1st Dept., 1970) affirming Supr. Ct.

75. In *Curtis v. Child*, 1972, the Idaho Supreme Court ruled for the state to continue certain elderly women in the state's Medicaid program when the latter received increases in OASDHI. The court based its argument on the federal regulations which required the application of a "flexible measure of available income" for the "medically needy." CCH, *Medicare & Medicaid Guide*, par. 26,524. Also, in 1972, the Pennsylvania Supreme Court held that where a Social Security increase took a Medicaid recipient out of the "categorically needy" (whose services included drugs) into the "medically needy" (whose services did not include drugs), if the medical expenses of the recipient were so large that she would inevitably reach the "categorically needy" there was in fact no need to "spend down" before being eligible for drugs. *Crammer v. Commonwealth, ibid.*, par. 26,526, and see Chapter 12, footnote 26. The California Supreme Court took a similar position with respect to recipients pushed up to the "medically needy" category by the Social Security increases. (The "medically needy" in California now have to pay the first $225 of expenses in any one quarter.) See *Dils v. Genduldig*, 1973, *ibid.*, para. 26,618.

76. *State ex.rel. Rebel v. White,* 26 Ohio St. 2d 707, 271 N.E. 2d 282 (S. Ct. of Ohio, 1971) involved claims for vendor payments by two operators whose licenses had been revoked by the Ohio Department of Health but then ordered reinstated by the courts. While these revocations were in effect, the state welfare department made money payments directly to welfare recipients in the nursing home, and the homes collected from them an amount smaller than the Medicaid vendor payments they had received prior to revocation. The homes sought a *mandamus* to compel payment of the difference, but the Ohio Supreme Court summarily rejected their claims. In *Department of Public Health v. Perry,* CCH *Medicare & Medicaid Guide,* par. 26.306 (Ga. Ct. of App., 1971), Georgia successfully sued a nursing home proprietor for the refund of some $5700 erroneously paid after termination of eligibility as a Medicaid provider. *Sigety v. Ingraham,* 311 N.Y.S. 2d 678 (N.Y. Supr. Ct.), 34 A.D. 2d 316 (App. Div., 1st Dept., 1970), 29 N.Y. 2d 110, 324 N.Y.S. 2d 10, 272 N.E. 2d 524 (N.Y. Ct. App. 1971) reversed the New York Commissioner of Health, who was empowered to ascertain whether nursing home rate schedules for Medicaid were reasonable and had ruled that they were not to exceed 50 percent of the average adjusted inpatient cost at proprietary hospitals. The plaintiff, alleging that his reasonable costs exceeded this amount ($29 per day in April 1969), challenged the authority of the Commissioner to determine "reasonable costs" on other than an individual, home-by-home basis in cases such as his. The Court of Appeals found evidence to support the defendant's conclusion that nursing homes exceeding the regulatory maximum were not being efficiently run, and it ascribed the plaintiff's high costs to his "predilections for a fashionable neighborhood" (his nursing home was in the Upper East Side of Manhattan).

77. See, for example, *Rhodes v. Harden,* 1973, where the Supreme Court of Kansas refused to enforce a 25 percent cutback for providers, CCH *Medicare & Medicaid Guide,* par. 26,643; and *Shady Acres Nursing Home v. Canary,* 1973, where the Ohio Court of Common Pleas held that a SNF was entitled to a hearing before Medicaid payments were cut off. *Ibid.,* par. 26,646.

78. In *Maxwell Nursing Home v. Wyman,* CCH *Medicare & Medicaid Guide,* par. 26,456 (2d Circuit, 1972), the Second Circuit granted 148 nursing homes, 75 percent of whose patients were Medicaid recipients, preliminary injunctions against termination of Medicaid payments. The New York Social Service Department had terminated their eligibility because of various violations of the Life Safety Code of the National Fire Protection Association. This termination had taken place in spite of the provision in the applicable federal regulations [45 C.F.R. §249.33] that some requirements could be waived in hardship cases as long as the safety of the patients was not endangered. The Department had refused to make any determination as to whether the specific violations in any of the nursing homes were waivable and had not held hearings prior to termination. The court ordered such hearings to be held as quickly as possible for each home. An important factor in the court's decision was that these homes had been eligible for Medicaid payments for some time under temporary waivers, and the requirement that homes conform with the Life Safety Code was relatively new. In 1973 the Second Circuit again intervened to ensure that the New York Medicaid authorities complied with both state law and HEW regulations in its attempt to terminate provider agreements. *Maxwell Nursing Home v. Wyman, ibid.,* par. 26,665.

79. There had, however, been some improvements in the system, especially with respect to the "fair hearings" procedures. For a useful outline of the revised procedures, see DHEW, MSA, *Fair Hearings: Summary of Federal Regulations,*

mimeo., August 1971. Nationwide, over a 6-month period, there were 3200 fair hearings in connection with medical assistance. DHEW, National Center for Social Statistics, *Fair Hearings in Public Assistance January–June 1971*, May 1972, Table 4. See also, Director's Column, *Clearinghouse Review*, vol. 4 (1971), p. 404.

It should be noted, however, that in August 1973, regulations were proposed (*Federal Register*, vol. 38, p. 22042) to dispense with the necessity of a fair hearing where fraud was involved.

80. A study of AFDC recipients undertaken for HEW in 1969 had, for example, found that welfare symbolized to them not so much a welcome relief but "the worst life"; the welfare stigma was more widely experienced in states which paid larger grants and where caseworkers were more client-oriented; and there was an over-all lack of self-esteem. Leonard H. Goodman, Samuel M. Meyers, Jennie McIntyre, *Welfare Policy and Its Consequences for the Recipient Population: A Study of the AFDC Program*, Dec. 1969 (Contract No. 405-WA-OC-67-07). U.S., Department of Health, Education, and Welfare, Social and Rehabilitation Services.

81. Kent Rice, Arkansas Health Planning Program, "Survival in Adversity—A Study of Family Health and Poverty," reported in *National Health Insurance Proposals, supra,* note 9, p. 1867.

82. For a series of views on urban medicine, see e.g., *Medicine in the Ghetto*, ed. John C. Norman (New York, 1969).

83. U.S., Congress, Senate, Committee on Government Operations, Subcommittee on Executive Reorganization, *Health Care in America, Hearings* before the Subcommittee on Executive Reorganization, 90th Cong., 2nd Sess., 1968, pp. 79–80. In earlier hearings Senator Thaler of New York had quoted an example of an elderly man who walked into his office, took out a billfold, and opened up a long line of glass-paned envelopes: his card for Medicare Part A, his Blue Cross Card, his union health card as a retired member of the bricklayers union, and his Medicaid card, which provided limited coverage to back up the other coverages. "I said, 'What is your problem?' He said, 'I got a bellyache, what do I do?' "

84. E.g.: "What is the goal of the program? The program's ultimate goal is to make medical care of high quality readily available to those unable to pay for it." U.S., Department of Health, Education, and Welfare, Medical Services Administration, *Questions and Answers—Medical Assistance*, 1968, p. 1.

85. Connecticut State Welfare Department, Application for Medical Assistance, Form W-80, 5/70. This form also informs a prospective client that if he or she wants services his wife or her husband will have to be contacted, together with the parents of an applicant under 21, to determine these relatives' ability to assist in payments.

86. Sarah A. Butts, *Public Assistance Social Services Related to Medicaid*, U.S., Department of Health, Education, and Welfare, Social and Rehabilitation Services, Publication No. (SRS) 72–23011, 1972, pp. 15–16.

87. *Ibid.*, p. 11 and *passim.* The suggestions for improvement made by the caseworkers point up some of the basic deficiencies in Medicaid information: provision to clients of a list of local doctors who accept Medicaid patients, client orientation programs about Medicaid, simple and concisely written material for clients, more direct intervention by caseworkers on behalf of clients with health problems, more follow-up on referrals, and utilization of volunteers for "friendly visiting."

88. Charles L. Schultze, Edward R. Fried, Alice M. Rivlin, and Nancy H. Teeters, *Setting National Priorities: the 1973 Budget* (Washington, 1972), p. 219.

89. California, Connecticut, D.C., Guam, Hawaii, Illinois, Kansas, Kentucky, Maryland, Massachusetts, Michigan, Minnesota, Nebraska, New Hampshire, New York, North Carolina, North Dakota, Oklahoma, Pennsylvania, Puerto Rico, Rhode Island, Utah, Vermont, Virgin Islands, Virginia, Washington, and Wisconsin. Montana was scheduled to begin coverage of the medically needy on July 1, 1973.

90. Additionally, home health services must be provided to any eligible person entitled to skilled nursing home services, and state Medicaid plans must assure transportation of recipients to and from providers of services.

91. Medical Services Administration, personal communication.

92. For the implications of this, see Henry J. Aaron, *Why Is Welfare so Hard to Reform?* (Washington, 1973) pp. 14–15.

93. U.S., Congress, Senate, *Social Security Amendments of 1972,* Senate Finance Committee Report, 92nd Cong., 2nd Sess., 1972, p. 220.

94. In Arkansas, for example, a total of 95 persons in 56 disadvantaged families studied (32 white families, 24 black), were found to have some seeing, hearing, or speaking disorders; Kent Rice, *National Health Insurance Hearings, supra,* note 9, p. 1853. Over the whole country, the American Speech and Hearing Association reported a quarter of a million deaf persons, together with some 8.5 million Americans with auditory problems which impair communication, 2.1 million with central communication (neurological) disorders, and 10 million with other kinds of speech disorders; Statement of Dr. Hayes A. Newbig, *Ibid.*, p. 1459. Medicaid was not equipped to deal with such disorders or to provide aid at all unless the individual was seriously in need; it was, indeed, a "catastrophic" program.

95. State of New York, *Report from the Governor's Steering Committee on Social Problems, on Health and Hospital Services and Costs,* New York, 1971.

96. The House Ways and Means Committee hearings of 1971 sparked contributions from organizations such as the Georgia Committee for National Health Care, the California Council for Health Plan Alternatives, the Arkansas Committee for National Health Insurance, the Pennsylvania Committee for National Health Security, the Oregon Committee for National Health Care, the Northeastern Wisconsin Citizens Committee for National Health Insurance, and other similar groups.

14

New York, California, and Illinois

Developments in New York and California, by far the largest Medicaid programs, continued to dominate Medicaid from 1970 to 1973, as in the early periods. For this reason alone, they deserve emphasis. But the specific forms of their Medicaid problems, joined with those of Illinois, provide independent studies of difficulties inherent in all the states. New York showed what happened when money was poured into a medical care system that almost defied administrative control; California in this period is a classic example of concern over costs overshadowing concern for medical care; while Illinois provides an almost perfect example of the tragic institutional battles that swirl around Medicaid programs in the states. An efficiency-minded governor, hoping to cut costs, found himself faced with entrenched bureaucrats and political machines, with a hostile legislature, judges, and welfare rights organizations, as well as dissatisfied providers.

New York: The Same Old Story

In New York, the destructive disputes between Albany and New York City left the program particularly vulnerable to fraud—of both the sophisticated and the unsophisticated variety. The absence of effective administration, moreover, was emphasized by the complex array of both public and private health services in the state, notably in New York City. The dual system of public care for the poor and private care for the nonpoor was, if anything, hardened through the contribution of Medicaid funds to the city's hospital and health system—perhaps thereby delaying its collapse, but also undoubtedly delaying reconsideration of its role in the total complex of services in the city. As the voluntary hospitals and private professionals had also been shored up by the rapid infusion of Medicaid funds into the network, the city could not control the activities of providers as a whole. Although continuing efforts were made to audit the Medicaid program and ferret out its grosser errors, the reaction from Albany was predictable. Eligibility levels were threatened once again. The limit of $5000 for a family of four survived 1970, but it was at once under attack in the 1971 meeting of the legislature.

The budget battle in Albany in the spring of 1971 was similar to many earlier battles. Governor Rockefeller proposed a state budget of $8.45 billion, reflecting "an austerity program to maintain state services at existing levels." The Reform Democrats alleged that secretly the Governor was trying to work out $703 million worth of cuts. As 10 percent of these cuts were alleged to be in the area of welfare, the liberal Democrats talked about making sure there was no quorum on hand for a vote.[1] In fact, the fiscal year began on April 1 without a budget. Mayor Lindsay, irritated by what he felt was the Governor's broken promise of revenue sharing with the localities, announced that "no budget is better than the budget that has been proposed."[2] The Mayor was wrong. When a budget did emerge, $760 million had been slashed from the Governor's package; and many of the cuts came in the welfare and Medicaid area. As one Democrat Assemblyman put it, the cuts were made by "ruthless Republicans" who would "if they could, repeal the 20th Century."[3] In turn, the Republicans accused the Democrats of thinking of "hearts and flowers" while forgetting that it was "the guy with the lunch bucket who pays the tab on all this."[4]

The budget that was passed ensured cuts both in eligibility and services under Medicaid. The income limit for a family of four was henceforth to be set at $4,500, and the medically needy were limited to physician services. They were no longer to be eligible for dental care, home nursing, optometry, drugs, sickroom supplies, glasses, prosthetic devices, physical therapy, laboratory, and x-rays. It was perhaps fortunate that there were few of the medically indigent left on the rolls.[5]

The cutbacks led to litigation almost at once,[6] even before the amending legislation went into force. Two class suits, *Brasher v. Rockefeller*[7] and *Bass v. Rockefeller*[8], were brought, and they led to temporary restraining orders. The courts found that New York had failed to comply with section 1902(d), which forbids cutbacks without the approval of the Secretary of HEW. Indeed, shortly thereafter, the *Bass* court went still further and gave an injunction against implementation until the Secretary's approval and the other requirements of 1902(d) were met.[9] In September 1971, however, the Secretary gave his approval, and the Second Circuit of Appeals remanded the case and ordered it dismissed.[10]

The result of this decision was that the full cuts ordered by the legislature went into effect by the fall of 1971.[11] It was expected that some

165,000 persons would be struck off the Medicaid rolls, with over-all savings in the neighborhood of $165 million out of a budget of $1.3 billion. Before that could happen, the Center on Social Welfare Law began new suits with the same plaintiff,[12] further challenging the legality of the cuts. *Bass v. Richardson*[13] called for a roll-back in the Medicaid cuts because the other statutory requirement, on which cut-backs are conditional, had not been met, namely, the requirement for utilization and cost-control procedures.

This time the City of New York, which claimed it would be forced to spend an extra $40 million annually in order to provide essential services to recipients, was allowed to intervene as plaintiff; and the plaintiffs were once again successful in enjoining implementation. The court found the record "overwhelming—top heavy in favor of the plaintiffs." Looking, for the purposes of a temporary injunction, at what the plaintiffs could probably prove, the court opined that the state had not implemented the strict utilization review procedures required by federal legislation (as indeed a confidential report from the Regional Office of HEW had so found), that the state had not demonstrated its commitment to the broadening of services by 1977, as required by section 1903(e), and that the Secretary could not reasonably have concluded that these requirements had been met before he approved the cutback.[14] In short, the state's new restrictions were illegal; and they were thus disallowed.

But, while the 1971 cutback in eligibility was thus delayed, the city had, by this time, capitulated and followed the remainder of the state in implementing the 20 percent co-insurance provisions, for the medically indigent, which had survived challenge in the courts. The impact, chiefly on recipients, was inevitable. It became less easy to find physicians,[15] dentists, and other providers prepared to service Medicaid patients. By 1973, for instance, the vice-president of the State Dental Society noted that a combination of the 20 percent co-insurance premiums and the 20 percent cut in professional fees had led to a "skidding" decline in participation by dentists in Medicaid—from 85 percent to 15 percent.[16]

Meanwhile, almost every other problem reappeared during this period. By no means everyone was losing from cuts in Medicaid. Fraud, for instance, seemed to make as good news as ever, especially in New York City. In the fall of 1971, Robert Rustin, the City Commissioner of Investigations, charged in a television interview that $1.5 million had been unjustly billed by transportation companies for taking Medicaid patients to hospitals.[17] During the same period, when the special allowances for clothing and footwear were deleted from the welfare cash assistance schedule, podiatrists were substituting up to 17,000 pairs of orthopedic shoes a month, at a far higher cost.[18] It also emerged that one of the leading figures in one of the Medicaid factoring firms, which the City had been trying to put out of business since 1967, was guilty of a $2 million fraud.[19] Eventually

12 persons connected with the factoring firm or the City's Department of Social Services were found guilty of fraud.[20]

In the meantime, there were internal disputes about the efficacy of New York City's Medicaid audit system. Councilman Carter Burden claimed that not only were Medicaid patients being exploited by "shoddy treatment and profiteering in storefront medical centers," but that the City Department of Social Services had been "blandly paying every bill received." While Dr. Bellin took some umbrage at the suggestion of sloppiness in his Department, he admitted that 10 percent of reported services under Medicaid were "unacceptable," a fact he attributed to low fees.[21]

More dramatic in their own way were the investigations into the City's Medicaid administration. Early in 1972, a Grand Jury indicated that nearly $1 billion "went down the drain" because of fraud and waste in the department. District Attorney Hogan went so far as to characterize the City's Medicaid administration as "completely disorganized, if not chaotic." The grand jury found nursing homes billing the city for the care of patients who were dead and dentists and pharmacists guilty of excessive and fraudulent claims, as well as city employees working with factoring firms to defraud the City. Abuses were said to be "not only flagrant, but widespread." In addition, the sampling of Medicaid patients for eligibility was termed "inaccurate, wasteful and useless," while there was an allegation that the City had lost two and a quarter million dollars in state and federal funds because of inadequate record keeping. Some of the records, the grand jury said, were kept in "shoe boxes." So bad were the records, the Report added, that the City was unable to defend itself when a dentist demanded a further $358,000 in addition to the $1,312,752 he had already been paid in 1968 and 1969.

The reaction to the report was inevitable. Human Resources Commissioner Jules Sugarman said there was "not one scintilla of evidence to support the judge's near-billion dollar estimate." He put the losses at nearer $5 million. Meanwhile Governor Rockefeller termed the jury's findings "shocking" and referred the report to the then recently created State Welfare Inspector-General (George Berlinger). In response, the City somewhat pathetically claimed that $1.6 million had been saved by Medicaid audits.[22] But the propensity of such allegations to recur was remarkable.

Towards the end of the year, for instance, a physician whom Mayor Lindsay had imported to become his first Addiction Services Agency Commissioner and who had gone on to private practice was accused of billing Medicaid $28,000 for patients he had never seen.[23] Early in February 1973, the Welfare Inspector-General singled out nursing homes and the incompetence and dishonesty of the New York City Medicaid Administration as particularly venal.[24] Shortly thereafter, $150,000 was set aside to begin an "exhaustive investigation" of misuse of Medicaid funds in the City's hospitals.[25] Four days later the City responded by opening a computer center to check on the eligibility of Medicaid recipients.[26] Early in 1973 Councilman Katz introduced a bill to curb Medicaid abuses in the City.[27]

It was, indeed, business as usual. By early 1973, the City was running a deficit of $75 million in its Medicaid budget.[28] At the same time, auditors from the City's Health Department uncovered the fact that physician kickbacks to and from laboratories had been costing the City $4 million a year.[29] The *Daily News* featured such headlines as "Pair of Medicaid Kings With a Midas Touch," "Foot Docs Wearing a $35-Million Golden Slipper," and "How Medicaid Paid $457,000 for Sesame Oil."[30] The only difference seemed to be that for once the state was not facing a deficit in its budget, and Governor Rockefeller was even talking about putting some people back on the Medicaid rolls.[31]

Certainly administration in the medical care field was not New York City's strong point; indeed, the Deputy Director of the Human Resources Administration conceded that "the present system doesn't make any damn sense."[32] Even the Health and Hospitals Corporation had difficulty implementing its plans, for example, the attempt to test all black youngsters for sickle cell anemia.[33] And the failings of the Medicaid administration seemed ever more glaring. Doctors again complained about the slow payment of bills, the State Medical Society alleging "chaotic" administration.[34] But at least the City moved to expedite payments to hospitals when it emerged that some hospitals had more than $2 million in backed-up claims.[35] Finally, in July 1972, the State Commission of Social Services established a new division to administer medical assistance, headed by a former Connecticut Welfare Commissioner, Bernard Shapiro, to emphasize utilization.[36]

This last move, however, was not seen solely as a cost-cutting move, and here perhaps was the beginning of a new direction. The other goal of Deputy Commissioner Shapiro was to "pay special attention to preventive medical care and to the encouragement of health maintenance organizations within the State, which could improve the quality of care and at the same time cut down on costs." Such an approach was in keeping with the urge to experiment with the delivery of health services, and mirrored, to some degree, the "health" concerns at the federal level. What was happening by 1973 was that New York's long championship of medical services to the needy was both corrupted and eroded to a meagre level, but without any cost reduction. The only logical new step was to encourage better organization in the health care system.

In other respects, too, New York stressed health service needs. From the late 1960s, Governor Rockefeller had been talking of some form of state health insurance, and in 1971 the Democrats called for a comprehensive state health insurance program.[37] The Grand Jury Report suggested setting up a federal-state-city task force to examine the possibility of health centers for the poor in place of the system of contracting with individual providers, an idea taken up by the County Executive of Suffolk County.[38] The concept did not, however, commend itself to local physicians; as a group they were at least in theory committed to the idea of a "personal physician" for all Medicaid patients.[39]

Although in this regard the possibility for movement seemed to exist, its full implementation would require massive changes in health care organization, including the raising of additional capital for developments such as health centers and HMOs; and such demands were beyond the resources of the Medicaid program. The situation at the beginning of 1973 was thus a stalemate. Inspector-General Berlinger greeted the New Year by reiterating the charge that Medicaid was responsible for an annual waste (through fraud and for other reasons) of $1 billion.[40] But it was beginning to seem that some large degree of waste was inevitable as long as Medicaid continued to operate in its existing framework. Cost-saving followed its hallowed path, although in December 1972 the City was finally allowed to switch to the dispensing of drugs by generic names.[41] All that one can say is that at best the passage of the 1972 Social Security Amendments increased the pressure for administrative consolidation. The logic for a state takeover of total responsibility for Medicaid,[42] perhaps as a step to total federalization, was increasingly clear. But it was also clear that the underlying problems of Medicaid, resting as they did on an unreformed health system, would not thereby go away.

The California Scene: History Does Repeat Itself

In California, too, history tended to repeat itself in the early 1970s. California's wide range of services and "mainstream" approach were, again, to be threatened by cost considerations. The economic crisis and hysteria that had characterized 1968 and 1969 had apparently died down; indeed, in August 1970, the eligibility levels were in fact raised; and in September 1970 the scope of benefits to welfare recipients and the medically indigent were made uniform. But behind this apparent complacency, trouble was brewing.

Governor Reagan and his cost-conscious administration did not look with favor on Medi-Cal. Not only were costs rising but the projected number of recipients was increasing rapidly. The program thus apparently encouraged "pauperization." For fiscal year 1970–71 the projected number of recipients was originally 2,119,600, but this was later revised upward to 2,294,000; the legislature was asked for a further $60 million. By December, however, Dr. Earl Brian, Director of the Department of Health Care Services, estimated a caseload of 2,402,900 persons. A $200 million deficit was in sight.[43]

This was the background to the announcement that, with effect from December 15, 1970, there would be a cut of 10 percent in physicians' fees and in fees to all other providers (except hospitals for inpatient care). Additionally, prior authorization was introduced for some drugs, price ceilings were put on others, while certification was required even for emergency hospitalization.[44] Governor Reagan then asked doctors "to again pull in their belts," a request the California Medical Association (CMA) described as "absolutely unfair." The President of the CMA declared "optimum care for Medi-Cal patients simply is no longer possible under these new regulations."[45] Nevertheless, the projected cuts were laid before the state's Health Review and Program Council for approval on December 2nd. They were expected to save some $111 million. When the Council asked about the possibility of the cuts being delayed until the legislature met, Dr. Brian was adamantly opposed, reminding the Council its function was only advisory.[46]

As in New York, litigation was as inevitable as it was swift. During December the California Association of Nursing Homes filed suit to enjoin the cut-backs; although a temporary restraining order was denied on December 14.[47] By that time, however, the Association, representing 900 out of the 1,300 homes in the state, had called on its members to boycott Medi-Cal with effect from February 1, 1971.[48] This in turn produced litigation of a different kind. On January 31, 1971, Judge Avakian of the Superior Court granted a temporary restraining order to prevent nursing homes boycotting Medi-Cal or transferring their patients to county hospitals.[49]

In the meantime other providers had gotten into the business of litigation. The president of the California Dental Association, Dr. R. Neil Smithwick, warned that many ghetto-area dentists' practices would collapse with the cuts in fees.[50] Dr. Vertis Thompson of the predominantly black National Medical Association claimed that physicians practicing in ghetto areas could not afford a ten percent cut in fees.[51] Innovative medical programs, like "Crisis Intervention," an emergency program of psychiatric care in the San Francisco area, were threatened by the requirement of prior authorization.[52] In January, the CMA President, Dr. Ralph Burnett announced "C.M.A. will be suing to restore the necessary medical care and medications that are essential to the health of the poor—not the question of fees. We challenge and do not accept the December 15 emergency regulations. They are in direct contradiction of the legislature's intent in enacting Medi-Cal."[53]

The California Medical Association instituted its suit on January 13, 1971, seeking a restraining order against the state on the ground that the emergency regulations were inconsistent with the Medicaid legislation. This suit was joined with one brought by California Rural Legal Assistance, alleging that the program was in fact operating within its budget and therefore the legislative mechanism allowing cutbacks had not been lawfully triggered. Indeed, as with the earlier Medi-Cal crisis, there were conflicting views about whether or not there was a budget deficit.[54] By February 1, the legislative staff suggested that Dr. Brian had overestimated the Medi-Cal deficit by approximately $100 million.[55] Meanwhile, a legislative hearing in Los Angeles revealed that massive backlogs of paperwork were developing by reason of the prior authorization provisions.[56] Yet when the *Los Angeles Times* suggested that the December crisis had been brought on by an overload of paperwork rather than any real deficit, the Governor was extremely displeased.[57]

By February, the legislature's Special Committee on Medi-Cal had reported, finding generally in favor of the Reagan position. It was estimated that there would have been a deficit of $100 million had the emergency cuts not been made. At the same time, the Committee felt there had been little coordination with other departments and that the impact on other medical programs had not been considered.[58] Other defects emerged. In an effort to cut costs, for instance, only one drug was authorized for treating psychiatric cases.[59] Indeed, by March, Assemblyman Gordon Duffy, a Republican, who had brought in a bill to cancel the cutbacks, announced that the Governor was prepared to rescind some of the cutbacks,[60] which were in any event due to expire on June 30. Meanwhile the litigation was dragging on. Eventually, in June 1971, the Sacramento Superior Court determined that Director Brian had failed to establish that an emergency had existed and the cutbacks had therefore been unlawful.[61] Once again the courts had thwarted the Reagan administration with respect to Medi-Cal.[62]

But the underlying situation was unsatisfactory. As Dr. Brian said in legislative hearings:

> *If there is no restructuring, this program will continue to gyrate wildly in the years to come, either with an embarrassing surplus or a cataclysmic deficit.*[63]

And the CMA, in an editorial noted:

> *The realistic solution is quite simple. The State should either reduce the numbers of persons eligible for care, or increase the funding for the program or both. But usually neither of these logical alternatives is politically palatable, so other alternatives are apt to be tried. These other alternatives seem somehow always to deprive patients of medical services. When either the quantity or quality of needed services becomes reduced by law or by fiat not only havoc but injustices are created. The further these unhappy alternatives to a realistic solution are pursued, the worse becomes the problem and the greater the suffering and injustices to the poor patient and often the poor providers as well.*[64]

California as Innovator

Such pious hopes probably spurred the writing of bills to reform Medi-Cal during 1971. In particular, the Administration proposed a comprehensive Medi-Cal Reform Program.[65] Under the revised Medi-Cal program, those on general assistance were to be included, but, with HEW's approval, beneficiaries would have to contribute to their care (supposedly to discourage wanton use, raise funds, and make recipients generally more aware of costs): Co-insurance would be applied to all recipients. There would be cutbacks in the amount of services that could be used in any one year and increased formalization of utilization procedures. The bill also encouraged Medi-Cal to make use of prepayment programs. Some of the proposed bills would have gone even further. Assemblyman Craig Biddle proposed a medical insurance program, along the lines of FHIP. With premiums ranging from $18 to $50 a month, the "recipients would purchase their insurance from a private company which would be reimbursed by the state."[66]

Meanwhile the CMA added their proposals. Under their bill, introduced by Senator Anthony Beilensen (Democrat), administration of Medi-Cal would be given to a public corporation run by a Board of Governors appointed for 6-year terms. Such a corporation would then negotiate a statewide prepayment contract with physicians.[67] The "mainstream" approach would thus be maintained. But Governor Reagan planned to keep Medi-Cal in the welfare field. Indeed in May 1971 the Governor was able to announce a different type of experiment. With what many believed was the blessing of the White House, the Governor had persuaded HEW Secretary Richardson to allow California to "experiment" by requiring co-payment by all recipients, including those receiving cash assistance: this had to be labelled as an experiment as Title XIX basically did not allow co-payment to be applied to the categorically needy. The Secretary was reported as saying: "It's hard for us to refuse a waiver to test something we believe should be in the law anyway."[68] Senator Alan Cranston, however, one of California's two Democratic Senators, bitterly attacked the move, and announced he would press for federalization of Medicaid to take "away from governors like Ronald Reagan the power and temptation to cut Medicaid budgets at the expense of the aged, infirm and sickly poor."[69] Yet there was obviously widespread support for the Reagan measure, which received legislative form as the Campbell Bill.[70]

The statistic that the average Californian spent $312 a year on medical care while Medi-Cal cost an average of $517 had an attractive political hue outside California as well.[71] And the Governor was prepared to go on the offensive. Early in 1972, he announced his own program of catastrophic health insurance.[72] The liberals countered this by introducing their compulsory comprehensive health insurance proposal, covering virtually all

Californians.[73] In this respect then, New York and California appeared to be moving in similar directions.

But with respect to Title XIX, the future lay in the Medi-Cal Reform Act, approved on August 18, 1971.[74] In some respects the legislation broadened the coverage of the program. In the future, medically indigent adults between 21 and 65 would be eligible for Medi-Cal (even though federal matching grants were not available for this group), and indigents under 21 were formally included for the first time. But while coverage was increased, services were curtailed. For instance, special duty nursing was no longer available. Moreover, for other services, a schedule of basic benefits was laid down: there were to be only two outpatient visits a month and drug prescriptions were limited to two a month. After such basic entitlements were exhausted, certain benefits on a supplemental schedule would be available. Co-payment was to be required under all the basic schedule services, and it was assumed that some 35 to 45 percent of those eligible for Medi-Cal would be required to make co-payments.[75] It was not however clear how the money was to be collected, as the CMA successfully lobbied against physicians having to collect the co-payment amounts.

The rub was that the new program was not expected to cut costs. The projected budget for 1972–73 was $1,688,656,545—a 12.6 percent rise from the previous year.[76] The prior-authorization procedures were already operating under pressure, as some 237,135 authorizations were being processed each month, with about 10 percent being denied.[77] An amending bill passed in the fall of 1971 increased the eligibility levels for the non-categorically related groups and added a few services. Meanwhile the new program was under attack in the courts. *Roberts v. Brian*,[78] decided in November 1971, threw doubt on whether special-duty nursing could be withdrawn, at least for those in nursing homes. A suit was also instituted challenging the Secretary's grant of permission to undertake the experiment requiring co-payment for welfare recipients, on the ground that this was not a bona fide experiment, for which the Secretary had authority to waive the regulations, but rather a cut in services without lawful authority.[79] But in a decision in September 1972 the attempt to enjoin co-payment failed.[80]

California was, like other states in these years, facing other problems. A group of state employees alleged that the use of fiscal agents for administering Medi-Cal was a violation of Article XXIV of the State Constitution —the so-called "civil service amendment." The court held that exemptions were permissible and that not every new state program required an extension of the civil service.[81] In the meantime, Blue Shield, one of the fiscal agents, was engaged in litigation with the Department of Health Care Services about the right of Blue Shield to charge the department for public relations activities.[82] The federal General Accounting Office was once more complaining of the overpayment of physicians in California;[83] while the

GAO also produced an extensive report on the many failings in the nursing home industry in California, suggesting fraud, substandard homes, false advertising, and a host of other issues.[84] Perhaps to crown everything, the recipients, as they organized, achieved the distinction of having the support of President Nixon's first cousin. Mr. and Mrs. Philip Milhous founded the Low Income Welfare Rights Organization in Nevada City. Said Mrs. Milhous: "There isn't a doctor in this town who'll make a pair of glasses for Medi-Cal patients. . . . People in rest homes can't get medication. You have no idea of how many people are actually suffering over this."[85]

Administratively, however, innovation was in the air. The new 1971 California legislation, for instance, provided a framework for stimulating the development of prepaid health insurance under the aegis of Medi-Cal; and the state was soon the focus of such programs. The idea of using such devices was not new: The San Joaquin Foundation's prepayment program had been under way for some years. But from 1971 onwards, the thrust towards prepayment was a broad one, with detailed codes and requirements; yet—in an almost inevitable cycle—providers proved cannier than administrators. In December 1972, the *Los Angeles Times* headed a report: "New Gold-Rush—Prepaid Medi-Cal Franchises Sought."[86] It reported that while some of the contracts for prepaid group insurance for Medi-Cal patients had gone to nonprofit organizations, most had gone to profit-making organizations who boasted to their investors that they hoped to produce a 2500 to 3000 percent return on their money. While the claims were probably inflated, it was clear that some of the contractors hoped to "make a killing" by providing totally inadequate services, and the *Times* did not hesitate to name names, including some persons close to the state administration.

Perhaps as the result of these disclosures, there was a flurry of legislative activity. The governor signed a bill prohibiting any prepayment health contract going to any firm in which a legislator, state officer, or employee had a direct or indirect financial interest.[87] Moreover, when it emerged that profit-making concerns were moving into prepaid programs, the CMA argued that this was illegal, as the unlawful practice of medicine. A bill was then rushed through the legislature in its dying hours of the 1972 session to allow profit-making organizations to sell prepaid health plans, only to be vetoed by the governor.[88]

Even then the situation was obscure. Some profit-making firms, following a policy of honesty-is-best, withdrew. The Whittaker Corporation, which had hoped to add health care for the poor to its conglomerate interests in biomedical research, boat building, steel, and textiles, dropped its plan for a prepayment plan in Fullerton. But other *de facto* profit-making plans were alleged to be lurking under *de jure* nonprofit facades.[89] Substance appeared to be added to that report when the *New York Times* reported that the

Mafia was moving into the HMO business in California.[90] A "pluralistic" solution was obviously in the making.

Illinois: A Clash of Giants

Medicaid's dilemmas of divided responsibilities were, however, nowhere more evident than in Illinois.[91] Medicaid had begun in that state in 1966, with coverage both for welfare groups and for the "medically indigent," the latter group being eligible for the same broad range of services available to welfare recipients. Thus Governor Richard Ogilvie, who came into office in 1969 on a plank of streamlining state government[92] and making it more administratively efficient,[93] found himself confronted by ever-expanding budgets. Indeed, state appropriations (as a whole) rose from $3.5 billion in 1969 to $7.3 billion for fiscal year 1973. Within that budget, not only had the welfare component doubled, but the cost of Medicaid had risen 280 percent in five years. There was an obvious incentive to streamline the program and to improve administrative efficiency; otherwise, major cuts would be necessary.

With gubernatorial elections looming in 1972, 6500 physicians received warning letters in January 1971 urging restraint in treating Medicaid patients, as there was a possibility that there would be insufficient funds to carry the program through June. While a Democratic State Representative from Chicago, Robert Mann, protested that "any medical system geared only to costs and not to quality care is bound to fail,"[94] there was no lessening of interest in wielding the economy axe.[95]

The program survived fiscal 1970. But the budget published in July 1971 provided for a $25 million cut in Medicaid funds.[96] Finally, in October 1971, Governor Ogilvie produced a five-point program for curbing Illinois welfare payments—four of the proposals being directly related to Medicaid.[97] Of these latter changes, the Governor said they called on the providers of care "to account for the services they deliver to Medicaid recipients," but at the same time recipients would be required "to have more responsibility for their actions in obtaining health services."[98] There were thus to be curbs on both providers and recipients.

Of the two parts of the program designed to apply to providers, the more innovative was called the Hospital Admission and Surveillance Program (HASP). The Program, administered by the Illinois State Medical Society through the Illinois Foundation for Medical Care, was designed to lay down specific lengths of hospitalization for specific illnesses, "based on recognized medical standards," and to develop systems of certification for various processes and procedures. This arrangement was apparently worked out during six weeks of intensive negotiation between the physicians and the state, and the President of the Foundation noted that "originally the administration planned a cost-cutting program that would have put doctors and hospital administrators under government control." But the Governor was apparently satisfied with the compromise, noting that "this health reform is the first of the kind in the country." By establishing norms, the length of stay of patients in hospitals could be routinely flagged (for over-extensions) and individual treatment plans evaluated. After all, if the stay of each Medicaid patient in hospitals could be shortened by one day, there would be an estimated saving of $12 million.[99]

Second, providers were to be subject to a more widespread reimbursement freeze. Although hospital room rates had been frozen as of January 1971, the new Director of Public Aid (Edward Weaver) claimed that, including x-rays, drugs, and lab tests, the state paid an average of $159 a day, while the average patient cost in hospital was $88 a day. In future, the state announced, it would pay only actual costs. Additionally physicians' fees were to be frozen with effect from June 30, 1971.[100]

As far as recipients were concerned, Illinois was to follow California's example: The major cutback was to be a "token payment" by recipients of $1 a day for hospitalization, as well as for an outpatient visit, $1 per visit to a physician, and 50 cents per prescription. This co-payment proposal, like California's would, however, have to be designated an experiment under section 1115 of the Social Security Act and required approval from HEW. It was expected to save $5 million a year. Additionally, medically indigent recipients were to have their entitlements cut. In particular, this group would no longer be eligible for drugs, physician services, dental care, optometrists, and podiatrists unless they were hospitalized. There were also to be certain cuts in optometrist and dental services for all groups. These cuts were estimated to save $14 million.

Finally, there was to be a change in welfare that, indirectly, might be expected to help the Medicaid budget. Unlike many states, Illinois still had a significant number of persons on general assistance, in other words, persons on welfare but for whom no federal categorical aid was claimed. This was especially true in Cook County which had hung on to its general assistance programs, even though at least some of the recipients would have been eligible for welfare through the state's categorical assistance programs. The exact reason for this was unclear, but it was widely thought to be related to the Democratic machine's reliance on the welfare vote.

The situation was further complicated by the fact that the state, in any event, largely footed the bill. Indeed, the arrangement cost the state dearly, for 85 percent of Cook County's general assistance grants were picked up by the state and only 15 percent by Mayor Daley's administration. Governor Ogilvie calculated that by taking over the general assistance grants and putting the recipients into federal categorical programs, the state might attract almost $40 million of federal money. As in New York, then, though for different reasons, there was a direct confrontation between state and city administrations.

It was clear from the moment of the October announcements that opposition to the changes in Chicago would be fierce, particularly on the recipients' side. Operation Breadbasket warned that the cuts would cause hospitals to close,[101] while the Chicago hospitals were talking of a $40 million deficit.[102] Meanwhile Cook County announced its intention of suing the state over cuts in general assistance[103] and actually began withdrawing Medicaid "green cards" from 10,000 general assistance recipients in Chicago.[104] In the meantime, there were battles in the state legislature in Springfield about work requirements in welfare.[105] Once again, Medicaid was in the thick of battle, and compromise seemed a long way off.

Illinois: "The Winter of Our Discontent"

Meanwhile, the Illinois Department of Public Assistance had to seek HEW's approval of the proposed cuts in Medicaid and, in particular, for approval of co-payment for cash recipients, which as noted required a waiver. The director of the department put the matter bluntly in his request to Washington: "Briefly, the alternatives are twofold: either to curtail the program's content even more drastically than do the current amendments or to discontinue the program to the medically needy altogether."[106]

Although cutbacks in services raised delicate issues of state effort, the co-payment question was more difficult. Since there was *prima facie* no way of obtaining HEW's general approval of a program-wide cost-sharing proposal (which was forbidden by the federal legislation), following the Reagan pattern the plan was presented to HEW as an "experiment" or "demonstration project" within the meaning of section 1115. But such a move was becoming transparent. Thus while the cutbacks seemed likely to be approved, the Associate Regional Commissioner of HEW was reported as saying of the co-payment proposals that Illinois "appears to be attempting to change its current State plan for Title XIX by means of a project and to thereby subvert the purposes and thrust of Section 1115 legislation."[107] California had already plucked the plum, and approval for Illinois was delayed.

By the end of October, however, the action had moved to the courts. Cook County was seeking an injunction to prevent the cut-off of state funds for general assistance on the ground that the new proposals were being applied only to Chicago and therefore were a violation of "equal protection."[108] At the same time hospitals in the state planned a suit, alleging that the new reimbursement regulations violated the statutory obligation to reimburse hospitals for their reasonable expenses. On the 31st, Chicago actually obtained a temporary restraining order in its suit,[109] and three days later the state Supreme Court let the trial judge's order stand.[110]

In the meantime, the recipients had begun their own court actions through the Chicago Legal Aid Society—an OEO-funded legal services program.[111] As soon as Governor Ogilvie had announced plans for the cuts, the Society had sought to intervene in the decisions being taken by HEW on the Illinois requests both for the cuts and for the approval of the co-payment experiment. As the Governor had already sent out letters to the 750,000 Medicaid recipients telling them of the cuts in services, the Legal Aid Society asked for a temporary restraining order against the cuts in Federal Court on November 1.

The argument made by the plaintiffs was that the state was attempting to make the cutbacks without the prior approval of HEW. But when Judge Will began an emergency hearing on the petition at 10:30 a.m. on November 2, it emerged that HEW had approved the cuts that very morning, at 8:30 a.m. According to the *Chicago Daily News*, "U.S. District Court Judge Herbert L. Will was visibly irritated about the time of Federal approval."[112] In the end, the judge gave a preliminary injunction because the 15-day notice of cutbacks required by the Federal regulation had not in fact been given.[113]

The decision undoubtedly upset the state's leaders. Governor Ogilvie stressed the rise in Medicaid costs from $81 million in 1966 to a projected $435 million in 1971–72.[114] Meanwhile the Attorney General of the State (Scott) disagreed sufficiently with the Governor's stand that he took himself out of the welfare cases.[115] At the same time Welfare Director Weaver insisted that the cuts would be made in December, after the appropriate notice had been given.[116] But already, on the general assistance issue, there was evidence that Ogilvie and Daley might be prepared to do a deal,[117] with Democrats in Springfield seeking to take money from one state pot or another and Republicans suggesting the money should come from the funds for Mayor Daley's Crosstown Expressway project.[118] Governor Ogilvie, however, still saw the solution to the general assistance crisis in terms of cuts in Medicaid.[119] If HEW would approve his cuts, the Governor felt sure he could assure general assistance money to Cook County.[120]

The various political moves left the providers somewhat divided. Particularly poignant were a series of journalistic interviews with ghetto doctors, practicing "volume medicine." Dr. Edward Regal and his brother-in-law, Dr. Michael Trubitt, had had their clinic destroyed in the riots following Martin Luther King, Jr.'s death. But they had rebuilt. As Dr. Trubitt put it: "We are not Dr. Schweitzers. . . . We prefer this type of medicine because we have a chance to see many different kinds of pathology. We see people who are very sick. And we give them good medical care." The Ogilvie cuts, especially HASP and co-payment, would in the view of the doctors, "leave ghetto doctors with dwindling practices. If patients didn't come, the doctors will close up and move."[121] The neighboring Chicago School of Business economists would not have dissented.

Meanwhile, notices of cuts in services to begin in December had been given,[122] and HEW's permission for the co-payment experiment was still being sought. By mid-November, the legal services lawyers were back in court again with further attempts to prevent the cuts, joining HEW, and arguing that the cuts were unlawful in the light of the "comprehensive care" provision and the absence of effective utilization review and fair-hearings procedures in the state.[123] To a limited extent, the legal services pleas were successful. On December 1, Judge Will refused to dissolve the temporary injunction until the merits of the case had been heard, finding at least a *prima facie* violation of federal law;[124] and a week later the Seventh Circuit Court of Appeals upheld the temporary order.[125]

Thus, in mid-December 1971, the action for a permanent injunction came before Judge Will. With the same points argued by the plaintiffs that had been put forward in the trial on the preliminary injunction, there was increasing evidence that Illinois had little in the way of utilization review. After Judge Will had refused motions for a directed verdict for the state, however, HEW lawyers began to imply he might be guilty of bias.[126] Judge Will therefore took himself out of the case.[127] The case was then assigned to a newly appointed judge, William Bower, but he had to withdraw because he had formerly been U.S. attorney and had participated in some of the pre-trial stages of the case. The case was then assigned to Judge Julius Hoffman—best known for his role in the "Chicago Seven" case; but after prevaricating and refusing to dissolve the injunction, he announced his retirement. The case eventually appeared in Judge Richard McLaren's docket.[128] Such, then, were the judicial vicissitudes.

Indeed, one way and another the state was having an uphill battle. Under court pressure, the Governor had acceeded to Chicago's request and released general assistance funds,[129] although it was recouping some of this by transferring Cook County's general assistance recipients to AFDC.[130] Nevertheless, by February, Governor Ogilvie was predicting a state deficit of $111 million by the end of June,[131] a state of affairs which was somewhat alleviated by the promise of a federal advance of $60 million in the following year's categorical welfare grants-in-aid.[132] There were other ways, too, in which the situation was alleviated. Illinois also cashed in on another federal "boondoggle," which was to exceed Medicaid in its rapid expansion. By "consolidating social service" programs, the federal government became liable to Illinois under Title IV(A) of the Social Security Act to pay three quarters of the cost of social services to welfare recipients.[133] This meant an extra $27 million in Federal funds.[134] And by April, the deficit in Medicaid itself was said to be declining because case loads were declining.[135]

With these changes in fortune, not to mention the eternal delays in court proceedings, it seemed a good moment to compromise the cutback proceedings.[136] After negotiations lasting most of the spring of 1972, Judge McLaren was able to enter an order which effectively restored most of the cuts that had been threatened the previous October. Even the Director of the Department of Public Aid seemed satisfied.[137] Of course, settlement of the cutback case did not end the war. In December of 1971 it had been reported that, because of the hospital cutbacks, "Several hospitals have said they will have to close down."[138] But the hospitals too were saved by Judge McLaren.

One matter remained outstanding: the co-payment experiment. The co-payment proposal required the specific approval of HEW under section 1115; and late in 1971 the legal services office set to work to discourage approval from being given. The legal aid lawyers alleged that the state application was "a badly veiled device to allow the state to avoid its statutory obligations, placing further burden on the population designed to be aided by Social Security legislation."[139] In short, the argument was that Illinois was interested not in experimenting but in saving money, and it is true that the Illinois proposal was thin on the articulation of the hypotheses which would be tested by the experiment. HEW was reluctant to move. It was in a difficult position. Under White House pressure it had caved in to a virtually identical proposal from California. Commissioner Newman urged alternatives on Illinois and was clearly frustrated by the attitude of the state's negotiators.[140] It was scarcely surprising that on March 17, 1972, the Regional Commissioner of SRS finally wrote to inform the state that its application had been denied.

By this time, of course, the financial situation did not seem quite so bad. By March the Governor was talking positively about using Medicaid dollars most effectively through HMOs.[141] And in April, the *Chicago Sun-Times* engaged in some investigative reporting on the efforts to find out what had really happened.[142] Once again, an apparently dramatic Medicaid crisis had fizzled out. In short, it was found that things looked better because Washington was providing more money from different pockets, the courts were slow and obstinate, and providers had discovered a natural affinity of interest with recipients.

It was typical of this crisis—as in other Medicaid battles in New York, California, and other states—that the protagonists were representatives of powerful groups, the rhetoric shrill on all sides, and the issues based on technical interpretations. In the various moves to obtain power and money, the necessity for care to recipients was—at least temporarily—a side issue. It was, after all, more dramatic to envisage the sudden closing of hospitals than to inquire about the effects of co-payment on recipients of care. But in Illinois, as in New York and California, the health care questions remained perplexing, incapable of permanent solution within the existing framework.

By May, 1972, the Illinois story was coming to its logical conclusion. Governor Ogilvie announced his own health care program, with emphasis on health care for children.[143] The legislature voted a supplementary grant to cover the welfare deficit,[144] and it emerged that by transferring 8500 Chicago welfare cases from general assistance to a categorical program the state was getting $3 million a month more in federal aid.[145] But Medicaid looked much in July 1973 as it had in July 1971. It was not about to wither away; and, as elsewhere, its major headaches remained.

NOTES

1. *New York Times,* February 2, 1971, p. 26.

2. *Ibid.,* February 2, 1971, p. 26. The actual cost of welfare and Medicaid in New York in 1971 was $4.1 billion, an increase of $876 million over 1970. *Ibid.,* March 26, 1972, p. 121.

3. *Ibid.,* April 3, 1971, p. 26.

4. *Ibid.,* April 6, 1971, p. 44.

5. Jo Ann Silverstein, *Medicaid in New York: A Play in One Act,* 1972 (paper presented at the Yale Medical School).

6. *New York Times,* May 11, 1971, p. 28. The changes had been signed into law on April 14.

7. CCH *Medicare & Medicaid Guide,* Par. 26.293 (E.D.N.Y., 1971).

8. *Ibid.,* Par. 26.296.

9. 331 F. Supp. 945 (S.D.N.Y. 1971).

10. CCH *Medicare & Medicaid Guide,* Par. 26.373 (2d Cir., 1971).

11. For adverse reactions of the Medical Society of the State of New York, see *American Medical News,* October 11, 1971.

12. *New York Times,* September 30, 1971, p. 1.

13. 338 F. Supp. 945. The defendants were HEW, its secretary, and the Commissioner and Department of Social Services in New York.

14. *New York Times,* October 28, 1970, p. 53.

15. *Ibid.,* December 7, 1972, p. 57.

16. *New York Post,* May 8, 1973, p. 9.

17. *American Medical News,* October 4, 1971, p. 2.

18. *New York Times,* September 27, 1971, p. 1. Dr. Bellin put an end to the practice by requiring prior authorization for such shoes. Requests for such shoes then dropped to 7,000 pairs a week.

19. *Ibid.,* February 15, 1972.

20. *Ibid.,* February 26, 1972.

21. *Ibid.,* August 4, 1971.

22. *Ibid.,* January 9, 1972, p. 30.

23. *Ibid.,* November 10, 1972, p. 1. He was later accused of using his proprietary hospital to bilk a further $250,000 from Medicaid. *Ibid.,* April 4, 1973. All told it was reported that Medicaid had paid some $8½ million to his proprietory hospital, some $1½ million of which was said to be by way of overpay-

ment. These payments had been made to Dr. Matthew despite his many and various troubles with the federal tax authorities and a finding by state inspectors that his hospital was "filthy—deteriorated—destroyed by addicts." *Ibid.*, April 24, 1973, p. 43.

24. *Ibid.*, February 8, 1973.
25. *Ibid.*, February 24, 1973.
26. *Ibid.*, February 28, 1973.
27. *Ibid.*, January 27, 1973, p. 1.
28. *Ibid.*, January 7, 1973.
29. *Ibid.*, January 11, 1973, p. 1.
30. *Ibid.*, February 4, 1973, p. E7.
31. *Ibid.*, December 31, 1972, p. 32.
32. *Ibid.*, February 4, 1973, p. E7.
33. *Ibid.*, November 7, 1971, p. 72.
34. *Ibid.*, February 6, 1972.
35. *Ibid.*, July 11, 1971, p. 41.
36. *Ibid.*, July 14, 1972.
37. *Ibid.*, February 11, 1971, p. 38.
38. *Ibid.*, February 23, 1972, p. 1.
39. *Medical Tribune*, December 21, 1970.
40. *New York Times*, February 8, 1973.
41. *Ibid.*, November 30, 1972, p. 1.
42. *Ibid.*, December 18, 1972. New York City was anxious to get out of the Medicaid business. *Ibid.*, February 4, 1973, p. E7.
43. Ruben Brooks, *The California Medical Assistance Program—Budget Crisis and Reform*, 1972 (paper presented at the Yale Law School). We have relied on this paper for the data in succeeding paragraphs.
44. For a full explanation of the cuts, see U.S., Congress, Senate, Special Committee on Aging, Subcommittee on Health, *Hearings* before the Subcommittee on Health of the Special Committee on Aging, Senate, 92nd Cong., 1st Sess., 1971, p. 45.
45. *California Medical News*, December 11, 1970, p. 1.
46. *San Francisco Chronicle*, December 3, 1970, p. 30.
47. *Ibid.*, December 15, 1970, p. 9.
48. *Hospital Week*, December 11, 1970, p. 1.
49. John McKee Pratt, *An Information Bulletin on the Probable Effects of the Cutbacks in the Medi-Cal Program*, The Community Relations Education Foundation, February 12, 1971. See also *American Medical News*, February 22, 1971, p. 8.
50. *San Francisco Chronicle*, December 4, 1970, p. 12.
51. *Ibid.*, p. 1.
52. *Ibid.*, December 19, 1970, p. 14.
53. *Ibid.*, January 10, 1971.
54. *American Medical News*, February 8, 1971.
55. *San Francisco Chronicle*, February 2, 1971, p. 1.
56. *Ibid.*, February 2, 1971.

57. *Ibid.*, January 28, 1971.

58. California Legislature, Assembly Special Committee on Medi-Cal, *Preliminary Report*, February 22, 1971, p. 3.

59. *San Francisco Chronicle*, January 16, 1971.

60. *American Medical News*, March 15, 1971.

61. *O'Reilly v. Brian*. Not reported, but see *American Medical News*, June 14, 1971. In particular, the court held that the director was not entitled to rely on §11422(c) of the Government Code, authorizing cutbacks.

62. In 1973, the California Court of Appeal (3rd Div.) affirmed the decision in *C.M.A. v. Brian*, holding the 1970 cutbacks partially invalid. 30 C.A. 3d. 637.

63. Dr. Earl W. Brian, Jr., *Statement to the Legislature Subcommittee on Medi-Cal*, February 1, 1971, p. v.

64. "Some Lessons from the Medi-Cal Crisis," *California Medicine*, vol. 114 (1971), p. 31.

65. State of California, Department of Health Care Services, *Medi-Cal Reform Plan*, April 1971, incorporated in AB 949.

66. *San Francisco Chronicle*, April 29, 1971, p. 11.

67. *California Medical Association News*, May 25, 1971.

68. *San Francisco Chronicle*, May 3, 1971, p. 1.

69. *Ibid.*, May 5, 1971, p. 7.

70. *American Medical News*, August 9, 1971 (AB949).

71. *New York Times*, March 4, 1971, p. 1.

72. *American Medical News*, February 28, 1972, p. 10.

73. The Consumers Health Protection Act, introduced by Sen. George Moscome (Democrat, San Francisco).

74. Chapter 577 of 1971.

75. State of California, *Analysis of the Budget Bill 1972–1973*, p. 630.

76. *Ibid.*, p. 622.

77. *Ibid.*, p. 626.

78. CCH *Medicare & Medicaid Guide*, para. 26.397.

79. *Health Law Newsletter*, July 1972.

80. *California Welfare Rights Organization v. Richardson* (N.D., Ca., 1972). CCH *Medicare & Medicaid Guide*, para. 26.519. On the other hand, in *Wing v. Brian* (Ca. C.A., Sacramento, 1972), the new property limitations in Medi-Cal were struck down.

81. *California State Employees Ass'n v. Williams*, 86 Cal. Rptr. 3d 309 (Ct. App., 3d Dist. of Calif. 1970).

82. *California Medical Association News*, May 25, 1971, p. 1.

83. *Washington Post*, February 5, 1971, p. 11a.

84. U.S., Office of the Comptroller General, *Continuing Problems in Providing Nursing Home Care and Prescribed Drugs under the Medicaid Program in California*, August 1970. A significant part of the blame for this state of affairs was laid at the door of the Regional office of HEW, *ibid.*, pp. 36–37.

85. *Newsweek*, April 17, 1972, p. 57.

86. *Los Angeles Times*, December 10, 1972.

87. *Ibid.*, December 27, 1972. Needless to say the bill had been vigorously opposed in the legislature.

88. *Los Angeles Times,* December 29, 1972.

89. *Ibid.,* January 23, 1973.

90. *New York Times,* May 2, 1973, p. 1.

91. On Illinois, see Michael L. Millman, *The Legal Aid Lawyer as Health Advocate: A Case Study of the Illinois Medicaid Reductions* (a Master's Thesis in the Department of Epidemiology and Public Health, Yale University, 1973). We are also grateful to William Robinson, Class of 1974 at the Yale Law School, who undertook research for us on Medicaid in Illinois. In this section we have also relied on personal recollections of those involved with the program in that state.

92. E.g., "State government must be reorganized to become a management tool for accomplishment," *Chicago Sun Times,* September 10, 1972, p. B 2. Cited Millman, *supra,* note 91, p. 13.

93. "The solution is management. I proposed to manage this state government as it has never been managed before." *Ibid.*

94. *Chicago Daily News,* January 29, 1971.

95. In June, Rep. Mann introduced a bill to take the administration of Medicaid away from the Welfare Department. Governor Ogilvie responded by urging the establishment of HMOs run by physicians. *Chicago Tribune,* June 24, 1971, Section 1, p. 5. The League of Women Voters also entered the fray, urging the Governor to bring the state in conformity with federal standards by providing a higher cut-off level for Medicaid. *Ibid.,* June 16, 1971, Section 1A, p. 12.

96. *Ibid.,* July 14, 1971, p. 1. The new budget provided $336 million for Medicaid. The Illinois public aid director estimated that $430 million would be needed to keep the program going at existing levels. *Ibid.,* September 6, 1971 § 1, p. 7. A week later the Director resigned. *Ibid.,* September 15, 1971.

97. *Ibid.,* October 7, 1971, p. 1.

98. Cited, Millman, *supra,* note 91, p. 30.

99. *Chicago Sun Times,* October 12, 1971.

100. *Chicago Tribune,* October 7, 1971, p. 1.

101. *Ibid.,* October 19, 1971.

102. *Ibid.,* October 21, 1971.

103. *Ibid.,* October 27, 1971, p. 1.

104. *Ibid.,* October 29, 1971, p. 1.

105. *Ibid.,* p. 5.

106. Letter dated September 9, 1971. Cited Millman, *supra,* note 91, p. 33.

107. F. P. Godwin, October 12, 1971. Cited Millman, *supra,* note 91, p. 35.

108. *Chicago Tribune,* October 30, 1971, p. 1.

109. *Ibid.,* p. 5.

110. *Ibid.,* November 3, 1971, p. 1.

111. For a detailed study of the politics of the litigation, see Millman, *supra,* note 91, p. 39 *et seq.*

112. *Chicago Daily News,* November 2, 1971.

113. *Chicago Tribune,* November 2, 1971, p. 2.

114. *Ibid.,* November 5, 1971, p. 2.

115. *Ibid.,* p. 1.

116. *Ibid.,* November 6, 1971, p. 3.

117. *Ibid.*, November 8, 1971.

118. *Ibid.*, November 10, 1971, p. 14; *Ibid.*, November 11, 1971, p. 1.

119. *Ibid.*, November 17, 1971, p. 1.

120. *Ibid.*, November 30, 1971.

121. Patricia Korval, "Ghetto Doctors React to Ogilvie Medical-Aid Plan," *Chicago Sun-Times*, November 4, 1971.

122. There were efforts to avoid compliance with the regulations. Governor Ogilvie wrote the Secretary of HEW, Elliot Richardson, on November 5, complaining that compliance would be an "administrative nightmare" and that:

> *Compliance with the regulation, as interpreted by the Court, completely eliminates the possibility of introducing orderly change into the welfare system, provides an unlimited opportunity to haress the welfare system, and diverts an already overburdened staff to more bureaucratic formalities and paper work. Ironically, this harassment cannot possibly provide any relief to recipients in cases such as ours in which there is no issue of fact.*

Secretary Richardson's response, however, was not particularly sympathetic: "It is clear from the regulations that the advance notice requirement is applicable to any proposed actions to terminate, suspend or reduce assistance." Cited Millman, *supra,* note 91, p. 43.

123. *Ibid.*, p. 44 *et seq.*

124. *Chicago Tribune,* December 1, 1971. This argument centered around the conflict between s.1903 (e)—the requirement of movement towards comprehensive care—and s.1902 (d)—the cutback provision.

125. *Ibid.*, p. 50. Millman, *supra,* note 91, p. 50.

126. *Ibid.*, p. 51.

127. *Chicago Tribune,* Jan. 7, 1972.

128. Millman, *supra,* note 91, pp. 51–52.

129. *Chicago Tribune,* November 30, 1971.

130. *Ibid.*, December 29, 1971, p. 1.

131. *Ibid.*, February 10, 1972, p. 1.

132. *Ibid.*, February 11, 1972, p. 1.

133. It was during 1972 that a large number of states discovered the open-ended funding potential of Titles IV(a) and XVI. For the crisis that this created see U.S., Congress, Joint Economic Committee, *Open-Ended Federal Matching of State Social Service Expenditures Authorized under the Public Assistance Titles of the Social Security Act, Hearings* before the Subcommittee on Fiscal Policy of the Joint Economic Committee of the Congress, Sept. 12, 13 and 14, 1972.

134. *Chicago Tribune,* February 16, 1972.

135. *Ibid.*, April 11, 1972.

136. Millman, p. 43. Something, it is said, ultimately achieved in Berghoff's Restaurant in Chicago.

137. *Chicago Tribune,* July 6, 1972.

138. "Illinois Medicaid: Problems are Cash Flow and Welfare Load," *Modern Hospital,* Vol. 117, No. 6, Dec. 1971, pp. 40–41.

139. Millman, *supra,* note 91, p. 55.

140. He wrote on January 28, 1972: "Illinois roundly rejected any suggestions to improve their utilization review. Their stated reasons were that they did not

wish to alienate providers who had already expressed dissatisfaction with the Illinois methods of reimbursements under Medicaid. It was also evident that Illinois was reluctant to consider any method of improving their utilization review measures on the grounds that such action might be considered an admission that their current UR methods might be deficient." Cited Millman, *supra,* note 91, p. 58.

141. U.S., Department of Health, Education, and Welfare, *Manpower Report of the President,* March 1972, p. 132.

142. *Chicago Sun-Times,* April 2, 1972.

143. *Chicago Tribune,* May 16, 1972, § IA p. 6.

144. *Ibid.,* May 26, Sec. 1A, p. 4.

145. The only major surviving change was HASP, which had reduced the average Medicaid hospital stay to 5–6 days, thereby saving the state $1.7 million monthly. *Hospital Week,* Sept. 29, 1972, p. 2.

15
The Courts and the Congress

In the continuing bureaucratic interweavings of Medicaid, the question constantly arose: Who was responsible for Medicaid's difficulties? The question, implying as it did the identification of various villains, was relatively simple to approach, if not always easy to answer. But the search for scapegoats obscured deficiencies in Medicaid, which were to be the base for extensive litigation in the courts. While administrators, politicians and the press were chasing fraudulent providers and recipients, Medicaid's goals and policies were still largely unresolved. Sometimes the program seemed a large and complex superstructure with no clear political commitment or philosophical foundations. Over the years the need for a set of common assumptions on which Medicaid policy could be built became self-evident. State legislatures were developing their own goals and assumptions for welfare medicine, based on budgetary politics. But as has been seen, state attitudes toward Medicaid did not always reflect congressional intent. While the question of who ought to have government-sponsored medical care in the American welfare state was one ultimately for Congress, the question of who was allowed care under the Medicaid legislation fell to judicial interpretation; and if the Supreme Court had not been moving away from its activist phase, policy-making by the judges might have been dramatic indeed.

Role of the Courts

The initial vagueness in the Medicaid legislation compelled the courts to play a significant role in the various battles surrounding Medicaid. There was a continuing ambivalence about whether Medicaid benefits were firm entitlements or "rights." The fragmentation of responsibility for the program provoked arguments and boundary disputes among providers and administrators, and the attempts to cut back on eligibility and services led, as has been seen, to continuing challenges from both recipient and provider groups. As a result, decisions about Medicaid's form, benefits, and development were frequently made in isolated decisions in the courts rather than by HEW regulations or program administrators. Such a process has sometimes been inconvenient from the administrative point of view: States have moved to change policies (usually through cutbacks in the program), and the courts, on behalf of recipients, providers or other government agencies, have blocked them. From the more general view of program development and clarification, the system has had some advantages, albeit cumbersome, costly, and roundabout administratively: at least a decision-making process developed. The federal government created the initial legislation; the states have tested its limitations; and in a number of important cases, the courts have made the ultimate decision on what, indeed, was the program's intent.

While these actions are in part a reflection of the lack of clear goals built into Medicaid, they also represent conflicting views as to what those goals should be. Direct conflicts could be avoided in Congress by creating deliberately vague legislation: the lack of consensus and the lack of goals were the cause and effect. But there could be no such avoidance in actually running the program. The most notable cases have thus represented direct clashes or confrontations around questions of power and interest; the Illinois and Cook County dispute is a case in point. City has fought state, providers have rallied to protect fees, and representatives of consumers have pushed for what they felt were their entitlements. In the absence of clear goals in the legislation, the courts have ultimately provided the focus for settlement. As a result, during the period this book covers, there have been times when policy-making sometimes seems to have passed to the judiciary rather than to have been outlined by the legislature and developed by the executive; and during the period covered by this section the judges have toyed with making major changes in direction of the program.

Examples of the day-to-day problems in the Medicaid program and their resolution—generally by state courts—have already been discussed, and it is not our purpose to re-analyze this aspect of the judicial function. The use of the courts as a device for social welfare planning does, however, invite special scrutiny. In this regard, the Medicaid program is not, of course, unique. That the courts should be involved in delicate, complex policy-making is by no means unusual in America. One has only to look back to the much-quoted phrase of de Tocqueville to the effect that "scarcely any political question arises in the United States that is not resolved, sooner or later, into a judicial question."[1] But, while de Tocqueville's words are widely cited, the implications of his approach are rarely fully comprehended. They go to the root of who should make vital social decisions. De Tocqueville himself was, in many ways, scornful of democracy; he saw the bench and bar as "the American aristocracy" who acted as a counterpoise to the "vices inherent in popular government." While the government, then, might pass sweeping legislation, the lawyers and judges would bring it within the bounds of reason and reality: "When the American people are intoxicated by passion or carried away by the impetuosity of their ideas, they are checked and stopped by the almost invisible influence of their legal counselors."[2]

One could scarcely call the Medicaid legislation the product of legislators "intoxicated by passion." Nevertheless, with Medicaid, as with other legislation, the perspectives of the legal profession itself were important. Congress might favor cost controls which, in turn, implied cutbacks; but the courts might take an opposing tack—protecting recipients, for example, and thus denying the basic policy of restrictionism. As there was some tendency on the part of the courts to favor recipients, at least in the initial interpretation of the legislation, the courts provided another arena of potentially conflicting decision-making. Moreover, for a period in the late 1960s the courts seemed prepared to re-engineer social welfare programs: the ghost of de Tocqueville, even if this time the judicial policies were liberal rather than conservative, seemed once more abroad.

Legal aid offices funded under federal anti-poverty programs had led to the development of "poverty law" as a specialty in the 1960s and they provided a focus for a significant series of class actions and test cases. While this is certainly not the place to attempt a serious analysis of the virtues of judicial activism and judicial restraint, it is perhaps fair to hazard the opinion that if liberals in the 1930s were right to castigate the Supreme Court of that period as "nine old men" seeking to substitute their notions of right in place of those of Congress, critics in the 1960s may have been justified in seeing some of the claims of poverty lawyers and at least some of the decisions of the Supreme Court as an attempt to impose the will of a minority in an area of broad social policy.

In terms of practical politics, however, as far as Medicaid was concerned, the will of the majority was not always clear. Did Congress intend the needy to have comprehensive medical care irrespective of cost? Did state cost crises override that intent? Should the definition of welfare eligibility stay fixed, or should it move up and down according to the varied burden on taxpayers? What rights in the system were vested? Some of these questions went beyond the Medicaid legislation to wider social questions and constitutional issues. A written constitution, judicial review, and the idea of fundamental laws may be undemocratic in the pure sense, but it is the price we pay for protecting minorities. To the courts go questions of reconciling conflicting interests. It requires judicial restraint, however, to ensure that the protection of minorities is not transformed into control and abuse by minorities.[3] As a welfare program crippled by rapidly rising costs, Medicaid was a fertile field for focusing these political and constitutional tensions.

But the inherently undemocratic element in judicial lawmaking beyond what Holmes described as the "interstitial" is matched by an equally unsatisfactory element: the fact that, in making law, courts may have to manipulate complex issues of policy, a task for which they are frequently institutionally incompetent. Courts are excellent institutions for preventing things from going wrong; they are far from satisfactory as instruments for developing new programs. It was this problem of institutional incompetence that became especially obvious as the courts moved into social welfare and ultimately Medicaid issues. The fact that the legislative and executive seemed unable to resolve the policy issues underlying welfare medicine should have been a sufficient warning that the courts were even less well equipped for the task.

Equal Protection

It was inevitable, given the political structure and the problems which have been described, that, as efforts were made to cut back on Medicaid programs, there would be battles in the courts. Had this not been totally inevitable, the form of the legislation insured that it was bound to happen. First, while the 1965 legislation provided that Medicaid should move forward to ever more comprehensive services [section 1903(e)], the 1967 Amendments included procedures for cutting back services [section 1902(d)]. There was thus an apparent direct conflict between initial intent and second thoughts, both part of the same legislation. Competing doctrines are the life-blood of a lawyer's work, but this conflict was an invitation to litigation, and it was an invitation that the second factor in the situation —the Welfare Rights Organization and OEO legal services—was not about to ignore.

The first order of business for recipients had been to put pressure on the courts to insure they were included. In these battles about eligibility there were some notable victories, such as *Triplett v. Cobb,*[4] where the court held that mothers of AFDC children had to be included in Mississippi's Medicaid program. Of great visibility and political notoriety were the "cutback" cases, which have already been described and discussed.[5] In general the courts insisted they were only testing the cutback legislation by the standards of Title XIX or state enabling acts. As Mr. Justice Sullivan put the formal narrow judicial role in the 1967 California cutback litigation: "Our function is to inquire into the legality of the regulations, not their wisdom. Nor do we superimpose upon the Agency any policy judgements of our own. . . ."[6] In practice, however, the cutback cases also provided a forum for raising the much wider issue of who in fact *ought* to be eligible for services under Medicaid. It was in these cases, especially those in New York and California, that the idea of mounting an assault on inadequate medical care for the poor through various constitutional arguments gradually took shape. In other words, rather than use the courts to prevent the states from cutting back their existing programs, the judicial process was to be used to expand welfare programs by arguing that existing programs violated various constitutional guarantees. The courts were to become a sword as well as a shield.

The idea that the different Medicaid categories were so irrational as to amount to a denial of equal protection under the Fourteenth Amendment of the Constitution was first floated before Judge Motley in *O'Reilly v. Wyman,*[7] although when a three-judge court was empanelled they were far less sympathetic to the concept, noting that such categories were "borderline cases" that arise "whenever classifications are established by law."[8] But the idea that the various categories in Title XIX might attract the taint of unconstitutionality had been launched. The willingness of any federal courts, however, to look with favor on such arguments made clear the potential of the Fourteenth Amendment's Equal Protection clause with respect to Medicaid; and the potential was considerable in view of the changes which had overtaken the concept of Equal Protection.

After being established during Reconstruction, the Amendment remained largely dormant in the late nineteenth century[9]; the concept of "equal protection" was rarely used in comparison with "due process,"[10] being, as Justice Holmes noted, "the usual last resort of constitutional arguments."[11] It was, however, from this period that the rationality argument or "reasonableness" test emerged.[12] Despite this slow start, the use of equal protection gradually gained a remarkable foothold in the post-New Deal Supreme Court. In a series of cases, beginning with a testing of Oklahoma's Habitual Criminal Sterilization Act,[13] and the Japanese Internment cases,[14] the breadth of the protection was widely expanded, while the "compelling state interest" test emerged as the limit of equal protection. The new test achieved favor (or notoriety) in the Warren Court's desegregation[15] and reapportionment[16] cases, as well as in a series of cases concerned with criminal procedure where the defendant was indigent.[17] Neither the "reasonableness" test nor "compelling state interest" would prevent the operation of the Fourteenth Amendment where there were classifications based on race or violating the idea of one-man, one-vote.

It was particularly with these last lines of cases that the idea that poverty might itself raise Fourteenth Amendment problems was stressed, and here was some further ammunition for welfare recipients and their legal advisers. Mr. Justice Black noted in *Griffin v. Illinois* that, "In criminal trials a State can no more discriminate on account of poverty than on account of religion, race or color."[18] The idea of poverty as a "suspect classification" was carried still further in the Virginia poll tax case in 1966.[19] Mr. Justice Douglas in the majority opinion noted: "Lines drawn on the basis of wealth or property, like that of race . . . are traditionally disfavored."[20] The Supreme Court seemed poised to move into the area of public assistance law, and hence into the area of Medicaid.

In 1969, in *Shapiro v. Thompson*[21] the Court struck down the residency requirements for categorical welfare assistance programs on equal protection grounds, the Court finding no "compelling state interest" to justify the burden on interstate travel, which itself was held to be constitutionally protected. Two years later, the Court invalidated state statutes that denied categorical welfare benefits to resident aliens.[22] At the same time, outside the equal protection area, the Court seemed to be on the verge of a willingness to restructure welfare law. In *King v. Smith* (1968),[23] the Court unanimously held that Alabama's regulation denying AFDC payments to the children of a mother "cohabiting" with an able-bodied man was invalid. In *Rosado v. Wyman* (1970),[24] although with a good deal of inbuilt flexibility, the Court held the 1969 New York welfare cutback violated that portion of federal law which required that "determination of need" levels reflect changes in the cost of living. As already noted, in *Goldberg v. Kelly* (1970),[25] the Court laid down due-process procedures for "fair hearings," a decision in which Mr. Justice Brennan even talked in terms of welfare as a "property" entitlement.

All of these decisions promised a definition of welfare much more akin to that of Social Security, i.e., the automatic entitlement to benefits provided one fell into the appropriate category.[26] Yet, just as the Court appeared poised for a rapid transformation of the traditional concepts of Equal Protection,[27] which would presumably have coincided with the increased interest in restructuring welfare programs, a transformation of a different sort occurred, for the Warren Court began to give way to the Burger Court. There was also a serious intellectual questioning of the attempt to transform the political concept of Equal Protection into a kind of minimum economic protection.[28] Even liberals questioned whether the courts were constitutionally equipped to attempt to develop those fundamental protections against poverty which seemed perpetually to elude Congress.

The Burger Court was obviously increasingly satisfied that the Supreme Court was not the place to make such fundamental social changes. When Maryland put a $250-a-month ceiling on welfare payments to a family, in the pivotal *Dandridge* decision, this was held to have a "reasonable basis" and not to discriminate unfairly against larger families.[29] Said the Court: "So long as its judgements are rational, and not invidious, the legislature's efforts to tackle the problems of the poor and needy are not subject to a constitutional straightjacket."[30] In *Jefferson v. Hackney*, in a decision directly relating to public assistance programs, the Court refused to intervene when Texas passed legislation providing that henceforth in the categorical assistance categories, AFDC recipients would receive 75 percent of the legislatively defined need level, while other categorical groups would receive between 95 and 100 percent.[31]

Medicaid just failed to get itself considered until after the federal courts, especially the Supreme Court, began to have doubts about the rapidly broadening scope of Equal Protection in the field of welfare law. That did not mean there were not a series of attempts to bring Medicaid within what seemed for a short time to be a limitless willingness by the Supreme Court to restructure welfare and related fields. In theory, the Court was available to develop those policies which Congress was reluctant to clarify and to implement effectively those policies which state welfare departments implemented with conventional caution. While various lines of attack were tried, all were in the end to prove fruitless.

In one series of decisions, the courts chose to decide the cases on "pure" statutory grounds rather than face the Equal Protection issue which plaintiffs often raised in order to justify federal jurisdiction. Perhaps the most dramatic example of this was *Dimery v. Iowa Department of Social Services*,[32] a decision which was ultimately to provide an almost perfect case study of the difficulties inherent in judicial policy-making. There a disabled minor who was too young for APTD and ineligible for the State's version of AFDC, as there was no absent parent, failed to persuade the court to hear the constitutional issue, namely, that there had been a denial of Equal Protection by reason of a failure to include a disabled child in the State's Medicaid program, either because the State's categorical assistance programs were not as extensive as they might be or because the State had not developed a "medically needy" category.

Dimery was, in fact, successful in his action before the three-judge federal court but not on Equal Protection grounds, the Court preferring not to raise the issue. Instead the Court decided the case on the ground that there had been an unlawful delegation under the Iowa Constitution in that the delegation by the legislature to the State Welfare Department of the decision about who was to receive medical assistance was without sufficient guidelines or standards. One can perhaps understand the court's reluctance to be drawn into the Equal Protection argument, as, effectively, in *Dimery* the court was being asked to strike down the whole concept of categorical assistance welfare programs. No doubt the court felt itself institutionally incompetent (or was politically unwilling) to destroy the basic structure of the 1935 legislation without at least some congressional assistance.[33]

Some of the problems of categorical assistance were, however, brought up in other Medicaid cases where equal protection arguments were unavoidably faced, almost invariably without success. Many of these cases, such as *Wilczynski v. Marder*,[34] involved a claim that parts of different states' Medicaid eligibility standards violated the equal protection clause.[35] There were, however, other attempts to use Equal Protection effectively to rewrite either the Medicaid programs or even all categorical programs. *United Low Income, Inc. v. Fisher*[36] grew out of Maine's decision, in 1971, to terminate its two-year participation in the AFDC-UP program and the related medical assistance program. After finding that this action did not require the prior approval of the Secretary of HEW, as it did not directly involve a cutback in Maine's Title XIX plan, the court reached the plaintiffs' Equal Protection argument, namely, that Maine's action had created an "invidious discrimination between needy children whose need stemmed from death, absence or incapacity of a parent and those whose need resulted from the unemployment of their father." The plaintiffs further argued that because the right to welfare affected the integrity of the family and even the right to life itself, the state had to show a compelling interest in sustaining such a revised classification. In rejecting this test, the court cited *Dandridge* and stated that the distinction could rationally be related to the goal of "maximum self-support and personal independence." Among other things, it might encourage gainful employment as an alternative to welfare and hence conserve state funds. Thus again a federal court refused to expand a state Medicaid program by invoking the Fourteenth Amendment.

A considerably more sweeping constitutional attack on a Medicaid scheme was made in *Fullington v. Shea.*[37] Colorado limited Medicaid eligibility to the categorically indigent and hence determined income levels on the basis of gross income rather than net income (i.e., gross income less medical expenses). This suit was brought by a group of former welfare recipients who had become ineligible for categorical assistance and Medicaid due to the 1969 Social Security increases. As a result, they were receiving less total assistance than before the Social Security increases. Among other things, the plaintiffs argued that Colorado's failure to include the "medically needy" in its Medicaid program violated the Equal Protection clause.[38] The plaintiffs' situation, it was argued, was similar to that of those eligible for Medicaid, yet they did not receive enough assistance to come up to the minimum subsistence level while the categorically needy did. They argued that the fundamental right to food, shelter, and other necessities was at issue. Citing *Dandridge,* the court accepted Colorado's "rational basis" argument that implementation of plaintiffs' demands "could conceivably create much administrative difficulty and uncertainty" and might "encourage excessive medical expenses and resultant waste" and hence would burden the state fiscally.[39] The court admitted that "gross inequity is apparent," but the decision was affirmed *per curiam* by the Supreme Court, with only Justice Douglas calling for the case to be set down for hearing.[40]

Indeed, in 1972, the Supreme Court may have put the final nail in the coffin of any possible application of Equal Protection to Medicaid. This was the Court's *per curiam* affirmation of *Cloud v. Dietz,*[41] a three-judge district court decision.[42] In *Cloud,* the challenge was to an amendment to Kentucky's public assistance regulations, which defined as "employed" persons working at minimum wage for over 30 hours per week in U.S.

Department of Labor vocational and training programs. Persons in this class were denied Medicaid benefits. This amendment was part of a general retrenchment in the state's Medicaid program due to unexpectedly high utilization and expenditures. The district court found that this classification was allowed by the federal regulations and, according to the state Medicaid Commissioner, had been pre-authorized by HEW. The court also held, citing *Dandridge,* that the exclusion of this class of persons, even though some of them needed Medicaid as much as those who were eligible, was relevant to the goal of affording the widest possible scope of coverage to the neediest under the prevailing fiscal circumstance. Since the Supreme Court reaffirmation of the position it had taken in *Fullington,* it seemed that the federal judiciary's excursion into fundamental policy-making in the area of Title XIX was, for all practical purposes, over.[43]

Although *Shapiro v. Thompson* and *Dandridge v. Williams* are, in some ways, not easily distinguishable, recent decisions suggest that the doctrine underlying the *Dandridge* decision (where the Supreme Court upheld Maryland's right to put the limit on the amount paid to any one welfare family) has foreclosed strict Equal Protection scrutiny of the states' Medicaid rules, so long as those rules do not fall into the "fundamental right" and "suspect classification" pits (i.e., in short, if they do not contaminate their restrictive actions with racial considerations). Poverty is not, then, after all a suspect classification *per se.* There are several sound considerations that may lie behind this movement. Most fundamentally, Medicaid, like all welfare programs, produces classifications favoring the poor. If poverty alone were to trigger the Equal Protection doctrine it might also be argued that welfare was discriminatory in that it discriminates against the "unpoor." Could the entire system survive the "compelling state interest" test? Second, the push for economic equality could overrun itself if not kept within doctrinal limits. If poverty *per se* were a suspect classification, there might well be serious attacks on the constitutionality of regressive taxes like the sales tax. While that might have much to commend it, in political terms it would be an unthinkable act by the judiciary in the 1970s. Indeed the basic question must be asked whether the courts can really do much of value, except in a negative way, short of striking down the concept of categorical programs—something even the most ardent judicial activist might eschew.

Some of the inherent, or at least practical, limitations on judicial policy-making may be grasped by looking at the history of Iowa's statute after *Dimery's* assault on categorical public assistance. After the plaintiffs won before the three-judge federal court on the ground that the discretion granted to the state welfare department violated the Iowa Constitution, in 1970 the legislature enacted new legislation to give the same powers, but with appropriate safeguards. Thus, when the case once more came before a three-judge federal court in 1972, the Equal Protection argument could not be avoided.[44] But the court, which three years earlier had found a substantial constitutional issue, had no difficulty in rejecting the Constitutional arguments. It was not about to accept the plaintiff's argument "that once a state decides to participate in a categorical assistance program, it is arbitrary and discriminatory to provide benefits for less than all the potentially eligible." After all, *Dandridge* had put narrow limits on any economic concept of Equal Protection; the moves had to be "so palpably arbitrary that the court cannot conceive of any constitutionally permissible objective."

The second *Dimery* decision was much blunter than its predecessor:

> *Because budgetary constraints make clear that all of the needy could not be adequately helped, it may reasonably have been the purpose and policy of the Iowa legislation to adopt eligibility standards which, instead of providing token benefits to all of the needy, provide full benefits to the poorest and those least able to bear the hardships of poverty. . . . Surely it is not irrational for the state to believe that those of the young who are blessed with healthy parents are more adaptable and better able to obtain the basic necessities of life than those who, for whatever reason, are without parental support, care and influence.*

The change in the judicial attitudes to poverty law could scarcely have been more marked.

Welfare activists may be able to win court battles, but the wars have to be fought in the legislature. Basic policies in the area may just not be amenable to judicial policy-making; as Justice Harlan in the opinion of the court in *Rosado v. Wyman* pointed out, conflicting welfare policies represent a "highly complicated area . . . that should formally be placed under the supervision of HEW."[45] The courts are not, of course, required to be eunuchs. They may have no choice but to determine whether cutbacks meet tests laid down by Congress and state legislatures. They may have no alternative but to strike a balance between recipients and the states or providers and the states.[46] But when it comes to restructuring the categorical programs or massive expansions of Medicaid, the judicial statesman may legitimately opt for caution.

It may be that Congress and the state legislatures have so far failed to come to grips with the basic problems of medical policy. It may be that MSA and the congeries of empires making up HEW have a long way to go in implementing effective medical policies. No doubt the courts are inevitably faced with disputes arising in the area of the federal provision of health care which involve some important element of policy making. No doubt the courts are a legitimate forum for welfare rights groups and others to put pressure on "the system." The courts, for instance, undoubtedly played an important role in preventing hasty cutbacks in programs as well as insuring that programs such as EPSDT were implemented, but some oversold the competence of the courts. In the last analysis, the courts cannot develop the health care policy which Congress and the Executive have so far failed to develop. Institutional competence is required of the courts as well as the other organs of government.

The Congressional Role

While HEW and the states were struggling to administer Medicaid, and the courts were attempting to define its provisions as well as being tempted to expand its coverage, Congress, responsible for initial obscurities in the legislation, was engaged, once again, in the creation of further wrinkles in the Medicaid program. From 1970 through 1972 there was a continuing round of hearings and reports that eventually led to new legislation: the Social Security Amendments of 1972 (P.L. 92–603). The struggle to define Medicaid thus moved back to the legislature, more precisely to its watchdog tax committees. But here, too, as in the courts, there was a reluctance to confront the larger social questions of who ought to have public medical care. The emphasis continued to be on Medicaid's cost, structure and administration.

The powerful and unique position of the two major tax committees of Congress with respect to Medicaid has already been noted. By mid-1970, the beginning of the period under review, the Senate Finance Committee was well entrenched as the federal overseer for both Medicaid and Medicare. But in the House, Congressman Wilbur Mills, Chairman of the Ways and Means Committee, was becoming increasingly interested in the health programs for which federal taxes were raised. The interests of both Senator Long and Congressman Mills were further stimulated when Senator Edward Kennedy became chairman of the Senate Health Subcommittee (a subcommittee of the Committee on Labor and Public Welfare) in 1971, providing an alternative showcase for hearings on national health insurance (in 1971) and on federal aid to assist health maintenance organizations (1971 and 1972). But whatever the underlying reasons, these were years packed with Congressional hearings that in one form or another affected Medicaid.

In one general area there was agreement. "Pluralism" had become a word much used in describing a basic tenet of the health care system. Presumably this was intended to represent the antithesis of "socialized medicine," a term by then rarely appearing. No one seemed to doubt that the future of American medical care lay in some form of public-private mix. The experience of Medicare and Medicaid had clearly shown that reliance on the private sector as a major dispenser of public funds had to be accompanied by some form of public regulation, if only to stem rising costs. Finally, the idea of the health maintenance organization also proved appealing to Congressional leaders who were otherwise of different health care persuasions.[47] But beyond this, there was no general agreement as to what forms any type of federal funding and federal regulation should take.

Once again, as in the passage of the Medicare legislation, the process was one of reconciling divergent views, so that eventually a single health financing policy would emerge in Congress, couched in appropriately conciliatory rhetoric. The period under review here—mid-1970 through mid-1973—reflects, however, only part of this process, for in mid-1973 there was still no general agreement in Congress over the necessity for national health insurance, irrespective of what particular form it might take. But during the period the conflicting views became evident. The Nixon Administration's concern was to keep a lid on total federal spending. The Congressional tax committees, meanwhile, were continuing efforts to make Medicare and Medicaid more productive and effective, and numerous proponents of national health insurance were suggesting schemes which differed radically among themselves, but which, without exception, would add to health care expenditures. Cutting across these attitudes were conflicting economic and humanitarian views of the purposes of welfare and of whether medical care was to be approached as a problem in its own right or continue as an appendage to debates on fiscal policy and the needs of special interest groups.

Medicaid appeared in two guises in these debates: first, as a program to be either continued or swallowed up under the various schemes of national health insurance; second, as an ongoing program in need of trimming and control in the face of state and federal fiscal constraints. The prospect of national health insurance formed a constant backdrop to Medicaid debates. But it was Medicaid's latter guise which proved more immediately important, leading as it did to legislation in the passage of the 1972 Amendments. While the courts had moved to protect recipients, Congress appeared more concerned with demands on the taxpayer and with cutting back on domestic federal expenses.

The Battle Commences: New Perspectives on Basic Philosophies

The tone of Congressional events in the period to mid-1973 was set early in 1970. This was the year of the Presidential veto, which was in turn responsive to the President's commitment to hold the line on federal spending. In his veto message on HEW appropriations (for fiscal 1970) in January, President Nixon struck a chord which could not but appeal to all fiscal conservatives:

> *There are no goals which I consider more important for this nation than to improve education and to provide better health care for the*

American people. The question is: How much can the Federal Government afford to spend on those programs this year?[48]

It was a good question, implying as it did a concrete philosophy to be embodied in the ultimate answer. If Medicaid's budget was to be a set amount, for example, perhaps apportioned in advance by state, one important definition of welfare medicine would be set. The question, however, was one Congress as a whole still seemed unwilling to face.

In the absence of any other single or integrated health policy, the focus inevitably remained on costs. Thus the Presidential veto was eventually sustained, and the appropriations bill was signed by the President on March 5, eight months to the day after the start of the 1970 fiscal year.[49] But the broad issues remained. How much was the nation willing to spend, and on what? Congressional debates shed little light on this area. In the event, the year ended, as it had begun, with a Presidential veto. By not signing the bill establishing departments of family practice in medical schools (S 3418) before Congress recessed, the President exercised a "pocket veto." Again, the President justified his action in terms of the lack of an over-all health policy for federal efforts.[50] Clashes between the President and Congress were to become a familiar aspect of the Nixon Administration, inevitable as they are under a constitutional system which enables one party to be in control of the Administration and another of Congress.

Yet in the health area, at least, Congress seemed loath to approach the substantive issues. While Senator Ribicoff's subcommittee report in 1970 raised serious questions about the federal role in health,[51] including abundant evidence of waste and overlap afforded through federal funding patterns, those very same patterns of federal funding were, at the same time, being extended. Hill-Burton funds for hospital construction were, for example, extended for three years in June 1970, despite an initial Presidential veto—the first time for ten years that Congress had overridden a Presidential veto of any legislation.[52] New pieces of legislation were constantly appearing, each providing only partial solutions to specific problems and ultimately adding to federal spending.[53] Meanwhile other *ad hoc* programs of the 1960s were being extended.[54] Rumblings of discontent from the White House about the contributions of these programs to federal costs were, however, again in evidence. In signing the Comprehensive Health Planning Agencies bill, the President stated that the authorization of $1.8 billion over three years was fiscally irresponsible and that efforts would be made to limit appropriations. The stage was thus set for continuing appropriations battles and administrative budgetary limitations from fiscal 1971 onwards.

In large part, the continuance of a patchwork approach to health services, all of which in some degree affected the recipients of Medicaid, reflected the special interests of individual senators and congressmen and various lobbying groups. The National Health Service Corps, for example, which might have been expected to provide a major boon to Medicaid beneficiaries in short-staffed areas, was the brainchild of the two Senators from the sparsely doctored state of Washington, Henry Jackson and Warren Magnuson.[55] Senator Edward Kennedy became a symbol for the national health insurance proposals endorsed by organized labor.[56] Senator Russell Long, with the encouragement of the health insurance industry, became a major proponent of catastrophic health insurance, introducing his own proposals to subsidize large family and hospital bills in the closing days of the 91st Congress,[57] at least in part to take some of the limelight from Senator Kennedy. Senator Wallace Bennett of Utah was pressing the idea of "professional standards review organizations," an idea developed from the American Medical Association's growing commitment to review of governmental medical services by medical associations.[58] Senator Moss, chairman of the Senate Subcommittee on Long-term Care, continued, with Representative Pryor, as the spokesman for improvement in nursing homes.

At the same time, those who sought comprehensive solutions to health care questions were no more closely in agreement. The Nixon Administration's commitment both to cost control and to a comprehensive approach to health care reform ran afoul of the Kennedy-Griffiths proposals for generous national health insurance benefits for all, organized through the Social Security system. These proposals were opposed from the beginning by the Nixon Administration on the grounds that the expected cost of $77 billion was the "equivalent to a Federal health tax of over $1000 per year for every household in the United States."[59] No accurate cost projections were, however, available in 1970 for the Administration's own comprehensive health plan for needy children, FHIP; nor, indeed, were full details of this plan ever made available. The year ended with a White House Conference on Children that became unruly but did at least endorse the idea of "comprehensive care" for children.[60] But the rhetoric of comprehensive care obscured quite different tactical approaches.

The cost emphasis, together with the sheltering of divergent views and special interests under the same rhetorical umbrella, formed the basic theme of HR 17550, the would-be Social Security Amendments of 1970. Although committee work had begun beforehand, HR 17550 was officially introduced by Chairman Mills and Representative Byrnes (the ranking Republican on the Ways and Means Committee) on May 11, 1970, and was reported out of Ways and Means three days later.[61] But it was to become bogged down in the Senate under the burden of amendments, to die in the last days of the 91st Congress, and to be resurrected as HR 1 in the 92nd Congress. As such it was finally passed, in emaciated form, in December 1972 as the 1972 Amendments.

The analysis of HR 1, which forms the substance of our final chapter, highlights the redoubled efforts to develop a policy or even a rhetoric which might command a majority in Congress and the approval of the White House in the area of income security, with its attendant problems of health maintenance. The compromise eventually underlined costs rather than service; and this in turn emphasized the essential element of consensus or compromise in all legislation. The Medicaid litigation had already underlined the limitations of the judicial process in the development of a strategy for welfare medicine; at least by default, Congress made basic policy. Yet Medicaid's primary aim was, it seemed, not to provide health care as a right to needy groups but to provide services only to the extent that medical bills would not defeat the purpose of programs for income assistance.

NOTES

1. Alexis de Tocqueville, *Democracy in America,* ed. Phillips Bradley (New York, 1954), vol. I, p. 282.

2. *Ibid.,* pp. 288–289.

3. The Thayerian-Frankfurterian argument in favor of judicial restraint is most eloquently restated in Alexander M. Bickel's *The Least Dangerous Branch* (Indianapolis, 1962).

4. 331 F. Supp. 652 (N.D. Miss., 1971). This was a class suit brought by mothers and other caretaker relatives of AFDC families to enjoin Mississippi from refusing them Medicaid assistance and providing it only for their children. The state argued that AFDC payments were made to support needy children and hence it was proper that Medicaid should likewise support them and only them. The court found this interpretation of the program's purpose at variance with a variety of enunciated policies. First, Mississippi itself considered the needs of the adults in setting levels of AFDC payments. Second, the state's Work Incentive Program regulations specified parents in AFDC families as "adults in the ADC budget." Third, the intent of the federal AFDC program was to aid families, not individual family members. Therefore, as long as Mississippi participated in Medicaid, it had to provide medical assistance to plaintiffs for the same period as it did for their children.

5. The 1967 cutbacks in New York, focusing on *O'Reilly v. Wyman,* 305 F. Supp. 228 (S.D.N.Y., 1969), were referred to in Chapters 7 and 9, at the same time as the mention of *Catholic Medical Center v. Rockefeller,* 305 F. Supp. 1256 (E.D.N.Y., 1969); 39 U.S. 820 (1970); remanded, see 430F. 2d 1297 (2d Cir. 1970); 400 U.S. 931 (1970)—the case growing out of the hospital "freeze" of 1969, which was held to be inconsistent with the legislative requirement to pay hospitals their "reasonable costs." The 1971 New York cutbacks, which led to *Braster v. Rockefeller,* CCH *Medicare & Medicaid Guide,* para. 26.295; *Bass v. Rockefeller,* CCH *Medicare & Medicaid Guide,* para. 26.296; 331 F. Supp. 945 (S.D.N.Y., 1971) (rehearing), *vacated as moot,* 464 F. 2d 1300 (2d. Cir., 1971) and *Bass v. Richardson,* 338 F. Supp. 478 (S.D.N.Y., 1971) were discussed in Chapter 14. The 1971 cutback in Illinois, which led to *Chicago Welfare Rights Organization v. Ogilvie,* CCH *Medicare & Medicaid Guide,* par. 26.405 (N.D. Ill., 1971) *CCH Poverty Law Reporter,* par. 1505.74 (7th Cir. 1971) was also described in Chapter 14; while *Kansas Hospital Association v. Mander,* CCH *Medicare & Medicaid Guide,* par. 26.420 (D.C. Kansas) was a similar decision where yet another federal court refused to allow a cutback in inpatient hospital services until approved by HEW. Cf. *Harmony Nursing Home v. Anderson,*

CCH *Medicare & Medicaid Guide*, par. 26.426 (D.C. Minn., 1972), where the court refused as a matter of discretion to enjoin Minnesota's freeze on rates of payment to skilled nursing homes, even though this freeze had not been approved by HEW, which the court apparently believed was necessary. The court argued that by the time of the hearing the plaintiff had dropped out of the Medicaid program and hence could not show the likelihood of irreparable damage necessary to warrant a preliminary injunction. California's 1967 cutback attempts, centering on *Morris v. Williams* 63 Cal. Rptr. 689, 67 C. 2d 733 (1967), were discussed in Chapter 7. The later California cutbacks, including the five "emergency" amendments of 1970 which led to *California Association of Nursing Homes Inc. v. Williams,* 4 Cal. 3d 800, 84 Cal. Rptr. 490; 85 Cal. Rptr. 73 (Cal. Ct. App., 3d Dist., 1970) and *O'Reilly v. Brian* and the December 1970 10-percent cutback were discussed in Chapter 14.

6. *Morris v. Williams,* 67 Cal. 2d 733, 737; 433 P2d. 697, 700; 63 Cal. Rptr. 689, 692 (1967). And see Chapter 7, footnote 30.

7. Unreported. For some other early attempts to introduce similar arguments see *Hunt v. Shapiro,* 258 A. 2d 100 (Cir. Ct. of Conn., App. Div., 1969), a plaintiff in person unsuccessfully argued that the Medicaid program was so arbitrary as to amount to a violation of due process and equal protection. The Connecticut Supreme Court of Errors, however, refused to certify the case for appeal. 257 A. 2d 44 (S. Ct. Conn., 1969). In *Horowitz v. Brian, CCH Poverty Law Reporter,* para. 1530.20 (Cal. Super. Ct., L.A. Co., 1970), a California case, the court similarly rejected an argument that the requirement that a Medicaid patient be certified by a doctor as needing emergency treatment was not a violation, *inter alia,* of the Fourteenth Amendment.

8. 305 F. Supp. 228, 232 (S.D.N.Y., 1969).

9. After the *Slaughter House Cases,* 16 Wall. 36 (1873) and *Plessy v. Ferguson,* 163 U.S. 537 (1896) in the late nineteenth century, with a limited exception in the sphere of economic regulation, see the line of cases beginning with *Santa Clara County v. Southern Pacific R.R. Co.,* 118 U.S. 394 (1886).

10. On the history of the Equal Protection doctrine, see especially J. Tussman and J. ten Broek, "The Equal Protection of the Laws," *California Law Review,* vol. 37 (1949), 341, pp. 380–381.

11. *Buck v. Bell,* 274 U.S. 200, 208 (1927). Indeed perhaps the only significant concept to emerge from this period was the idea of a standard of "reasonable classification." Some such test was almost inevitable in developing this clause of the Fourteenth Amendment, as the command is not to discriminate, yet almost all legislation is inherently discriminatory.

12. As the Supreme Court put it in 1920, "the classification must be reasonable, not arbitrary, and must rest upon some ground of difference having a fair and substantial relation to the object of the legislation, so that all persons similarly circumstanced shall be treated alike." *F. S. Royster Guano Co. v. Virginia,* 253 U.S. 412, 415.

13. *Skinner v. Oklahoma,* 316 U.S. 535 (1942). Opinion of Mr. Justice Douglas. On Douglas' contribution to the new equal protection, see Kenneth L. Karst, "Invidious Discrimination: Justice Douglas and the Return of the 'Natural-Law-Due Process Formula,'" *U.C.L.A. Law Review,* vol. 16 (1969), p. 716.

14. See especially *Korematsu v. United States,* 323 U.S. 214 (1944).

15. See especially *Brown v. Board of Education,* 347 U.S. 483 (1954); and *Brown v. Board of Education,* 349 U.S. 294 (1955), implementing the former decision.

16. *Baker v. Carr,* 369 U.S. 186 (1962); *Reynolds v. Sims,* 377 U.S. 533 (1964), and *Avery v. Midland County,* 390 U.S. 474 (1968) applying the principle of "one man-one vote" enunciated in the prior cases to local as well as state government.

17. E.g., *Griffin v. Illinois,* 351 U.S. 12 (1956); *Douglas v. California,* 372 U.S. 353 (1963). Both these cases were decided primarily on Equal Protection grounds, although most of the leading criminal procedure cases of the period were decided on other constitutional grounds.

18. 351 U.S. at 17.

19. *Harper v. Virginia Board of Elections,* 383 U.S. 663 (1966). But see the vigorous dissenting opinion of Mr. Justice Harlan.

20. 383 U.S. at 668.

21. 394 U.S. 618 (1969). Again see the articulate dissent of Mr. Justice Harlan.

22. *Graham v. Richardson,* 403 U.S. 365 (1971). This decision undoubtedly influenced the Florida authorities in opening the Medicaid rolls to 18,500 Cuban refugees who were bringing an action, through legal services, challenging the Florida statute requiring American citizenship or over 20-year residence in Florida before admission to Medicaid. *New York Times,* Dec. 10, 1972, p. 66, col. 6.

23. 392 U.S. 309 (1968). Mr. Justice Douglas, in his concurring opinion, invoked the Equal Protection Doctrine.

24. 397 U.S. 397 (1970).

25. 397 U.S. 254 (1970).

26. For the argument that welfare should give "rights" see Charles Reich, "Social Welfare in the Public-Private State," *University of Pennsylvania Law Review,* vol. 114 (1966), p. 487. For an articulative critique of that position, see Richard M. Titmuss, "Welfare Rights, Law and Discretion," *Political Quarterly,* vol. 42 (1971), p. 113.

27. For a bullish view written at that time, see Rand E. Rosenblatt, *Litigation Under Title XIX: The Eligibility Question,* 1970 (paper presented at the Yale Law School).

28. See especially, Frank J. Michaelman, "Foreword: On Protecting the Poor Through the Fourteenth Amendment," *Harvard Law Review,* vol. 83 (1969), p. 7.

29. *Dandridge v. Williams,* 397 U.S. 471 (1970).

30. *Ibid.,* p. 485. On rather similar grounds, the Court later upheld California's constitutional requirement of a local referendum before low-cost housing was built in an area. *James v. Valtierra,* 402 U.S. 137 (1971). For the majority Mr. Justice Black held there was no "suspect classification," since the California law was based on a "devotion to democracy, not to bias, discrimination, or prejudice." *Ibid.,* 141. In dissent, Mr. Justice Marshall called the state's provision—"an explicit classification on the basis of poverty—a suspect classification which demands exacting judicial scrutiny." *Ibid.,* 144–145.

31. *Jefferson v. Hackney,* 406 U.S. 535 (1972). Although blacks and Mexican-Americans formed a far higher percentage of AFDC recipients than in the other categories, Mr. Justice Rehnquist held that as racial motivation had not been proved, the "traditional standard of review" was applicable.

More recently still the Burger Court has refused to interfere in what some lower courts had held was the unequal protection inherent in the method of financing public education in the U.S. In *San Antonio Independent School District v. Rodriguez,* 93 S. Ct. 1278 (1973), the Supreme Court held that the local tax method of school support, although "imperfect" has a rational relationship to a legitimate state purpose.

32. 320 F. Supp. 1125 (S.D. Iowa, 1969).

33. The case was vacated and remanded by the Supreme Court, 398 U.S. 322 (1970). In so doing, the Supreme Court relied on an intervening decision that in such cases the doctrine of abstention required an authoritative state court interpretation of state issues prior to a decision on federal issues.

34. 323 F. Supp. 509 (D. Conn., 1971). The Connecticut Welfare Department, in regulations promulgated in 1970, had lowered to $250 the maximum value of liquid resources allowable for an individual, but the department had excepted a home and car (of any value) and U.S. Government veterans' life insurance. Plaintiffs, in this class action, claimed that this regulation—particularly with respect to veterans' insurance—arbitrarily created two distinct classes of recipients. After disposing of various related statutory claims, the court reached this equal protection argument. Citing *Dandridge,* it posited the "reasonable basis" rather than the "compelling state interest" test as the applicable standard, in rejecting the equal protection argument. The home exemption was found to be reasonable, as it is in the state's interests not to have to provide shelter for recipients who already have it; the state could rationally conclude that it is cheaper to allow recipients to keep their home than to divest them of it and later have to shelter them itself. Allowing a recipient to keep his car was held to be reasonably related to the state's interest in encouraging him to become self-supporting, as transportation facilitates the search for employment. The court added that even the lack of limits on the allowable value of a home and car was not enough to compromise this rationality. Finally, it held that veteran's insurance was different from ordinary life insurance, which Connecticut did not exempt, in that government insurance was "in the nature of a gift" given to veterans for "human and patriotic reasons." Therefore, even this distinction in the regulations did not create invidious discrimination. *Ibid.*

35. In *Schaak v. Schmidt,* CCH *Medicare & Medicaid Guide* par. 26.385 (E.D. Wis., 1971), another federal court took jurisdiction, on the ground that Wisconsin's exclusion from the "medical indigent" category of anyone with an equity in excess of $7500 in a home and the land "used and operated in connection therewith." The decision, however, turned on a formal interpretation of HEW's regulations (45 CFR ¶ 248.21), which stated, "Resources which may be held must, as a minimum, be at the most liberal level used in any money payment in the State on or after January 1, 1966. . . ." As Wisconsin had no homestead limitation on its OAA, AFDC, AB, or APTD programs, it was clearly in violation of the regulations. And the HEW regulation, because it was promulgated pursuant to Title XIX, had the force of law, and again the constitutional argument was not reached.

In *Roberts v. Brian,* 484 P.2d 1378 (Calif. Supr. Ct., 1971), a nursing home patient, who was a myoclonic epileptic and whose physician prescribed a personal attendant during working hours, alleged, *inter alia,* a violation of equal protection when this was denied by Medi-Cal authorities. The Supreme Court of California avoided the constitutional issue in deciding for the plaintiff, by interpreting Medi-Cal regulations in her favor. *Boisvert v. Zeller* was handled in a similar way, 334 F. Supp. 403 (D.N.H., 1971). There a severely mentally retarded person was not eligible for Medicaid in New Hampshire since that state's APTD regulations included only the physically disabled within the definition. By the use of somewhat tortuous reasoning, the Federal District Court avoided passing on the constitutional issue by deciding that the New Hampshire regulations were inconsistent with the Federal regulations.

36. 40 F. Supp. 150, 154 (D. Me., 1972).

Nursing home inmates also attempted to use equal protection claims. A class action by Medicaid recipients in skilled nursing homes, *Waier v. Schmidt*, involved Wisconsin's refusal to "pass along" to them part of the Social Security increases of 1969. Plaintiffs and other such nursing home patients were allowed to keep $9.00 per month to cover personal needs; they contended unsuccessfully that the applicable federal statute intended this to be increased by $4.00. More broadly, they argued that this was a vastly smaller amount than other categorical recipients were allowed to keep and that this distinction constituted invidious discrimination. The court twice held that this constitutional argument was insubstantial, as other categorical assistance recipients had to provide themselves with numerous necessities while nursing home patients did not. 316 F. Supp. 407; 318 F. Supp. 22 (E.D. Wis., 1970).

In fact, an earlier case, *Catalano v. Department of Hospitals of the City of New York*, 229 F. Supp. 166 (S.D. N.Y., 1969), had involved a similar equal protection attack on the "endorse-over" rules imposed on nursing home patients receiving Medicaid. The plaintiffs' complaint was that in-patients were allowed to keep only $180.00 annually for personal needs, while other Medicaid recipients could keep $2300.00 as maintenance income. Without citing *Dandridge* (but only, one may be sure, because it had not been decided), the Court cited the obvious rational basis for the distinction and dismissed the claim, refusing, as the *Waier* court had, to empanel the three-judge court which would be necessary were a "substantial" constitutional attack on a state statute involved.

37. 320 F. Supp. 500 (D. Colo., 1970).

38. For a criticism of the court's interpretation of plaintiffs' claims as well as of its statutory interpretation, see University of Pennsylvania Law School and U.C.L.A. Law School, Health Law Project, *Preliminary Materials on Health Law*, Part V, *Medicaid*, 1971 edition, p. 161.

39. Plaintiffs' initial argument, according to the court, was that Colorado was required by Title XIX to implement Medicaid for the medically needy, even if the maintenance income level for this class was set at a level equal to that for the categorically needy. The obvious benefit for plaintiffs would be that, under the "spend-down" requirement, net rather than gross income would be determinative. The argument that Title XIX required inclusion of the medically needy was rejected in the light of construction of the statutory provision.

40. 404 U.S. 963 (1971), *rehearing denied*, 404 U.S. 1027 (1972).

More easy to reject was the equal protection argument when claimed on the grounds that it was invidious to provide Medicaid methadone treatment at an approved center but not through a private physician. *Harris v. Rockefeller*, CCH *Medicare & Medicaid Guide*, par. 26.406 (E.D. N.Y., 1971); *ibid*, par. 26.419 (2d Cir. 1972). Both the trial and appeal courts saw this as a reasonable distinction in view of Methadone's classification as a dangerous drug.

More complex was the case of *City of New York v. Wyman*, where the City and two pregnant indigents challenged the State Department of Social Service regulations denying reimbursement for abortions unless "medically indicated," although the general law of the state had been changed to allow abortions for any reason. The trial court invalidated the regulation in a less than clear opinion, apparently on constitutional grounds, including, so it would seem, equal protection. 321 N.Y.S. 2d 605; 66 Misc. 2d 402 (N.Y. Supr. Ct., Special Term, New York County, Part 1, 1971). In the Appellate Division, the decision was upheld, but explicitly not on constitutional grounds, 322 N.Y.S. 2d 957; 37 A.D. 2d 700, Supr. Ct., App. Div., 1st Dist., 1971; while the Court of Appeals disagreed with both the lower courts, 30 N.Y. 2d 537 (Ct. of App. 1972). This decision was later reversed by a three-judge federal court apparently on equal protection grounds. *New York Times*, August 25, 1972, p. 1, col. 2 (And see now *Klein v. Nassau County Medical Center* (E.D.N.Y., 1972), CCH, *Medicare & Medicaid Guide*, para. 26.512.) The litigation may, however, have become moot as the result of the Supreme Court decision limiting the power of the states to prevent abortion. See *Roe v. Wade*, 410 U.S. 113 (1973); and see now *Nassau County Medical Center v. Kline*, CCH *Medicare and Medicaid Guide*, par. 26,669 (1973 U.S. S.C.).

Several other cases had dealt with abortions sought by Medicaid recipients. *Jedrezjewski v. Minter*, CCH *Poverty Law Reporter*, par. 15.464 (D.C. Mass., 1971), held that a woman had been properly denied payment for an alleged therapeutic abortion, because it had not been proved that the proposed abortion was actually needed to save her physical or mental health. In *Alice v. State Department of Social Welfare*, CCH *Medicare & Medicaid Guide*, par. 26.277 (Cal. Supr. Ct., Sacramento, 1971), Medi-Cal officials were restrained from refusing to issue a Medicaid card to a pregnant, emancipated minor without parental notification of the pregnancy. The applicant had medical permission for a therapeutic abortion and was otherwise eligible for Medi-Cal.

41. 405 U.S. 906 (1972). Once again Mr. Justice Douglas noted that he was in favor of hearing oral argument.

42. CCH *Poverty Law Reporter*, par. 1225.52 (D. Ky., 1971).

43. Indeed, we were able to find only one case thus far in which a challenge to a state Medicaid practice has been sustained on equal protection grounds without being reversed later. This was *Loredo v. Sierra View District Hospital*, CCH *Medicare & Medicaid Guide*, par. 26.198 (Cal. Supr. Ct., 1969). There the defendant, a state district hospital, admitted all patients without reference to their source of income, with the exception of Medi-Cal recipients who sought elective surgery. The reason the hospital's board of directors gave for promulgating this policy was the fear that such patients would overtax the hospital's surgical facilities to the detriment of other patients.

Ginsberg J., found that this fear was unsupported by any evidence and, in a cursory holding, opined that as a governmental agency the hospital "may not discriminate between classes and groups of the public without substantial justification" and that the distinction in question was "discriminatory, unlawful and in conflict with the laws and constitutions of the State of California and the United States." It should be noted that this decision seems to have rested on statutory and state constitutional grounds as well as on the Equal Protection clause, although the Court cited no statutes or constitutional provisions. It should also be noted that this case was decided prior to *Dandridge*.

On the other hand, the federal courts have recently rejected at least three claims about allegedly unconstitutional aspects of the Medicaid program. In *Legian v. Richardson* (S.D. N.Y., 1973), a three-judge court, citing *Dandridge*, found nothing unconstitutional about the failure to cover those under 65 in a mental institution. CCH, *Medicare & Medicaid Guide*. par. 26.614. In *Florida v. Richardson* (N.D. Fla., 1973) it was held there was nothing *prima facie* unconstitutional in the federal regulation [252.10 (b) (3)] prohibiting nursing home administrators forming a majority of the state licensing body for nursing homes. *Ibid.*, par. 26.668. In *Opelika Nursing Home v. Richardson* (M.D. Ala., 1973) it was held that there was nothing unconstitutional in a regulation limiting payments to SNH's under Title XIX to the amounts paid for ECFs under Title XVIII. *Ibid.*, par. 26, 701.

44. 344 F. Supp. 1181 (S.D. Iowa, 1972).

45. 397 U.S. 397 at 422.

46. See Chapter 13 (c).

47. Some provision for HMOs (under a variety of titles) appeared in national health insurance proposals submitted to the 92nd Congress by such diverse groups as the Nixon Administration (S1623); proposals sponsored by Senator Javits for a gradual extension of Medicare (S836); proposals supported by the health insurance industry (HR4349); a split scheme of federal inpatient insurance and private outpatient insurance submitted by Republican Senators Scott and Percy (S1598); as well as in the most sweeping bill for national health insurance, endorsed by the AFL-CIO and sponsored by Senator Kennedy (S 3) and Representatives Griffiths and Corman (HR 22); and a variety of other less visible insurance proposals. But such proposals were relatively vague.

48. "Veto Message on the Labor-HEW-OEO Appropriation Bill," Jan. 27, 1970. *Public Papers of the Presidents, Richard Nixon,* 1970 (Washington D.C., 1971), p. 21.

49. See Congressional Quarterly Service, *Congressional Quarterly Almanac* 1970 (Washington, 1971), p. 139 and *passim*.

50. ". . . [T]he picemeal bill I am rejecting today simply continues the traditional approach to adding more programs to the almost unmanageable current structure of Federal Government health efforts." Memorandum of disapproval of a bill to promote training in family medicine, December 26, 1970, *Public Papers of the Presidents, Richard Nixon,* 1970 (Washington, 1971), p. 475.

51. U.S., Congress, Senate, Committee on Government Operations, Subcommittee on Executive Reorganization and Government Research, *Federal Role in Health,* 30 April 1970, S. Rept. 91-809, 91st Cong., 2nd Sess.

52. P.L. 91-296, *Congressional Quarterly Almanac 1970, supra,* note 49, p. 81.

53. While vetoes were apparently considered for both, the President signed a bill to set up a National Health Service Corps, to provide U.S. Public Health Service doctors for urban and rural shortage areas (P.L. 91-623), and a Comprehensive Alcoholism Bill (P.L. 91-616). A Communicable Disease Act, including grants for vaccination, was enacted (P.L. 91-464), although opposed by HEW on grounds that these grants should be funnelled through Comprehensive Health Planning Agencies. Reportedly the White House would not admit it was signed until five days after signature. *Washington Reports on Medicine and Health,* Oct. 26, 1970. A housing bill was also signed which included increased loan guarantees for hospital construction, including profit-making institutions (P.L. 91-609), as was a bill to give grants to state and local governments to eliminate the causes and incidents of lead-paint poisoning (P.L. 91-695). Legislation was also passed to coordinate family planning services and related research activities, with priority given to low-income areas (P.L. 91-572).

54. Mental retardation services received a boost with legislation to assist states in providing comprehensive services for those suffering from neurological disorders (P.L. 91-517), and other legislation was continued, notably federal assistance for educating health professionals (P.L. 91-519) and extension of the

"Great Society" duo of university-based Regional Medical Programs and state and local Comprehensive Health Planning agencies (P.L. 91-515). *Ibid.*, Nov. 9, 1970.

55. On this, see Eric Redman, *The Dance of Legislation* (New York, 1973).

56. S 4297 in the 91st Congress.

57. The Long proposals, pushed by the commercial health insurance industry, would have covered 80 percent of family health care costs over $2000 per year, together with 80 percent of all hospital costs after the first 60 days, to be financed through Social Security contributions. The proposals were endorsed by the Senate Finance Committee in December 1970 and were incorporated into H.R. 17550.

58. The House of Representatives passed H.R. 17550 in May 1970, including the Administration proposals for rather ill-defined "program review teams." The prospect of such community-wide utilization review mechanisms being established, with a primary object of cost control, and organized outside the traditional structures of the medical profession prompted the AMA to act. At its 119th annual convention in June 1970 the AMA recommended the development of a government-sponsored network of peer review organizations, established under the auspices of state medical societies, as part of a proposed "Health Insurance Assistance Act of 1970" (Medicredit). Senator Bennett's proposals were developed at his request by the staff of the Senate Finance Committee, which reportedly deemed them a "step in the right direction." *Washington Report on Medicine and Health,* July 6, 1970.

59. Testimony of HEW Undersecretary John Veneman, before the Senate Labor and Public Welfare Committee, September 23, 1970, reported in *Congressional Quarterly Almanac 1970, supra,* note 45, p. 605.

60. *Washington Report on Medicine and Health,* December 21, 1970.

61. House Report No. 91–1096.

16
Congress and the Future

All this, however, was not clear when Congress reconvened in 1971. Rather, it at last seemed as if the future of Medicaid might be clarified through the apparent willingness of the Nixon Administration to face the cash assistance issue head on. The President had attacked the piecemeal nature of medical programs; his counselor, Daniel Moynihan, had provided FAP and FHIP to respond to these directives. At last there seemed a serious chance of reworking cash assistance and welfare medicine programs. But the possibility was not to become reality. The low level of cash support and the threat of mandatory work provisions in FAP alienated liberals who in any event, as far as medical care went, preferred comprehensive National Health Insurance; cost and concern with "states' rights" alienated conservatives. The country was thus left with its traditional fragmented approach, and the immediate future seemed to hold only traditional fragmentary reforms.

"Once More Unto the Breach, Dear Friends"

As with the earlier Social Security Amendments, H.R. 17550 and its successor consisted of a variety of proposals falling under different titles of the Social Security Act. In its first incarnation, H.R. 17550 would have increased Social Security benefits by 5 percent, effected other changes in the OASDHI program, and altered the Medicare, Medicaid, and maternal and child health programs "with emphasis upon improvements in the operating effectiveness of such programs." In connection with Medicaid, the most obvious examples of this emphasis were the provisions allowing the Secretary of HEW to refuse or reduce reimbursement to providers for capital costs (e.g., depreciation, interest, return on equity capital) where such expenditures were not consistent with state or local health care plans and authorizing the use of prepayment and other experimental methods of paying hospitals and other providers.[1]

From the beginning, the emphasis with regard to Medicaid was cost-consciousness. H.R. 17550, as initially drafted, contained a number of relatively straightforward provisions. For example, payments were to be refused to any provider accused of abusing or defrauding Title XIX. And hospitals would no longer automatically be entitled to "reasonable costs," if their actual costs were lower.[2] Recipients, too, were to have their wings clipped. The bill would have allowed states to require flat deductibles or co-payments from the medically indigent (although not the categorically indigent), without the existing restriction that such deductibles be reasonably related to the recipient's income and resources. Not surprisingly, the bill abandoned the fiction that there was a 1977 deadline for the establishment of comprehensive care. As a partial palliative, the bill required (rather than merely allowed) states to extend coverage ex post facto to an otherwise eligible recipient for three months prior to his application for Medicaid.

Cost-consciousness was the watchword. The bill required hospitals and nursing homes to have utilization review (UR) committees, similar to those under Medicare; called on the federal government to pay 90 percent of the costs incurred by the states in setting up effective mechanical claims processing and information retrieval systems, together with 75 percent of the costs of operating such systems; and, in an effort to encourage uniformity, if not efficiency, gave the state health departments responsibility for certifying health facilities for participation in all programs which fell under Social Security legislation (Medicare, Medicaid, and Maternal and Child Health Services). This would end the practice in some states of having different bureaus certifying institutions for different health care programs. Such recommendations were in direct line with those made in the 1967 and 1969 Amendments.[3]

Of much more interest were direct attempts to rechannel the funding of Medicaid into more "desirable" directions. One such general attempt was to encourage schemes of prospective reimbursement, i.e., payment to providers for specified services to be given to Medicaid beneficiaries on a lump sum or per capita basis. The obvious advantage here was in budgetary control: budgets were set in advance rather than being reimbursed on an open-ended, retrospective basis, and any losses would be met by providers. The initial House version of H.R. 17550 also included a rather vague authority for experiments in prospective reimbursement and an option for Medicare and Medicaid recipients to receive care in a health maintenance organization (where prospective reimbursement could be assured). But in addition it sought to redress the institutional funding patterns of spending under Medicaid, by imposing dollar penalties on long-term institutional care and adding dollar incentives for ambulatory care.[4]

This proposal is interesting in that it attempted, however clumsily, to ascribe health priorities for Medicaid. There were, of course, some health priorities defined in federal legislation in the required services states had to provide in order to be eligible for Medicaid. But a relative ranking of the required services themselves had never been attempted. States were free to provide as much or as little hospital, nursing home, or doctor care as they wished, the patterns in large part being dictated by the availability of service and interest of providers in Medicaid recipients. Health maintenance organizations, too, were understood to re-order health priorities, by paying relatively more for preventive and ambulatory care and relatively less for hospitalization. But using federal leverage directly to influence the various types of payment was both bold and controversial.[5] Nevertheless this provision survived passage in the House, with the other elements of H.R. 17550, and was sent for consideration by the Senate.

The bill's history in the Senate is less straightforward. The House proposals had apparently been shaped by a series of hearings held by the Ways and Means Committee in October and November of 1969.[6] The changes in the bill proposed by the Senate were largely the result of the report written by the Finance Committee staff in February 1970,[7] shortly before that committee resumed hearings on Medicare and Medicaid.[8] Later in the year, the Finance Committee also held hearings on H.R. 17550, but little fresh testimony on Medicaid was elicited.[9] Strangely enough, with few exceptions, the McNerney Report appears not to have directly influenced the Senate or House version to any great extent; perhaps Congressional distrust of the Administration extended even to its blue-ribbon committees.

When H.R. 17550 emerged from the Finance Committee on December 11, 1970, after the November elections, it had become a conglomerate bill, including not only Social Security, Medicare, and Medicaid provisions, but also a watered-down version of President Nixon's Family Assistance Plan,[10] various protectionist trade provisions, and Senator Long's proposal for a federally-funded catastrophic health insurance program. These latter additions, all of which were controversial, were apparently added by the committee in a South Sea Bubble spirit, hoping that the amendments would slip through the Senate, which was likely to give broad support to the remainder of the bill.[11] The primary difference with respect to Social Security was that the Senate version called for a 10 percent hike in benefits. (Ultimately a 20 percent hike was to be approved, but this awaited pre-election largesse, in 1972.)

The numerous changes and additions made in the Medicare and Medicaid sections of H.R. 17550 showed that the Finance Committee staff had been busy. By this time, of course, Medicaid was being besieged on all sides. President Nixon had by then made his statement that it was "inefficient, inequitably excludes the working poor, and often provides an incentive for people to stay on welfare,"[12] an argument for replacing a large part of Medicaid with FHIP; and the McNerney Report's criticisms were being taken seriously, at least outside Congress. But while both of these sources envisaged a "new" Medicaid, the Senate Finance Committee's purposes were more immediately realistic. They proposed a series of modifications in the existing system.

Most of the House proposals for Medicaid were left untouched by the Senate. But the Senate Finance Committee went much further than the House in specifying fiscal controls, with a special emphasis on utilization review.[13] Indeed, a legacy of the Committee's hearings in the summer of 1970 was a clear recognition of three basic types of fiscal control which could be applied to Medicaid (and Medicare): direct controls over fees, prospective reimbursement procedures, and *ex post facto* audit techniques. Utilization review procedures were the most visible examples of audit techniques.[14] Utilization review was becoming so popular that it stood in danger of becoming yet another oversold panacea. Thus, while the Finance Committee weakened the House provision reducing federal subsidies for institutional care, by making any reductions apply only to states with inadequate medical audit and review procedures,[15] it added Senator Bennett's proposals for Professional Standards Review Organizations (PSROs). These were to provide a network of medical society (or other) audit groups covering each state, with responsibility for reviewing both institutional and noninstitutional services under Medicare, Medicaid, and other federally-sponsored programs.

The Bennett Amendment was to provide constant fuel for debate from 1970 to the present. In attenuated form it was included in the 1972 Amendments; the PSRO was to become yet another health care acronym. But the sweep of the initial proposal deserves emphasis. As originally proposed, the Bennett Amendment would have established professional standards review organizations in each geographical area, to review services given under Medicare, Medicaid, maternal and child health programs, and other designated programs. The PSRO would thus provide a central monitoring system over a substantial amount of the health services given in each area, including virtually all services to those over 65. Qualified organizations were to be designated as PSROs by the Secretary of Health, Education, and Welfare for each area; the medical society would be offered the first choice. Responsibilities for the new organization would be wide and would include approval in advance for all elective hospital admissions, a provision much resented and later deleted.[16]

But although PSROs provided an important new ingredient to the Medicaid[17] and Medicare debates, the Senate Finance Committee's recommendations also spread broadly in other respects. Notably, the House's provision for payments to HMOs was tightened, by the noticeably more sceptical Senate Committee, to ensure that specific quality standards were met and that HMOs would escape the exploitation by profitmaking organizations that nursing homes had experienced.[18] In addition, an Inspector-General for Health Administration would be appointed to check into the economy, legality, and effectiveness of federal health programs;[19] and criminal penalties would be made more stringent and more explicit for fraud and illegal acts by Medicare and Medicaid providers.

Another significant set of proposals among the host offered by the Senate Finance Committee related to the limits as well as the potentials of federal standard-setting. The 1970 hearings had pointed up the difficulties experienced in states such as Idaho, where federal nursing home standards were unenforceable because of lack of staff in rural areas. The Senate version of H.R. 17550 required HEW to develop means of testing the proficiency of health personnel, particularly nurses, not then qualified to render certain services because of failure to meet educational and training criteria. The goal was to mitigate the shortage of professionals by waiving rigid standards in appropriate cases, and by providing a 5-year period in which the persons whose credentials had been waived could attend training programs. This concern over staffing was to continue in subsequent debates, with the final version of the 1972 Amendments authorizing a special waiver, under specific conditions, of the requirement that an RN be available at all times for skilled nursing facilities in rural areas.[20]

Taken together, the Medicare and Medicaid provisons of the Senate Finance Committee's version of H.R. 17550 represented a potpourri of proposals rather than one integrated whole. Such was the usual fate of Social Security provisions. There was even some doubt as to how the various new structures would fit together. Were the PSROs, for example, to review medical procedures in the HMOs, thus demolishing the Administration's efforts to establish HMOs as decentralized, self-policing units? How did the catastrophic health insurance proposal mesh with the apparent intentions elsewhere in the legislation to refocus health care payments away from hospital care and on to preventive medicine? And where did the Inspector-General fit into all of this?

While such questions were of intense interest to all who would be immediately affected by the bill—Medicaid patients, medical societies, hospitals (which could become subject to review by PSROs, as the proposals were then drafted), health insurance companies—they were only part of the plethora of questions brought forth by the total Social Security bill. In the bill reported out by the Finance Committee, textile quotas and tariffs jostled with widows' benefits, welfare reform experiments, child care corporations, work incentives for public assistance recipients, family planning services, and veterans' pension increases. Debate in the Senate on H.R. 17550 began on December 16, 1970 but quickly bogged down in a series of complicated parliamentary maneuvers over the bill's welfare and trade provisions. This deadlock lasted until after the Christmas recess, by which time it was clear that no action would be taken on the bill unless the controversial sections added by the Finance Committee were deleted. On December 28 Senator Long won passage of an amendment to drop the trade, catastrophic health insurance, and most of the welfare provisions from the bill, including family assistance.[21]

The action left only the Social Security, Medicare, and Medicaid provisions in the bill, together with a few welfare provisions, including amendments intended to override specific Supreme Court decisions.[22] The next day, December 29, the Senate passed what was left of its version of H.R. 17550 by an 81–0 vote.[23] Chairman Mills, however, saying that it would be impossible to work out differences in the Senate and House versions before the end of the session, refused to take the bill to the conference committee. But, he promised, the bill would be resubmitted in the 92nd Congress, with top priority. With tongue in cheek, or misplaced confidence, he set the goal for passage as February 12, 1971.[24]

Thus died the proposed reforms in Medicaid, supported by the Administration and passed (with some differences) by both houses of Congress. Early in 1971, Congress passed a separate 10 percent increase in Social Security benefits,[25] but by then reform of Medicare and Medicaid had been incorporated into H.R. 1 of the 92nd Congress, which soon had a history even more complex than its predecessor.

The Warriors: National Health Insurance

If 1970 was the year of the veto, 1971, the first session of the 92nd Congress, was the year when welfare reform died and national health insurance came of age. Tussles continued between the cost-conscious Administration and a relatively profligate Congress.[26] But, as far as Medicaid and other health care programs were concerned, the spotlight was on reform of both welfare and governmental health care schemes. Reforms in the Medicaid program, primarily for the purposes of efficiency and economy, elicited perhaps the least controversy in the entire deliberations, but once more they became ensnared in the fights over other proposals and once more failed to win enactment.

National health insurance proposals got off to a quick start in the 92nd Congress with the reintroduction, in a somewhat modified form, of the "Health Security" proposals, introduced in both the House and the Senate in January.[27] These proposals, the widest of all those suggested, were a direct descendant of the Wagner-Murray-Dingell bills of the 1940s.[28] They endorsed the principle of health services provided to all as an entitlement under the Social Security system; the program would have no means test provision, would be federally administered, and would include a wide range of benefits, with no cost-sharing by recipients and few benefit limitations.[29] Funding was to be through payroll taxes and federal general revenues.

The Kennedy bill, as it came to be generally called, brought into the open questions which many members of Congress (and the public) were unwilling to face. If, indeed, there was a health care crisis and a need for more effective insurance coverage, here was a bill which unabashedly addressed itself to comprehensive national health insurance. Moreover, by replacing an array of public and private funding schemes by one relatively simple insurance system, regionally and locally administered, other questions would be faced—notably, the establishment of health planning agencies, local health care systems, and regulatory bodies to ensure that services were available and obligations met. Under such a scheme Medicare would be abolished; it would no longer be necessary. Medicaid would revert to the classic function of public assistance: a back-up program to pay for noncovered services for the needy (most notably, nursing home care over 120 days).

As in the earlier health insurance debates, opposition to the Kennedy proposals centered on its sweeping nature, its reliance on public agencies, its cost, and whether it was even necessary. As before, less drastic alternatives were suggested. Federal-state grants programs for the needy were no longer fashionable; Medicaid had at least had that negative effect. But other suggestions proliferated. Senator Javits introduced into the 92nd Congress his proposals for a gradual expansion of Medicare to cover the whole population.[30] Senators Pell and Mondale introduced a proposal to require employers engaged in interstate commerce and government agencies to provide specified health benefits through prepaid health plans or similar arrangements.[31] Senators Scott and Percy recommended a federal hospital insurance program administered through HEW regional offices, together with voluntary outpatient care through private insurance.[32] Senator Long's advocacy of catastrophic health insurance—designed as an alternative to the Kennedy proposals—appeared in its full glory as a separate bill.[33]

In the House, Representative Burleson presented the health insurance industry's answer to national health insurance: a voluntary program for employers to cover employees, a voluntary individual insurance package administered under state supervision, and a heavily subsidized state plan for the poor and uninsurable.[34] The AMA's solution, Medicredit, appeared under the sponsorship of Representatives Fulton and Broyhill.[35] The American Hospital Association's "Ameriplan" (a scheme based on an extended function for hospitals), while later to founder, was still extant. The U.S. Chamber of Commerce, apparently startled by Administration plans to unload the costs of health insurance onto employers, was reportedly developing its own proposals.[36] Nor were these by any means the full extent of the various proposals.

Central to all of the debates on national health insurance in the 92nd

Congress were, however, the Nixon Administration's own proposals. While the Kennedy proposals could be seen as standing at the radical end of the spectrum and Medicredit at the conservative end, the Nixon Health Strategy, announced in a health message to Congress in February 1971,[37] fell squarely in the middle. Indeed it was not one strategy but a veritable collection of strategies. The health delivery system was to be improved through the development of HMOs, FHIP was to take care of financing the health needs of poor families with children, standard health insurance benefits for the working population were to be developed, employers were to be required to subsidize employee benefits, and a series of proposals would help stimulate a better production and distribution of health professionals.

These proposals were expanded in a so-called White Paper in May 1971 and formed the theme of Administration proposals throughout the 92nd Congress.[38] The basic theme was clear. Preference was for "action in the private sector," based on the "fundamentals of our political economy—capitalistic, pluralistic, and competitive. . . ."[39] There was less emphasis on the single comprehensive solution than there had been in earlier proposals. In Congress, the proposals appeared piecemeal. Senator Bennett sponsored the legislation covering FHIP and the employers' subsidization plan; it also —not entirely coincidentally—included PSROs, by then being pushed as the Administration's solution to quality control.[40] Legislation for health maintenance organizations[41] and for health manpower education[42] was to be considered separately. Despite the rhetoric of comprehensiveness, then, the Administration proposals were inevitably fragmented.

The proposals, moreover, were handicapped in two vital respects. Without welfare reform, FHIP made little sense; thus one part of the health insurance proposals was doomed from the beginning. At the same time, proposals for health insurance for the middle class—compulsory employee coverage with a 75 percent employer subsidy—could not appeal to the employers themselves; and the private insurance industry was becoming concerned at the strange sight of a hard-line Republican administration seeking to regulate their operations and perhaps even to set up public insurance agencies.[43]

In one way or another, then, all of the health insurance proposals before the 92nd Congress had flaws for some influential sector. Medicredit had too few controls for health care reformers; the Kennedy proposals too many for the private sector. The Nixon proposals were piecemeal; the Javits solution extended a deficient system (Medicare) to a larger population. But Congress was engaged in the time-honored process of working toward some eventual form of consensus.

The record being built was impressive. Hearings before the Senate Health Subcommittee on national health insurance in 1971 resulted in eleven volumes of testimony;[44] these formed the source material for a book by

Senator Kennedy clearly designed to advance his position as a leader of the national health insurance movement.[45] Meanwhile, Chairman Wilbur Mills, whose political ambitions rose as the 1972 elections began to loom, was making the House Ways and Means Committee an alternative focus for insurance hearings; he capped Senator Kennedy by publishing 13 volumes of health insurance hearings in 1971.[46] The committee also began to rival the Senate Finance Committee in producing relevant reports, notably on the health care industry [47] and on the various proposals for health insurance.[48]

As the various proposals moved through the 92nd Congress in 1971 and 1972, some eventual changes in health financing appeared increasingly likely. National health insurance was a plank in the Democratic party platform in the 1972 elections, but the *idea* of national health insurance was no longer partisan.

"These Wounds I Had on Crispin's Day"

With national health insurance siphoning off much of the interest in health financing, and with welfare reform central to President Nixon's own interests,[49] the Social Security bill of the 92nd Congress, H.R. 1, was predominantly a welfare bill. In December 1970, some 20 lobbies representing organizations as diverse as the AFL-CIO, the National Association of Manufacturers, Common Cause, the National Association of Counties, and the National Welfare Rights Organization had formed a precarious coalition to press Congress into enacting some kind of welfare reforms.[50] Members of the Congress themselves, of course, had long been dissatisfied with the patchwork of programs that constituted the welfare system in the United States. It seemed that welfare reform was at last ripe. But, again, the primary bottleneck was action in the Senate.

As promised, H.R. 1 was introduced the first day of the new Congress by Chairman Mills, together with Representative Byrnes of the Ways and Means Committee. The bill provided the traditional "sweeteners"—OASDI benefit increases—and included many of the same changes in Medicare and Medicaid that had cleared the House in 1970. Most of the attention, however, focused on the bill's provision for reform of Titles I, X, and XIV, to be replaced by a new federal-state program of aid to the aged, blind, and disabled, and repeal of AFDC, to be replaced by a Family Assistance Plan similar in many respects to that which the Nixon Administration had been urging since 1969. If both were passed, there would be a virtual federalization of cash assistance.

The Ways and Means Committee went directly into executive sessions, to emerge in May 1971 with a bill even more sweeping than its 1970 effort. With an eye to conservative and blue-collar constituencies, the committee detailed a reformed assistance program that would set up a totally federal program to take over existing programs of aid to the aged, blind, and disabled; a federal-state work-oriented program (administered by the Labor Department) to cover families with an employable member who was able to work; and a federal Family Assistance Plan to replace AFDC for families with no member able to work. Generally the assistance emphasis was on federal administration and on the concept of "work rather than welfare dependency."[51]

It was these proposals, together with the basic income level of $2400 for a family of four, which were to spark the most controversy. Nevertheless, these provisions, together with the remainder of H.R. 1, were passed by the House, 288–132, on June 22, 1971, after two days of debates, centering primarily on the FAP.[52] Votes against the bill came primarily from a coalition of liberals, who thought the mandatory work provisions regressive, and conservatives, who thought the bill too costly. But H.R. 1 ran into a series of delays. In the Senate, the Finance Committee began hearings on H.R. 1 late in July 1971, but the hearings were soon curtailed in order for the Committee to consider President Nixon's "New Economic Policy." Indeed, Presidential enthusiasm for welfare reform, at least as an immediate measure, appeared to be waning, under a basic policy conflict; the wage-price squeeze could not easily be squared with passage of an expensive federal income program.[53]

In any event, it was becoming clear that H.R. 1 was in trouble in the Senate. By then, three rival welfare schemes were being mooted. The first was the House version, which was supported by the Administration. The second was sponsored by Senate liberals such as Senator Ribicoff, who opposed compulsory work requirements and wanted a $3000 per year guaranteed annual income for a family of four (later reduced to $2600, in an abortive attempt to compromise with HEW).[54] The third proposal, supported by Senator Long, represented the views of Senate conservatives who favored "workfare" and were basically against FAP. These three quite different views of what welfare was for had no common basis for reconciliation. The basic "sweetener" of Social Security—a 20 percent pre-election increase in OASDHI benefits—was removed from H.R. 1 and passed separately in June 1972.[55] But the remaining provisions of the bill, which had by then swollen to 989 pages, were in jeopardy, as long as the welfare deadlock remained.

The Senate Finance Committee finally released its report on H.R. 1, a closely-packed volume of 1285 pages, on September 26, 1972, three weeks before Congress was due to adjourn.[56] In an effort to pass H.R. 1 in some form, the Senate voted to approve a 2-year to 4-year test of *all three* rival welfare approaches. In such guise the Senate cleared H.R. 1, only to have all FAP provisions deleted in conference when the different sides could not agree. Thus no welfare reform provisions for the AFDC population were incorporated into the 1972 Amendments.

In the flurry, however, the companion piece to FAP and "workfare" was continued. The provision to federalize AB, OAA, and APTD survived the various turmoils as the recipients in those programs did not generate the hostility by this time associated with AFDC recipients. Thus the curious situation was reached whereby welfare reform was indeed achieved, but almost inadvertently and for the "wrong" population. Proposals to federalize AFDC actually resulted in federalizing all federal-state categorical cash assistance programs *except* AFDC.[57] That is not to say that such a radical reform may not be eminently desirable and highly significant. With three of the categorical assistance groups federalized, Supplementary Security Income (SSI) as the new "category" is called, is now administered by the Social Security Administration in Washington and closely integrated with OASDHI.[58] As the month for implementation (January 1974) neared, it was thought that twice as many persons would claim payments, since much of the welfare stigma would be gone. If this is so, not only will there be a profound effect on Medicaid,[59] but the very nature of cash assistance will have changed.

P.L. 92–603: Medicaid Provisions

The dramatic events surrounding welfare reform thus had obvious implications for Medicaid. But it was one of the many peculiarities of H.R. 1 that it did not regard medical assistance as an element linked to welfare reform. FHIP, for example, while appearing as part of the President's Health Strategy, was not included in H.R. 1; nor were there any provisions for federalizing Medicaid with respect to the federalized OAA, AB, and APTD categories. Although the 1972 Amendments, as passed, note that states are required to cover all existing cash assistance recipients under the local Medicaid program,[60] the Medicaid programs themselves will continue to vary from state to state, and the states have an option about covering those newly recruited to SSI. In practice, however, it is almost inconceivable that a state like New York, which is expecting that the effect of SSI will be to double the number of aged, blind, and disabled claiming cash assistance,[61] will deny this new group Medicaid.[62]

Specific changes in the Medicaid program proposed for H.R. 1 by the Ways and Means Committee, and subsequently modified, were an amalgam of proposals made by the two houses of Congress in 1970, with a few important additions. Among those which remained unchanged and were ultimately written into the legislation was the elimination of the 1977 deadline for comprehensive services.[63] But much that was new appeared in H.R. 1 as it moved through the Congress. The growing emphasis on HMOs by the Administration and other groups in the Congress[64] was reflected in H.R. 1's provisions.[65] The Act permitted states to waive Federal "statewideness" and comparability provisions for Medicaid recipients so that states could (with HEW approval) provide more generous health services than those in the state Medicaid plan through prepaid comprehensive health programs.[66] Elsewhere in the legislation, Medicare payments, too, were finally to be allowed to be made to health maintenance organizations under similar general arrangements.[67] The way was thus open for increased "buying-in" to relatively comprehensive health care systems for Medicare and Medicaid patients.

Besides such prospective reimbursement methods, utilization review once again raised its head. The plan for PSROs was again attached to the bill by the Senate Finance Committee and incorporated into the 1972 Amendments. Although far less sweeping than the original Bennett Amendment, this section provided for a totally new structure of review of services under both Medicare and Medicaid. Physician-sponsored organizations were to be designated as PSROs (usually including 300 or more physicians), with the responsibility of assuring that institutional services under the program were both medically necessary and professionally adequate. The most controversial aspects had been ironed out. Notably the PSRO could delegate hospital and HMO review functions to existing committees in those institutions, and review of noninstitutional care was made optional.[68] Nevertheless, the development of PSROs was one of the major innovations of the 1972 Amendments.

Linked with utilization review was the provision, inherited from H.R. 17550, of a reduction in federal matching payments for long-term stays in institutions. While attenuated, this provision also survived as an adjunct of utilization review. States having inadequate programs to control utilization of institutional services under Medicaid or failing to conduct independent professional audits of patients (required by law) would risk a one third reduction in federal matching payments for long-term stays in institutions.[69] Enforcement was, indeed, the theme. As we noted in discussing child health services, the 1972 Amendments also allowed the reduction of the federal share of AFDC payments for noncompliance with this provision.[70] In other cases, too, federal funds were to be limited. Notably, both Medicare and Medicaid payments were to be disallowed with respect to certain capital expenses disapproved as being inconsistent with state or local health care plans; and the federal share of nursing home costs under Medicaid, effective 1973, was to be held to 105 percent of the costs of previous years.[71] The Inspector-General, brought to life again by the Senate Finance Committee, was killed at the conference stage. However, disclosure of the ownership of intermediate care facilities was required, as was the requirement of publicity for reports of deficient institutions.[72]

As far as Medicaid recipients were concerned, there were certain changes. Family planning services were made mandatory services under state Medicaid plans; optometrists and chiropractors could henceforth be covered under the rubric "physicians' services"; and a 3-month retroactive coverage was required for patients (including deceased persons) found eligible for Medicaid. Medicaid recipients were also to be allowed to carry their benefits for four months after Medicaid would normally terminate because of increased family income, a partial solution to the vexing "notch" effect. But, as might be expected, the tone of the bill was not "consumer-oriented."

Recipients had, conversely, much to lose. Cost-sharing and deductible provisions, while perhaps the most controversial elements of H.R. 1, survived into the 1972 Amendments. The final provisions for cost-sharing required states to impose monthly premium charges on the medically indigent. Following the House version of the bill these could be graduated according to income, following standards to be developed by the HEW Secretary.[73] In passage through the Senate, however, the provisions were softened to provide that alternatively, states could require "nominal deductibles" and "nominal co-payment amounts," which did not have to vary by income. The conferees also agreed that such nominal amounts could also be levied on cash assistance recipients for nonmandatory Medicaid services.[74]

As a final glance at H.R. 1's Medicaid provisions, a number of other provisions should be rapidly sketched, to give the complex flavor of the bill as well as its substantive effect. Highly significant was the fact that the "maintenance of effort" concept was relinquished with the repeal of Section 1902(d). In the future, states could reduce expenditures on Medicaid from one year to the next. In perhaps the final divorce of Medicaid from Medicare and the general concept of "mainstream" medicine, states were also to be allowed to determine for themselves what were "reasonable costs" for inpatient hospital care under Medicaid. On the other hand, standards for extended care facilities under Medicare and skilled nursing homes under Medicaid were finally combined, as so-called skilled nursing facilities.[75] Full federal funding of nursing home inspections was allowed; and standards were to be developed, by diagnosis, for the minimum periods during which the post-hospital patient would be eligible for benefits.

Elsewhere in the legislation, Medicare was significantly extended to include for the first time OASDHI recipients below the age of 65. Not only was Medicare extended to the disabled under 65; in an interesting break with its earlier philosophy of Medicare, Title XVIII was also to cover an element of the catastrophic costs of middle-class medicine. Coverage was extended to all insured workers with chronic renal disease and to the costs of kidney transplantation or dialysis three months after the beginning of dialysis treatment. As the movement for national health insurance faded, it seemed that sops had been thrown, represented by eclectic expansions of Medicare. Catastrophic health insurance for other (middle-class) groups remains, as this book goes to press, as an area for future possible consensus—but again one offering a fragmentary approach to health care costs rather than a "solution" for welfare medicine.

Viewing them as one piece of legislation, what can one say of the 1972 Amendments? One obvious comment is that—as with previous Social Security legislation—P.L. 92–603 can be comprehended only as the sum of diverse parts.[76] There was no basic idea of Social Security, including health protection. In the absence of any clear commitment in Congress to a philosophy of either health or welfare, such an outcome should perhaps be expected. The demise of welfare reform in 1971, confirmed in 1972, was probably a good indication of the deep splits in the Congress over basic issues. Health, too, was bounded by constricted viewpoints. By 1973, there appeared to be a growing rhetoric of agreement about the need for health care financing (national health insurance) and health care delivery (health maintenance organizations), but not much willingness to tackle the practical realities of these allegedly shared goals.

Despite all the hearings in the 92nd Congress, the pendulum of events appeared to have swung back to a repressive view of welfare and a "magic bullet" approach to health: money for heart and lung research,[77] for discovering and treating venereal and other communicable diseases,[78] and for establishment of a national program to deal with sickle cell anemia.[79] In welfare, too, the real action was in the pieces rather than the whole: in the survival of OEO legislation,[80] in school lunch programs,[81] in meals and other nutritional and health services for older Americans,[82] and in the federalizing of cash assistance for the old, blind, and disabled, achieved in the 1972 Amendments. These were no mean achievements, but basic problems were not tackled.

Some of the weaknesses of Medicaid were direct outcomes of the ponderous, complex nature of the Congressional process, formulated as it is by a series of committees, individuals, and lobbying groups. But perhaps some of the strengths of the democratic process also emerged. As the 93rd Congress dawned,[83] however, and the numerous ramifications of the 1972 Amendments were being explored by Congressional staff, federal agencies, and state and local governments, it was clear once again that the major emphasis of social change would rest on financing rather than polemics. The last major battle of the 92nd Congress was President Nixon's request for a ceiling of $250 billion on federal spending for fiscal 1973. Although this was rejected by the Senate, the old questions remained. Whether couched in terms of tax reform or of the need for a balanced federal budget, there was still no solution to the President's earlier question: On what is federal money most profitably to be spent?

NOTES

1. U.S., Department of Health, Education and Welfare, *Task Force on Medicaid and Related Programs*, p. 37.

2. Cf. *Connecticut State Dept. of Welfare v. HEW* 448 F2d 209 (2d Cir. 1971). At the same time, payments to providers generally were not to exceed "customary charges" to the general public even where such "customary charges" were lower than "reasonable" or actual costs.

3. Also unsurprising were a sprinkling of minor provisions relating to specific interest groups. For example, Christian Science nursing homes would no longer be required to have licensed administrators to be eligible for Medicaid payments, and HEW was to study the feasibility of including chiropractic services under Medicare, based on the experiences of Medicaid with such providers; both provisions were to survive into the 1972 legislation.

4. Specifically, the federal share of payments to states for outpatient hospital services, clinic services, and home health care services would be increased by 25 percent, with a 95 percent maximum federal share; while the federal subsidy for Medicaid patients in general hospitals would be reduced by one third after 60 days and by a like amount after 90 days in skilled nursing homes or mental hospitals. After 365 days in a mental hospital, the federal share of reimbursement for any recipient would be eliminated. This last proposal was incorporated into H.R. 17550 almost intact from an earlier bill sponsored by Rep. Dawson, H.R. 16654 (Dawson, 25 March 1970).

5. Representative Pickle (Texas), who led the floor opposition to the reduction in payments for nursing home facilities, said that he and other congressmen had received considerable correspondence protesting this cutback. Yet an attempt to avoid the traditional House closed rule, primarily in order to amend this provision on the floor, failed on roll-call votes. Apparently most of the House agreed with Chairman Mills that "we have unlimited evidence that the skilled nursing homes are being overutilized." But, except for the Dawson proposal, none of the Medicaid provisions created much controversy in the House; and, after alteration by the Ways and Means Committee to include an Administration-backed cost-of-living escalator in Social Security benefits, the bill passed the House on May 21, 1970, by 344–32. *Congressional Record*, vol. 116, pp. 16552, 16554–58, 16587–88 (1970).

6. U.S., Congress, House Committee on Ways and Means, *Social Security and Welfare Proposals, Hearings* before the Committee on Ways and Means, 91st Cong., 1st Sess, 1969.

7. U.S., Congress, Senate, Committee on Finance, *Medicare and Medicaid: Problems, Issues and Alternatives*, Report of the Staff to the Committee on Finance, Committee Point (1970).

8. U.S., Congress, Senate, Committee on Finance, *Medicare and Medicaid, Hearings* before the Committee on Finance, 91st Cong., 2nd Sess, 1970.

9. U.S., Congress, Senate, *Social Security Amendments of 1970, Hearings* before the Committee on Finance, 91st Cong., 2nd Sess, 1970.

10. A stronger version, much closer to the Administration proposals, had been passed by the House in April, as H.R. 16311.

11. Congressional Quarterly Service, *Congressional Quarterly Almanac, 1971*, Washington, D.C., 1972, p. 1051.

12. *Weekly Compilation of Presidential Documents*, vol. 6 (1970), p. 748.

13. Often, in fact, the wording of the Senate Report accompanying H.R. 17550 was identical to that of corresponding sections of House Report 91-1096, which had accompanied the House bill out of committee. Those proposals, left virtually intact, included the elimination of the 1977 deadline for comprehensive programs, the new limits on levels of payments to providers, the elimination of the requirement that co-insurance or deductibles must be related to income, the requirement for utilization review in hospitals and nursing homes, the encouragement of experimentation with prospective payments, and the fiscal incentives for installation and operation of data-processing systems for claims control.

This last provision gives a good example of the interplay among the Administration and both houses of Congress in formulating much of this bill. The lack of efficient data-gathering and processing facilities in many of the states had been a recognized problem in Medicaid from its inception. The Finance Committee staff had recommended that penalties be placed on states that did not implement a claims control system approved by HEW. HEW, however, as the McNerney Report had suggested, recommended use of the carrot rather than the stick, and this was the approach that worked its way into the House bill and was approved by the Finance Committee. See *Medicare and Medicaid: Problems, Issues and Alternatives, supra,* note 7, pp. 130–131; *Medicare and Medicaid, Hearings, supra,* note 8, pp. 189–90.

14. The Senate Finance Committee's hearings on Medicare and Medicaid in April, May, and June had elicited detailed information on the operation of two medical society plans, that of the San Joaquin Medical Society Foundation (Stockton, Calif.) and the Certified Hospital Admission Program (CHAP) developed by the Medical Care Foundation of the Sacramento County Medical Society. The emphasis on utilization review was continued in the hearings on H.R. 17550, held in June and July 1970. See notes 7 and 8, *supra.*

15. The change was made under pressure from various constituencies, including the states. For example, the president of the American Nursing Home Association suggested that the House provision for federal reductions in institutional payments be deleted in view of various other utilization review proposals which, he argued, would solve the problem of overutilization of nursing home and inpatient facilities more equitably. The Senate compromise was an attempt to "differentiate between those states which are adequately controlling utilization and those which are not." See *Social Security Amendments of 1970, Hearings, supra,* note 9, p. 680; Senate Report No. 91-1431, p. 124.

16. These PSROs would have been designated by the Secretary of HEW to represent at least 300 physicians at the local level, with priority in designation being given to existing local medical societies. The purpose of PSROs would be to evaluate the necessity and quality of services rendered under federal programs. A hierarchy of PSRO councils would be established at the state and national levels as well, and the local PSROs would have to show their effectiveness during a trial period of two years. The PSROs would be empowered to report abuses to HEW, which would take appropriate action. The Amendment did not specify how the review itself would be carried out or how far the PSRO would be primarily a watchdog over professional fees. In other respects, though, the proposals were explicit. The Amendment laid upon health care practitioners the obligation of prescribing economical services, as well as those deemed medically necessary and of good quality. Any practitioner refusing to comply with the PSRO's standards in these respects might be reported to the Secretary; in turn, subject to a system of hearings and appeals, a fine could be levied on

practitioners of up to $5000, as well as possible exclusion of the offender from the payment program. This medicine was strong. Indeed, if it had been enacted as written, the Bennett Amendment could have set up a potentially powerful system of health service controls, enforced through national and local patient information systems. Presumably medical society review procedures would have absorbed the present utilization review committees in hospitals and nursing homes, and the role of the medical society would have been enormously strenghened.

17. On this see Howard N. Newman, "PSRO Implications for Medicaid," speech to the National Conference of Professional Standard Review Organization, Albuquerque, February 12–13, 1973. Commissioner Newman looked forward to the day when PSRO would be responsible for all Medicaid services, not merely institutional ones.

18. The House version had already specified that HMOs accepting Medicare patients should draw at least half of their enrollment from non-Medicare and non-Medicaid patients (section 239). The Senate added provisions whereby HMOs would, for example, have to have an open enrollment period at least annually, on a nondiscriminatory basis; include at least 10,000 enrollees; and meet certain performance standards. At the same time, however, the states would be permitted to make arrangements with neighborhood health centers and similar organizations to prepay them for comprehensive services to Medicaid recipients.

19. This person, who would be within HEW but would also make reports to Congress, would have broad powers, including the authority to suspend administrative regulations (subject to a veto by the Secretary). The proposal was Senator Ribicoff's, and followed his previous concerns over federal accountability.

20. Among other proposals, the sections of Title XIX added in 1969, forbidding a state to reduce its total expenditures from one year to the next, was to be repealed. The requirement that available services throughout a state be identical for all recipients, which had prevented many states from entering into prepayment agreements, would be modified to encourage use of more varied types of facilities. HEW would be authorized to implement the requirement for diagnostic and screening services for minors, with regulations establishing priority for services to the youngest groups. (At that time, HEW had hardly implemented this statute at all due to fiscal exigencies within the states.) Finally, Medicaid matching funds would be made available for eligible minors in public mental institutions.

21. Daniel P. Moynihan, *The Politics of a Guaranteed Income* (New York, 1973), Ch. VII.

22. *Congressional Record,* vol. 116, col. 43640 (1970). For instance, by reinstating man-in-the-house and residency limitations, which changes Senate liberals tried unsuccessfully to delete. One more Medicaid amendment was added to the bill on the floor—Senator Percy's proposal, which he had first introduced in 1969, that blind and disabled persons over age 21 have their eligibility determined without regard to parental resources. Attempts by Senator Curtis to delete sections providing for PSROs and for the use of health maintenance organizations under Medicare failed, as did an amendment by Senator Harris that would have reinstated the 1977 deadline for comprehensive services. *Congressional Record,* vol. 116, pp. 43662, 43649–43652, 43691 (1970).

23. *Ibid.,* p. 43868 (1970).

24. Congressional Quarterly Service, *Congressional Quarterly Almanac, 1970* (Washington, 1971), pp. 1042, 1048.

25. House Report 4690; P.L. 92–5.

26. The fiscal 1971 budget for HEW had been threatened by a Presidential veto, but last-minute trimming by House and Senate conferees brought down the total. While the appropriation was still more than $200 million over the President's request, it was signed in December 1970—again, halfway through the fiscal year. The fiscal 1972 budget, introduced in February 1972, brought the conflict to the fore again, assuming as it did the closing of USPHS hospitals, reduction in funds for Regional Medical Programs, no hospital construction grants, although including additional funds for cancer research, sickle cell anemia, and health maintenance organizations. Battles shaped up immediately around the PHS hospitals and the status of Hill-Burton funds.

27. H.R. 22 (Griffiths-Corman bill), Jan. 22, 1971; S. 3 (Kennedy), Jan. 25, 1971.

28. Not surprising, as both were largely written by the same pen—that of Isadore S. Falk, by then Professor Emeritus of Yale University and director of a new prepaid group practice scheme in New Haven, Connecticut.

29. Benefits included unlimited hospital care, 120 days of nursing home care, physician services, dental care for children under age 15 (later extended to age 25), services of other health professionals, lab and x-ray services, medical appliances and eyeglasses, and prescription drugs for chronic and other specified illnesses. The major items not covered were long-term institutional care, psychiatric care, and drugs for nonspecified conditions.

30. S. 836 (Javits) "National Health Insurance and Health Services Improvement Act of 1971," Feb. 18, 1971. Benefits would be the same as Medicare, plus dental care and drugs. The scheme was thus subject to similar kinds of limitations on benefits (e.g., 90 days of hospital care), deductibles, and other co-payment arrangements. Medicaid would have been unaffected for the over-65 age group and would have benefitted chiefly with respect to the AFDC-related groups, who would thereafter be covered for Medicare-type benefits.

31. S. 703 (Pell-Mondale) "Minimum Health Benefits and Health Services Distribution and Education Act of 1971," Feb. 10, 1971.

32. S. 1598 (Scott-Percy), "The Health Rights Act of 1971," April 21, 1971.

33. S. 1376 (Long), "Catastrophic Illness Insurance Act," March 24, 1971. This proposal provided for a federal program for persons under 65, for hospital and nursing home care after 60 days of hospitalization. It would have been administered through the Medicare program.

34. H.R. 4349 (Burleson) "National Health Care Act of 1971," Feb. 17, 1971, endorsed by the Health Insurance Association of America.

35. H.R. 4960 (Fulton-Broyhill) "Health Care Insurance Act of 1971," Feb. 25, 1971. Endorsed by the American Medical Association, this scheme would have allowed graduated credits against personal income taxes of between 10 and 100 percent of the cost of a qualified private health insurance policy, depending on the individual's taxable income. Thus it, too, provided an additional boost to private health insurance, with the usual features of limited benefits and co-insurance. Medicaid would have been largely unaffected.

36. *Washington Report on Medicare and Health*, February 15, 1971.

37. "Special Message to the Congress proposing a National Health Strategy," February 18, 1971, *Public Papers of the Presidents: Richard Nixon, 1971* (Washington 1972), p. 170.

38. U.S., Department of Health, Education, and Welfare, *Toward a Comprehensive Health Policy for the 1970's: A White Paper,* May 1971.

39. Elliot Richardson, Secretary of HEW, "Foreword," *Ibid.,* p. i.

40. S. 1623 (Bennett) "National Health Insurance Partnership Act of 1971," April 22, 1971. The provisions were virtually identical to the House bill sponsored by Representative Byrnes, H.R. 7741. The employer plan would require employers to provide coverage for employees and their families, through private health insurance. Health maintenance organizations would be made available as an option both for this plan and for FHIP.

41. S. 1182.

42. S. 1183.

43. This latter objection was met, rather completely, in the "White Paper," with assurances that private health insurance would not be abolished. *Supra,* note 38 at p. 26. But the question of regulation remained, as indeed it does today.

44. U.S., Congress, Senate, Committee on Labor and Public Welfare, Subcommittee on Health, *Health Care Crisis in America, Hearings* before the Subcommittee on Health of the Committee on Labor and Public Welfare, 92nd Cong., 1st Sess., 1971.

45. Edward Kennedy, *Crisis in American Medicine* (New York, 1971).

46. U.S., Congress, House, Committee on Ways and Means, *National Health Insurance Proposals, Hearings* before the Committee on Ways and Means, 92nd Cong., 1st Sess., 1971.

47. U.S., Congress, House, Committee on Ways and Means, *Basic Facts on the Health Industry,* Committee Print, June 28, 1971.

48. U.S., Congress, House, Committee on Ways and Means, *Analysis of Health Insurance Proposals Introduced in the 92nd Congress,* Committee Print, August 1971. This report was in fact prepared by HEW.

49. President Nixon in the State of the Union address called welfare reform one of his "six great goals" for Congressional action and in April cited it as "White House priority number one." "Annual Message to the Congress on the State of the Union," January 22, 1970, *Public Papers of the Presidents, Richard Nixon, 1970* (Washington 1971), p. 8.

50. *Congressional Quarterly Almanac 1970, supra,* note 24, p. 521.

51. U.S., Congress, House, Committee on Ways and Means, *Social Security Amendments of 1971,* House Rept. No. 92-231, 1971, p. 3.

52. Congressional Quarterly Service, *Congressional Quarterly Almanac 1971,* Washington, 1972, pp. 524–6.

53. Daniel P. Moynihan, *The Politics of a Guaranteed Income* (New York, 1973), Ch. VII. The rival proposals of some liberals and the outright hostility of some welfare groups (e.g., NWRO) killed what was the most radical welfare legislation proposed in a generation. For some background to the welfare rights viewpoint, see Frances F. Piven and Richard Croward, *Regulating the Poor* (New York, 1971). For a typical example of the opposition to FAP, see Milwaukee County Welfare Rights Organization, *Welfare Mothers Speak Out* (New York, 1972). For a more balanced viewpoint, see Joel F. Hadler, *Reforming the Poor* (New York, 1972), Chapters 6, 7 and 8.

54. *Congressional Quarterly Weekly Report,* vol. 30 (1972), p. 498.

55. P.L. 92-331 also included automatic increases in Social Security levels tied to rises in the cost of living.

56. U.S., Congress, Senate, Committee on Finance, *Social Security Amendments of 1972,* Senate Report No. 1230, 92nd Cong., 2d Sess., 1972.

57. As passed, AB, OAA, and APTD will be administered by the federal government as of January 1974. Supplementary Security Income will become Title XVI of the Social Security Act, as amended. A federal guaranteed income will be assured to persons in these categories of $130 per month ($195 for a couple), but up to $20 a month in Social Security benefits and $65 a month in earnings may be disregarded. P.L. 92–603, sect. 301; Social Security Act, sects. 1611 and 1612. In some states, therefore, benefits under these categories will be considerably higher than those of AFDC.

58. U.S., Department of Health, Education, and Welfare, Social Security Administration, *Supplementary Security Income: Introduction to the new federal program of aid to the aged, blind, and disabled.* April 1973.

59. The new program made another 2.8 million persons eligible for cash assistance. HEW, Office of the Secretary, News Release, May 30, 1973.

60. With the exception of newly eligible recipients of the federalized "Supplemental Security Income for the Aged, Blind, and Disabled" who qualify because of the new provision for a $130 minimum benefit, with a disregard of $20 of Social Security or other income. P.L. 92–603, Sec. 100.

61. *New York Times,* July 19, 1973, p. 46.

62. The new law allowed the states to limit their Medicaid coverage of the aged, blind, and disabled to the standards applied in January 1972. *New York Times,* July 10, 1973, p. 45, col. 1. But while legal, it was probably politically not possible to exclude the new SSI recipients from Medicaid benefits. *Washington Post,* June 27, 1973, p. A25, col. 1. For the regulations cataloging the alternatives open to states in covering SSI recipients under Medicaid, see *Federal Register,* vol. 38 (August 6, 1973) p. 21188.

63. Other House provisions which survived the 1972 Amendments included the limits on reimbursement to provide for capital costs where expenditures were in conflict with local and state plans; provisions for experimenting with prospective reimbursement to providers; and the elimination of statewideness and comparability requirements, where the Secretary of HEW approved, to encourage agreements between states and organizations which might provide care in excess of that generally offered under the state plan.

64. The Senate Health Subcommittee held hearings on HMOs in 1971 and 1972, and Senator Kennedy developed his own bill for HMOs (S. 3327). The Senate passed this bill in the 92nd Congress, authorizing $5.2 billion of federal money for development of HMOs in a 3-year period, but no House action was taken. Legislation sponsored by Representatives Roy and Rogers (H.R. 11728) was similarly unsuccessful.

65. The Ways and Means Committee had recommended a 25 percent increase in federal matching funds with respect to state contracts with HMOs or other comprehensive health care facilities. The Senate Finance Committee deleted this provision, reasoning that if HMOs are indeed more economical than other delivery systems, it would be in a state's interest to deal with them without any additional incentive. U.S., Congress, Senate, Committee on Finance, *Social Security and Welfare Reform: Summary of the Principal Provisions of H.R. 1 as Determined by the Committee on Finance* (1972), p. 21.

66. P.L. 92–603, Sec. 410. Payment to such organizations could not be higher on a per capita basis than the per capita Medicaid payments in the same general area.

67. P.L. 92–603, Sec. 226. Such payments were not to exceed 100 percent of Part A and Part B per capita costs in a given geographical area—with exact amounts being dependent on assessments of HMO efficiency.

68. The option is that of the PSRO. But since these must be physician-sponsored organizations (until January 1976, when other organizations may be considered), this really means the option of community physicians. P.L. 92–603, Sect. 249F. The legislation also states clearly that PSROs would not be involved in determining charges and fees.

69. P.L. 92–603, Sect. 237.

70. See Chapter 12, footnote 53.

71. P.L. 92–603, Sect. 221, 102, respectively.

72. P.L. 92–603, Sect. 225. This latter provision was added by the Finance Committee to provide incentives for such facilities to upgrade themselves and for patients and physicians to use institutions not on the "deficient" list.

73. According to the Senate Finance Committee, the expectation was that the states would fix such fees at whatever level was necessary to effect a savings of 6 percent in the medically indigent programs. Additionally, the states would be allowed to impose deductibles and co-payments on the medically indigent which might be unrelated to income. These provisions, together with the nominal deductible and co-payment requirements for the categorically needy, were later to be opposed by the Administration; but they were added, according to the Committee report, as a "cost control device" to introduce an "element of cost consciousness on the part of patients and their physicians." *Summary of Principal Provisions of H.R. 1 as determined by the Committee on Finance, supra,* note 65, p. 21. The tentative regulations have now been published, see proposed regulations 248.21 and 269.40. *Federal Register,* vol. 38 (1973), p. 17508. The emphasis appears to be on the nominal element in the charge.

74. P.L. 92–603 Section 103.

75. For details of the merging of Medicaid standards for SNH and Medicare standards for ECF, in SNF's, see 38 *Federal Register* p. 18620 (July 12, 1973) and p. 21437 (August 8, 1973).

76. At the same time, even legislation affecting Title XIX of the Social Security Act (Medicaid) could not be found solely in the Social Security Amendments. E.g., the incorporation of ICFs into Medicaid (P.L. 92–223); see Chapter 12. Another notable example of the 92nd Congress was a provision in a tax bill (P.L. 92–178) denying tax deductions for money gained through kickbacks, bribes, and referral fees under Titles XVIII and XIX, the burden of proof resting on the Treasury. *Congressional Quarterly Almanac* 1971, *supra,* note 11 at p. 457.

77. P.L. 92–275.

78. P.L. 92–449.

79. P.L. 92–294.

80. P.L. 92–424.

81. P.L. 92–433.

82. P.L. 92–258.

83. In June 1973, H.R. 8410 (the debt-ceiling bill) was reported out of the Senate Finance Committee with amendments designed to protect the Medicaid "rights" of those covered by Supplementary Security Income (SSI). U.S., Senate, Committee on Finance, *Press Release,* June 21, 1973. Chairman Russell Long

also proposed a basic federal health benefits program for low-income groups. The program would provide 60 days of hospital care and nursing home care without limitation, physician services subject to a nominal co-payment, all coupled with catastrophic health insurance. The nationwide standards would be $2400 for a single person and $4800 for a family of four. *Statement of Senator Russell B. Long before the Louisiana AFL-CIO*, Baton Rouge, Louisiana, April 16, 1973. The proposed program would include "spend-down" provisions for everyone, come into effect in 1976, and be expected to cost $5.3 billion more than existing Medicaid programs.

Epilogue

There are a number of messages to be drawn from Medicaid. First and fundamentally, there was the lack of clarity about what Medicaid was and for whom it was created. Was it to be regarded as a noncontributory health insurance program for the poor, thus a true "sleeper" of the 1965 legislation; or was it, rather, an extension of pre-existing vendor payment programs? The legislative history of Medicaid suggests that the latter approach was favored. Medicaid was a further step in a process begun by Kerr-Mills. In this respect, the new program was not so much innovative as incremental. Its broadening of services and eligibility, and its new administrative requirements (notably the requirements of single standards across welfare programs and across each state) were apparently seen as extensions and rationalizations of the previous programs. Indeed, Medicaid's political appeal in 1965 was partly based on this. Viewed as an alternative to contributory forms of health insurance, Medicaid's structure embraced the evident flaws of Kerr-Mills as the price of its political acceptability.

Yet at the same time, Medicaid was destined by its very extensions and rationalizations to establish a widespread system of government-guaranteed health benefits. Although virtually noncontributory, this system was not unlike earlier European forms of national health insurance, but it was locked into an administrative structure designed to provide cash assistance, not service benefits. And 400 years of history were not about to be undone by a new health "emphasis."

Title XIX of the Social Security Act, as drafted, was destined to be ineffective in its double heritage as a health service program and as an expansion of public assistance. Indeed, it was the mixing of a program of services and a program of cash assistance that provoked Medicaid's initial dilemmas. At base, the program depended on a definition of eligibility tied to the recipient's cash status, rather than to his medical needs. But more generally it was never made sufficiently clear whether Medicaid was to be regarded as one of an array of federal health care programs (the "health" side of HEW) or as part of a broader program of income maintenance (the "welfare" side). Although there is evidence that some legislators intended to provide a new concept in medical care, in which the poor would have equal treatment with the rich, there is ample evidence that other legislators, even among those who were in favor of Title XIX, saw no need for any radical change from earlier policies. Under these policies health care was purchased from private vendors on the same kind of peripheral basis as funds for specific goods such as bedding and pots and pans are authorized for cash assistance recipients.

The lack of clearly stated national goals for Medicaid in 1965 was a major and reverberating deficiency. Congress, in many ways, made a series of classic errors which were transmitted down the line as the programs were developed in the states. These errors led to conflict in interpreting Medicaid between powerful committees in Washington and the legislatures of major states (most particularly New York and California), almost tempted the judiciary to go into the business of trying to solve the crisis, and brought on state budgetary crises and the sometimes selfish behavior of the medical providers. In that sense the villains portrayed in these pages were themselves the victims of confusion in Congress.

Why was there this initial confusion about the purposes and goals of Medicaid? There can have been few legislators unaware in 1965 that Kerr-Mills was somewhat less than a success. Kerr-Mills had indeed received substantial publicity in the debates preceding the 1965 legislation. That program had already demonstrated the basic characteristics later to plague Medicaid: the transfer of funds by states from one public pocket to another under the stimulus of greater federal matching funds; the unevenness of programs from state to state; the implications of attaching a system of medical vendor payments to an administrative structure of grants-in-aid that relied on minimal federal direction; the interpretation of "medical indigency" as a rather rigid test of means, albeit at a somewhat higher average level than for cash assistance; the greater interest of state legislatures in balancing their budgets than in reorganizing medical care; and, in the state bureaucracies, the inadequate administrative expertise for running a major medical program. Yet Title XIX was developed under similar principles.

But although Medicaid has been beleaguered by structural and functional defects, its incremental approach to social legislation has had two major positive effects. These may be termed the principles of marginal gain and greater chaos. On the one hand, the identification of Medicaid with Kerr-Mills, rather than thrusting it forward as a new program, assured Medicaid of passage. As a result, Medicaid has brought medical care to many millions of persons, with less individual financial anxiety than had the program not been developed; in this sense, the gains are real, albeit expensive. On the other hand, by exaggerating the weaknesses in the health and welfare systems, Medicaid has had an intrinsic social importance in accelerating Congressional and general concern over the costs and provision of health services. Without a doubt, the Medicaid experience, coupled with some rather similar concerns over Medicare, has been a salient factor in the development of proposals for national health insurance. In retrospect, the muddle of Medicaid will undoubtedly be seen as a necessary forerunner of rationalization of health services in the United States in the 1970s or 1980s, part of what may be an essential chaos which precedes and precipitates major legislative reform. Under this argument, Medicaid's problems were inevitable, and the program itself was born to be transitional.

Whether one accepts these observations of Medicaid's long-term effects, the fact remains that Congress, or at least its leaders in the health and welfare areas, did not have a planned long-term objective for Medicaid at the time of the legislation. Medicaid was the culmination of a continuing thread of argument in Congress, going back at least to the 1940s, calling for an approach to medical care provision through welfare instead of through a general program of health insurance. Medicaid thus appears to have been as much built on the rhetoric of the past as on the realities of the present. It was a classic case of fighting the last war rather than the next one.

While lack of a well-thought plan is the first observation to be made of Medicaid, the second is that there were bound to be basic problems in a system of vendor payments designed to cover only a minority of the population. In its shape as well as its intentions, Medicaid began with built-in deficiencies. The assumption that effective and economical medical services can be provided through existing structures of health services and public assistance was challenged almost as soon as the program was implemented. The problem was in the legislation itself, not in the reactions of the various states; for Medicaid, nominally an assistance program, was blessed (or cursed) with attributes inappropriate to the welfare tradition. Unlike other forms of assistance, Medicaid was asked to do more than fill a gap or provide a back-up service for reasonably effective programs in the private sector. With respect to health services, the other programs themselves were insufficient.

If Medicare, designed to provide health care as an entitlement to the whole population over the age of 65, had been sufficiently comprehensive, Medicaid's substantial and growing commitment of services to the elderly would have been unnecessary. Similarly, if private health insurance had effectively covered the working population (including continuing coverage for survivors and dependents and in times of sickness and temporary unemployment), the concept of medical indigence need not have been invented. As it was, Medicaid, with its uncontrollable budgets and rising costs, has been a reflection of broader deficiencies in the health sector.

The progress of events might well have been foreseen. Medicaid's early "mainstream" connotations were bound to be inflationary. Payment of hospitals according to their "reasonable costs" ensured Medicaid's direct involvement in the rising costs of hospital care. Requests by physician groups for fee reimbursement at rates akin to those in the private sector and the massive construction and opening of nursing home beds were other elements in cost increases. Nor were the states anxious, at least in the early years, to offend the very providers on whom they depended. Four factors thus contributed to the rising costs: the expanded size of the covered population; the greater willingness by the covered population to seek and receive services, once these were subsidized; higher fees for health care (the result both of higher fees in the health sector as a whole and the linking of Medicaid reimbursement rates to private fee levels); and at least some waste and fraud on the part of providers.

As the states benefitted from the windfall of additional funds from the federal government through Medicaid's larger subsidies, there was also an initial generosity in the states toward their expanded vendor programs. Medicaid provided a remarkable opportunity for the states to provide services to their citizens at federal expense, while at the same time raising vendor reimbursement levels. States might go about this process in different ways—California, for example, stressed provision of services while New York emphasized eligibility levels—but the over-all message was the same. State budgets rose, and as they did, so did the matching grants required from the federal treasury under the Medicaid formula.

The impact of these movements was twofold. On the one hand, remedial measures had to be taken to control the cost of services through providers, whose role had shifted from the pre-Medicaid role of donors of care to a new role as exploiters of the system. On the other hand, reins were to be put on spending by the states, over whom the federal government had previously exerted relatively little authority with respect to assistance programs in general or vendor payments in particular. Neither providers nor the states took kindly to the new federal efforts, despite the fact that the new efforts were frequently ineffective. At times the providers found themselves working with state bureaucracies; at other times providers found a unity of interest with recipients against the states. New power relationships were developing.

The efforts to curb costs took a variety of forms. With the 1967 Amendments, eligibility levels were redefined in terms of cash assistance programs. Mandatory coverage was reduced, while the goal of comprehensive care was finally abandoned in 1972. Efforts at fee controls, including fee schedules and prepaid reimbursement schemes, were part and parcel of the same efforts, as indeed was the growing clamor for the review of the utilization of services. Each state approached its cutbacks and reviews in its own style. But the remedies were general and the problems created by those remedies fell equally on all the states, and ultimately on the recipients: the problem of the "notch" effect, the reluctance to inquire too fully what happened to persons removed from the rolls (or to sick persons denied health care for economic reasons), and widespread professional resistance.

Medicaid demonstrated that cost containment could not be left to the states; indeed, the federal grant formulae, designed to encourage the poorer states to develop programs, actually encouraged greed by the richer. Federal officials were, however, reluctant to move in on the states. In the early years, such reluctance could be ascribed to the traditional deferring of the federal welfare bureaucracy to the states, and to the lack of strong Congressional backing, even where specific legislative authority existed (for example the long delays in developing regulations). But even after Congressional concern over cost was self-evident from a spate of committee hearings, there continued to be foot-dragging from HEW. This process was later compounded by President Nixon's pronouncements on decentralization. Just as federal authority appeared to be poised for effectiveness, it transpired that it was to be subject to devolution. The present role of HEW, following a brief, relatively successful crackdown on substandard nursing homes, continues to be ill-defined; while more effective than in the earlier period, civil servants in MSA are still working in a kind of administrative limbo.

This lack of specificity in administrative roles has dogged Medicaid from its beginning. Attempts to clarify the various interrelationships among the federal government, the states, and the providers, however, have prompted action along two different fronts. One series of actions in Congress has been designed to make administrative functions more specific, in order to contain Medicaid's costs. The 1972 Amendments, for example, include provisions for peer review and other activities to tighten Medicaid's various bureaucracies. These arrangements, which basically take Medicaid one step further in its development, are evolutionary in nature. Regulation is extended to make the existing program more efficient.

At the same time, in reaction to the problems and complications following each effort to solve Medicaid's dilemmas and cost increases, there have been a series of reform actions, symbolized by Congressional hearings for national health insurance. The wide variety of political views held by those now espousing some form of nationalized, total-population, full-service, extensively regulated health plan for the country is an impressive indicator of the pervasiveness of the second approach. Rather than extend programs such as Medicaid a little further, the proponents of health insurance for the whole population would tackle some of the problems at Medicaid's roots, for national health insurance could put an end to eligibility difficulties, inequities, low-quality service, state greed, and subsidies for the providers of medical services.

Such an apparently sweeping solution will not, however, automatically eliminate such problems, unless careful heed is taken of those lessons, learned from Medicaid, which might be expected to apply to all forms of government health provision. One of the problems Medicaid faced, and all government health care programs will face, is the relationship between the government and existing medical structures. The purchase of services by a public agency in the private sector is an appealing prospect. It is one which is continuing to appear in proposals for health payment schemes. But the philosophy of the public-private mix contains its own dilemmas, not the least of which is the tacit assumption that the private sector itself is efficient. Yet by the very fact that the medical care industry is dominated by legalized economic monopolies, namely the health professions, there is reason to question this assumption. Certainly the Medicaid experience gives little ground for optimism that the private sector can regulate itself efficiently. Professions which have not felt the "chill winds" of competition for several decades are unlikely to emphasize efficiency of their own free will when the federal government begins paying the bill. Thus the long-time concern of the medical monopolies that federal funds would mean federal control were undoubtedly justified. If there is a desire to make use of the private rather than the public sector for providing medical care, then, ironic as it may seem, there may have to be more obvious and structured government control through regulation than if the services were provided by a governmental agency.

Thus any program with national goals that wishes to administer an effective program in the private sector as it presently exists will have to include (and to enforce) national standards and appropriate regulatory mechanisms over the operation and charges of providers who are themselves organized either as monopolies or oligopolies. If Medicaid, whether revised or replaced, is to be a national program, then the federal government is going to have to set standards and to take a major role in dealing with the providers. The restructuring of medical providers almost certainly calls for greater political strength and acumen than any single state can provide, and for a federal role which is immensely stronger than that yet developed for Medicaid. Only in this way can the federal government effectively deal with monopoly providers.

From the providers' point of view, the existence of a partial national health service (i.e., health insurance for some but not for all of the population) rather than a universal system, has been seen to have little to commend it. The combined impact of Medicare and Medicaid since 1965 has been one of rapid provider regulation. Indeed, this history of Medicaid is filled with accounts of fee reviews, audits, and publicity with respect to apparently high reimbursements. In the process, Congressional committees and government agencies have taken a watchdog role over what, in a universal scheme, might more properly be delegated to professional agencies. The development of PSROs is one attempt to utilize professional self-regulation in the public interest. But such organizational developments, even where they work successfully, will still only deal with part of the nation's health bills: politically, therefore, they will still not be central to the politics of health care administration.

Indeed, Medicaid's experience has shown a series of government units becoming more organized because of the cost implications of Medicaid. At the same time, the health sector has, politically, become *less* organized. The AMA is far less influential than it was in 1965. Physician unions are now developing, but these assume a negotiating rather than a managerial role. The power relationships between government and the providers thus have already begun to change. Paradoxically, universal health insurance, applying to virtually all health bills, could redress the balance, by encouraging the professional and institutional groups of medicine to become more highly organized as an essential concomitant of the program. Thus, while federal regulation would be strengthened, so also would the organized authority of providers. Ultimately, therefore, for the providers, reform may be a more conservative approach than the continuation of apparently minor program extensions.

Another important area for consideration as part of the broad legacy of Medicaid is the role to be played in future programs by the states. Medicaid provides an important case study of a national program administered by the states. Although there is absolutely no evidence that they were interested in being given the role, the states were put in the position of organizers of medical care programs through the 1965 legislation. In many respects, they had both Kerr-Mills and Medicaid thrust on them because it was not politically possible for the federal government to come out in the open and run its own program. Although Medicaid was technically a program of federal aid to states, there was a wistful notion that the graduated federal subsidies would lead to the best of all possible worlds; equal provision of care to the needy in all of the states.

As it has turned out, state control of Medicaid has led to continuing variations—indeed, gross discrepancies—in the level of care in different parts of the country. It has become increasingly self-evident that national problems must lead to national solutions. In this sense FHIP or the McNerney suggestions for the federalization of Medicaid were politically more courageous and intellectually more honest than the federal-state formulas. But the failure of Congress to federalize Medicaid, even for those groups now covered by federalized cash assistance (SSI) under the 1972 Amendments, underlines the reluctance to deal with a nationwide problem at a national level. This reluctance appears to continue even after these fundamental reforms in cash assistance programs.

How far the states could act as effective agents of a tightly run federal program remains as yet an unanswered question. In retrospect, it is scarcely surprising that states were unwilling or unable to control extensive medical care programs—even when a significant part of the "tab" was paid by Washington. Moreover, this reluctance appears to have continued. So far, at least, state response to regulations for early and periodic screening—involving, as it does, not only the control but *de facto* the running of some health programs—appears lukewarm at best. Even though this response may be an accurate gauge of the temperature of Congress, the augers for state initiative are not generally encouraging. The evidence of Medicaid suggests that if it is the purpose of Congress to bring medical care to every person in the country (or even to every needy person, whatever that may mean) control of these services cannot be left to the 50 states and to other governmental units.

Indeed, the present organizational structure of Medicaid raises vital political, if not legal, issues of equal protection. Even with respect to cash payments, the Nixon Family Assistance Plan moved toward nationwide standards and administration. These are being translated into SSI with respect to the old, blind, and disabled. It is notable, too, that SSI is a federal program organized through the regional and district offices of the Social Security Administration rather than through the states. Indeed, the option is one-way: States may contract with SSA for supplementary benefits under state assistance programs, but SSA will not delegate its basic programs to the states. *A fortiori* this central control will have to apply to the service aspects of the largely federally-funded Welfare State. These observations point to a federal program for Medicaid, or for whatever scheme replaces it.

Symptomatic of all Medicaid's dilemmas, however, has been a lack of decision about the paying of Medicaid's costs. This aspect of Medicaid, too, has implications that go beyond Medicaid to consideration of other health payment systems. Health services can be provided through very different cost mechanisms, ranging from government-owned and operated facilities with staff on salary (as in New York's municipal hospitals and clinics) to a completely unsubsidized private system. One major problem of Medicaid was its attempt to combine features of many different arrangements. It did not encourage government-owned and operated facilities. Indeed, where such facilities existed most extensively, in the county hospital system in California, efforts were made to dilute that system in the effort to provide the poor with "mainstream" medicine.

But Medicaid did not fully espouse the private market system either. If it had, the poor would have been given funds to use or not to use on medical care as part of their cash assistance benefits; or, alternatively, would have been given either a private health insurance policy or health vouchers. There have been flirtations with such arrangements, notably in the experiments in buying Medicaid patients into a prepaid group practice arrangement, but in general Medicaid has exercised controls neither through demand (coordinated consumer behavior) nor through supply (responsibility for health care practitioners and institutions). Recipients have never been clear about their "rights"; providers have not been clear whether they are to treat Medicaid patients as "real" patients or charity cases.

As a result of the present confusion, different parts of the cost have been loaded onto different groups in the population and different units of government with benefits distributed in various ways among providers and recipients. It is not surprising that Medicaid has been accompanied by cries alleging overlapping services, duplicate payments, fraud and waste, nor that its operation should seem so chaotic. The way in which the system of vendor payments was established led almost inevitably to a scramble by all concerned to get as much as possible while paying as little as possible, in money, service, political credit, or liability.

The familiarity of medical vendor payments as a means of providing public assistance health care in the states was understandably the strongest factor in the use of this mechanism for Medicaid. Underlying this political reality, however, there appear to have been three basic assumptions behind the adoption of medical vendor payments in Medicaid. The first was that services are more likely to be available and are of better quality through purchase in the private sector, rather than through the development of a publicly financed and controlled system of hospitals and clinics. Existing problems in public hospital systems (of which New York City is a notable example) would seem to bear out this assumption. The second was that many states and counties did not have a ready-made system for development. The third was the acceptance of a social ethic of equal opportunity in medical care. There was (and remains) a commitment by many reformers to provide medical services to the poor of roughly the same quality as those provided to other members of the population; this was interpreted as meaning provision of services through the same disorganized set of providers available to the middle-class population, rather than espousing a separate-but-equal philosophy of medical care.

The result of these assumptions has been the dissemination of money in a piecemeal fashion rather than its use to fashion deliberate policies. Thus, policies have tended to be made through program implementation rather than through planning or conscious choice. As we have seen, in the wake of the latest efforts at cost controls, one of the basic assumptions underlying Medicaid, that of providing for mainstream medicine, has broken down. It has proved impossible to overthrow centuries of poor-law mentality; and present philosophies, at least in terms of reimbursement levels, appear to accept the continuation of two classes of medical care.

The dispersion and dissemination of cost decisions is a critical factor to be considered in any program that builds on the Medicaid model, which in this respect is similar to the Medicare model. As long as decisions are made piecemeal in response to specific difficulties as they arise, rather than with the total design in mind, programs will be in constant difficulties. What comes out of Medicaid's experience is that without a design for a total health service program, with an appropriate flow of dollars, together with checks and balance to complete that design, the rhetoric of the program is largely meaningless. The abandonment of the mainstream approach to medical care for the poor was one of Medicaid's casualties of cost containment. In an equally cavalier spirit the concept of medical indigence was grossly attenuated. Yet these were the very principles of which in 1965 Medicaid was supposedly built. What happened? Either in 1965 the phrases were the mere mouthing of words without any serious commitment, or the need to control soaring costs appeared in the event a more important principle than social equity or alleviating indigence.

Our reading of events in general supports the latter proposition: the vague philosophies outlined in the legislature were overtaken by economic pragmatism which in turn generated other philosophies, if we may honor those attitudes with that name. But, if this is so, there is a simple lesson to be applied to current debates. However concerned and committed the proponents of national health insurance are to principles of social justice, comprehensive health entitlements, and better medical care, their rhetoric is meaningless unless the flow of money into their programs is designed to advance these aims, over and above the advancement of aims of the system's various other interest groups;[1] otherwise there will be a similar free-for-all exercise of self-interest on the part of providers, administrative agencies, and fiscal agencies that has distinguished the Medicaid experience. And the same old cycle will begin again: cost increases, the search for villains, retrenchments, the hope that some simple solution will appear in a scattershot of demonstration projects and organizational gimmicks, power plays, recourse to the courts, and new (restrictive) legislation. The heroic principles will be ditched.

If principles are to be translated into actuality, any further extensions of health benefits will have to tackle the structure and function of the health care system. This need has become increasingly evident in the Medicaid years. Report after report has emphasized the inefficiency and waste in the health care system; indeed, the new programs of the 1960s—Medicaid and Medicare being the foremost contenders—have added to the pre-existing overlaps and confusions. Both programs have emphasized institutional care (notably hospital care) rather than the maintenance of health, disease prevention, and rehabilitation. Both have injected additional funds into already wealthy states and institutions rather than attempted to fill gaps in services and areas. Both have added a new element of complication for the persons who are presumably the reason for the program and are its ultimate beneficiaries. Indeed, the beneficiaries sometimes seem caught in an organizational maze, being asked to cope not only with vagaries in the private system but with inconsistencies in the public sector. Medicare and Medicaid overlap in benefits for the elderly; while public hospitals and clinics, mental health centers, OEO health centers, and other government-sponsored activities, each of which acts more or less independently, add to a previously diffuse health care system.

The degree of influence Medicaid has had over the health care system must also not be understated. Our thesis is that it has had considerable influence; in addition to providing medical care, it has, for example, stimulated the building of profit-making nursing homes, added to increased demand and thus caused cost increases, made public attitudes much more skeptical toward health care providers, and thus caused stronger provider regulation. These are no mean changes in an 8-year period. But at the same time the influence has been largely unplanned and unexpected. It is quite clear that no health planning agency or professional group would have deliberately set out a design for a health system in 1965 that aimed to produce the over-all results which Medicaid has effected. Because history may repeat itself in the passage of some form of national health insurance, this point is worth considerable emphasis. Any large-scale infusion of funds will have important impacts on the health care system; the questions are whether these are planned or unplanned, and if planned, what goals are to be attained.

In contemplating national health insurance in the 1970s, Congress appears to be falling into the same trap of goal evasion as in 1965, or for that matter in 1960, when Medicaid and Kerr-Mills were being discussed. While the questions now go to the provision of health insurance for the whole population, rather than merely to the poor and the elderly, the general process is broadly the same. There is a similar concentration on conceptual issues rather than on what is to be attained and what will be the effects of any program. In the early 1960s, the debate centered on the insurance versus the assistance approaches to medical care. In the early 1970s, with the assistance approach out of favor, the argument is, instead, over the degree to which a national health insurance program would use the private insurance mechanism (e.g., as in Medicredit) or be a tighter governmental system (as in the Kennedy Health Security proposals). But, as in the earlier debates, the conceptual questions tend to provide a smokescreen of rhetoric behind which concrete administrative questions can be hidden, as well as an honest appraisal of the cost.

Medicaid's central dilemmas are thus in danger of reappearing in current debates. Once again, two separate processes are in conflict. On the one hand rhetoric may be politically necessary as a bridge enabling basically conflicting views to be at least temporarily reconciled so that legislation may be enacted. No one can be against "medical care" or "health" for all American citizens. If the terms are broad enough and sufficiently resilient, spokesmen for divergent interests can find a common niche: national health insurance, in its various guises, is a case in point. On the other hand, by conveniently obliterating the practical realities forming the real areas of anxiety—the effects of different forms of funding on the behavior of the health care system—national health insurance legislation will run into the same problems as Medicaid: administrative confusion, cost alarums, retrenchment. As with Medicaid, one paradoxical effect of current proposals is that national health insurance schemes, such as Medicredit, or programs for catastrophic medical expenses, are more likely in the long run to lead to strong federal regulatory controls, even "socialized" medicine, than are proposals that attempt to reform the system. Medicaid's experience is directly relevant.

Even without any form of national health insurance, the continuation of the present piecemeal approach to the funding of medical care will lead to stronger controls over providers, national standards of care and benefits, and greater administrative centralization (greater, perhaps, than the current proposals for national health insurance). The establishment of SSI will raise, again, the question of federal administration of the Medicaid program, at least for the old, blind, and disabled; and the federalization of AFDC programs will undoubtedly be reconsidered. The resulting federalization of Medicaid would give the United States a national health program for the poor. Administrative convenience would dictate that its shape be parallel to, if not merged with, the existing national Medicare system. Thus, in subsequent rationalizations, Medicaid would form the basis of a universal health care system.

At the time of writing, in 1973, these last possibilities seem the most likely. The movement for universal national health insurance appears, at least temporarily, to be on the wane. In the long run, however, some form of national health provision seems inevitable, either through new legislation or through continuing modifications of the current system. In the process, as with the development of national health insurance in Europe, the rhetoric may be of social justice but the rationale and implementation will be matters of practical economics. Although even conservative newspapers may deplore the social inequities of Medicaid—where, for example, the only way to get satisfactory medical care is to divorce a sick spouse[2] or go on welfare[3]—Medicaid policy will continue to be affected primarily by its cost elements. As we have noted, however, this process may in itself lead to major changes in health care provision. Indeed, in the long run, the pragmatic, incremental approach to health legislation—the extension of existing programs and controls until a major rationalization is inevitable—may turn out to be more radical than any of the health insurance options now being suggested.

In summary, whether one rates Medicaid as a failure or success, or somewhere between, depends on the touchstone used in such a measurement. The basic faults of Medicaid, epitomized by lax administration and unanticipated costs, were inherent in the legislation; a more effective design would demand the establishment of clear goals and priorities. The noble phrases embodied in the legislation, promising comprehensive care to the medically indigent, were not to be realized; in this respect, implementation was disappointing. The inequities of welfare medicine, with provisions of services based on a means test, have been amply demonstrated, both in respect to the "notch" effect (whereby low-income workers may have fewer medical services than those on Medicaid[4]) and in arbitrary definition of eligibility. It may be, of course, that nothing approaching "equity" is possible in the provision of medical services.[5] The problems of allocation (or tampering with the market, depending on your perspective) may be just so great that no matter how extensive the funding or how great the willingness to restructure providers, equity is just not possible, or other countervailing pressures may be there. Medicaid has shown, however, that there will be an absence of clarity about what is to be achieved in terms of the standards of care, an inability to define equity, and a basic reluctance to commit funds, until decisions are thrust upon Congress from apparent breakdowns in existing programs. If the long-term solution for health care in the United States is to be a success, then its architects would do well to study carefully the Medicaid experience.

NOTES

1. What is surprising, is that liberal politicians seem surprised, e.g., Senator John Tunney (Democrat, California): "There are now ominous signs appearing which seem to suggest that all which was gained for the poor and elderly may soon be lost under the guise of 'economy.'" U.S., Congress, Senate, Committee on Labor and Public Welfare, Subcommittee on health, *Health Care Crisis in America, Hearings* before the Subcommittee on Health of the Committee on Labor and Public Welfare, 92nd Cong., 1st Sess., 1971, p. 3; and per Senator Edmund Muskie (Democrat, Maine) "Now we seem to be turning back upon our commitments and, instead of pushing towards better health care, we are dismantling our first effort."

2. See a case in Florida, reported in *New Haven Register*, January 19, 1973 ("Divorce Only Answer for Man Aiding Sick Wife") and *ibid.*, February 21, 1973 ("Man Divorces Sick Wife to Get Treatment Paid"). There the divorce became necessary because Mr. Thomas earned $550 a month, $117 over the Medicaid maximum. Mrs. Thomas, suffering from terminal multiple sclerosis, was in a nursing home asking $500 a month. The couple had been married 32 years. And see editorial, "A Divorce that Challenges Society," *ibid.*, February 26, 1973, p. 22, col. 1.

In another case, from Georgia, Nathan Bichen was reported to be resisting suggestions from social workers that he divorce his paralyzed wife to qualify for Medicaid. Mr. Bichen had already sold his home and furniture to pay the nursing home bills, but was still having to find $300 a month. Mr. Bichen was quoted as saying: "I go to church, and live a Christian life, and I just wouldn't do a thing like that even if I have to dig ditches." *Ibid.*, April 21, 1973.

3. *In Pennsylvania*, a worker earning $7800 a year whose son had a hemophiliac condition needing $1000 of treatment a month, was advised by the welfare department to give up his job and take one that paid less in order to qualify as "medically indigent." *Ibid.*, November 1, 1972.

4. The Columbia study suggested that while the poorest had the greatest need of medical care, since Medicaid those on public assistance (and in certain respects the medically indigent) had greater access to all forms of medical care than those just above the Medicaid limits. Columbia University, School of Public Health and Administrative Medicine, *Effect of Medicaid on Health Care of Low-Income Persons*. See especially Table H.

These findings are important since most available data are too crude to make observations on the apparent effects of social programs. For example, it is known that, on average, low-income persons are hospitalized at a higher rate than other income groups, but this general observation may reflect the existence of Medicaid, higher morbidity rates, delays in seeking preventive care or early treatment, a lack of alternative health resources in low-income areas, other reasons, or a combination of all of these. See particularly the following two tables:

Persons Hospitalized per 1000 population: All Ages

	1962	*1966*	*1968*
Low income	94.7	106.6	114.5
Middle income	97.6	100.9	95.4
High income	86.7	88.9	81.8

Physician Visits per Capita: All Ages

	1964	*1967*	*1969*
Low income	4.3	4.3	4.6
Middle income	4.5	4.2	4.0
High income	5.1	4.6	4.3

Low income was defined as less than $4000 in 1962 and 1964, less than $5000 in 1966, 1967, 1968, and 1969. Middle income was defined as $4000–$6999 in 1962 and 1964; as $5000–$9999 in 1966, 1967, 1968, and 1969. High income is defined as $7000 and above in 1962 and 1964; as $10,000 and above thereafter. Taken from Charles L. Schultze, Edward R. Fried, Alice M. Rivlin, and Nancy H. Teeters, *Setting National Priorities: The 1973 Budget* (Washington, 1972), pp. 224–225.

5. See e.g., Bruce Stuart, "Equity and Medicaid," *Journal of Human Resources*, vol. VII (1972), p. 162; and Rashi Fein, "On Achieving Access and Equity in Health Care," *Milbank Memorial Fund Quarterly*, vol. 50, 1972, p. 157. For the comparative viewpoint, see Odin W. Anderson, *Health Care: Can There Be Equity?* (New York, 1972).

Appendix

Table 1. Medicaid (and Related) Program Payments to Providers of Health Care, Fiscal Years 1966–73 (Thousands of Dollars)

Fiscal year	*Medicaid*	*Kerr–Mills and related programs*	*Total*	*Percent increase over previous year*
1966	$ 362,578	$1,229,042	$1,591,620	— %
1967	1,936,753	334,243	2,270,996	42.7
1968	3,221,707	229,669	3,451,376	52.0
1969	4,126,380*	225,106	4,351,486	26.1
1970	4,977,585*	116,316	5,093,901	17.1
1971	6,345,199*	—	6,345,199	24.4
1972	7,825,000*	—	7,825,000	23.3
1973	8,802,000	—	8,802,000	12.5

* Payments to intermediate care facilities are included in the total for Fiscal Years 1969–72 even though they were administered under the cash assistance programs until January 1, 1972, when they were switched to Title XIX.

SOURCE: United States Department of Health, Education, and Welfare.

Table 2. Total Medical Vendor Payments in order of size of state programs, fiscal year 1973 (Millions of Dollars)

State	*Total benefits*	*Percent of National Total*	*Cumulative Percent of National Total*
New York	$1,749	19.9%	19.9%
California	1,441	16.4	36.3
Illinois	512	5.2	42.1
Texas	434	4.9	47.0
Massachusetts	416	4.7	51.7
Pennsylvania	402	4.6	56.3
Michigan	390	4.4	60.7
Ohio	268	3.0	63.7
New Jersey	236	2.7	66.4
Wisconsin	190	2.2	68.6
10 Largest States	*6,038*	*68.6*	68.6
Minnesota	181	2.1	70.7
Georgia	179	2.0	72.7
Virginia	168	1.9	74.6
Alabama	151	1.7	76.3
Florida	139	1.6	77.3

Maryland	132	1.5	79.4
Washington	127	1.4	80.8
Indiana	120	1.4	82.2
Connecticut	116	1.3	83.5
North Carolina	111	1.3	84.8
20 Largest States	*7,462*	*84.8*	*84.8*
Oklahoma	100	1.1	85.9
Tennessee	98	1.1	87.0
Kentucky	90	1.0	88.1
Louisiana	85	1.0	89.0
Colorado	80	.9	89.9
Puerto Rico	70	.8	90.7
Kansas	67	.8	91.5
Missouri	62	.7	92.2
Mississippi	58	.7	92.8
South Carolina	58	.7	93.5
Nebraska	57	.7	94.2
Rhode Island	55	.6	94.8
Dist. of Columbia	54	.6	95.4
Arkansas	43	.5	95.9
Maine	41	.5	96.3
Oregon	36	.4	96.8
West Virginia	34	.4	97.1
Hawaii	33	.4	97.5
Utah	31	.4	97.9
New Mexico	30	.3	98.2
Iowa	29	.3	98.5
Vermont	24	.3	98.8
Idaho	19	.2	99.0
South Dakota	18	.2	99.2
North Dakota	16	.2	99.4
Montana	15	.2	99.6
Nevada	14	.2	99.8
Delaware	13	.2	99.9
New Hampshire	12	.1	100.0
Wyoming	5	.1	100.1
Virgin Islands	1	—	100.1
Guam	—	—	100.1
*Total**	*$8,802*	*100.0%*	*100.0%*

* Columns do not add to totals due to rounding.

SOURCE: November, 1971 State estimates of their Medicaid expenditures. United States Department of Health, Education, and Welfare.

Table 3. Total Medicaid Benefits by State and by Assistance Status, Fiscal Year 1973 (Millions of Dollars)

State	*Total benefits*[a]	*Eligible for cash assistance*	*Medically needy*
Alabama	$ 151	151	—
Alaska	—	—	—
Arizona	—	—	—
Arkansas	43	43	—
California	1,441	1,218	222
Colorado	80	80	—
Connecticut	116	52	65
Delaware	13	13	—
District of Columbia	54	30	24
Florida	139	139	—
Georgia	179	179	—
Guam	—	—	—
Hawaii	33	22	11
Idaho	19	19	—
Illinois	512	396	116
Indiana	120	120	—
Iowa	29	29	—
Kansas	67	57	10
Kentucky	90	58	31
Louisiana	85	85	—
Maine	41	41	—
Maryland	132	62	70
Massachusetts	416	179	237
Michigan	390	249	140
Minnesota	181	126	56
Mississippi	58	58	—
Missouri	62	62	—

Montana	15	15	—
Nebraska	57	41	16
Nevada	14	14	—
New Hampshire	12	11	1
New Jersey	236	236	—
New Mexico	30	30	—
New York	1,749	1,084	666
North Carolina	111	72	39
North Dakota	16	15	1
Ohio	268	268	—
Oklahoma	100	74	27
Oregon	36	36	—
Pennsylvania	402	270	132
Puerto Rico	70	39	31
Rhode Island	55	30	24
South Carolina	58	58	—
South Dakota	18	18	—
Tennessee	98	98	—
Texas	434	434	—
Utah	31	24	7
Vermont	24	21	4
Virgin Islands	1	—	1
Virginia	168	105	62
Washington	127	109	18
West Virginia	34	34	—
Wisconsin	190	178	12
Wyoming	5	5	
*U.S. Total**	*$8,802*	*6,778*	*2,024*

* Columns do not add to totals due to rounding.

SOURCE: November, 1971 forecasts by States of their expenditures. United States Department of Health, Education, and Welfare.

Table 4. Number of Medicaid Recipients* and Percentage Change over Previous Year, Fiscal Years 1969–73

	Fiscal year 1969		Fiscal year 1970		Fiscal year 1971		Fiscal year 1972		Fiscal year 1973	
Eligibility category	*Number of recipients*	*Percent change*	*Number of recipients*	*Percent change over prior year*	*Number of recipients*	*Percent change over prior year*	*Number of recipients*	*Percent change over prior year*	*Number of recipients*	*Percent change over prior year*
TOTAL	12,060,000	—	14,507,000	+20.3	18,223,000	+25.6	20,632,000	+13.2	23,537,000	+14.1
Age 65 and over	2,900,000	—	3,200,000	+10.3	3,600,000	+12.5	3,800,000	+ 5.6	4,000,000	+ 5.3
Blindness	75,000	—	107,000	+42.7	123,000	+15.0	132,000	+ 7.3	137,000	+ 3.8
Disabled	960,000	—	1,200,000	+25.0	1,500,000	+25.0	1,700,000	+13.3	2,000,000	+17.6
Children under 21	5,900,000	—	6,500,000	+10.2	8,300,000	+27.7	9,400,000	+13.3	10,800,000	+14.9
Adults in AFDC type families	2,225,000	—	3,500,000	+55.1	4,700,000	+34.3	5,600,000	+19.1	6,600,000	+17.9

* "Recipients" means people who actually had at least some of their health bills paid by Medicaid (or related programs).

SOURCE: United States Department of Health, Education, and Welfare.

Table 5. Medicaid Recipients by Assistance Status, Fiscal Year 1973

	Categorically needy	*Medically needy*	*Total*
All recipients	19,677,000	3,860,000	23,537,000
Age 65 or over	3,128,000	872,000	4,000,000
Blindness	127,000	10,000	137,000
Permanent and total disability	1,740,000	260,000	2,000,000
Aid to families with dependent children	13,682,000	2,718,000	17,400,000

SOURCE: United States Department of Health, Education, and Welfare.

Table 6. Medicaid Benefit Expenditures, by Type of Service, Fiscal Years 1967–71 (Thousands of Dollars)*

Type of service	*Fiscal year 1967*	*Fiscal year 1968*	*Fiscal year 1969*	*Fiscal year 1970*	*Fiscal year 1971*
			Amount		
Inpatient hospital care	$ 912,662	$1,360,947	$1,586,092	$1,887,438	$2,288,384
Nursing home care	766,120	1,063,950	1,291,363	1,321,000	1,673,999
Physicians' services	222,543	379,551	516,404	577,745	717,104
Dental care	72,246	190,000	208,688	168,653	181,315
Prescribed drugs	179,424	235,218	301,341	395,402	473,020
Other services	115,261	220,970	369,298	457,153	604,414
Not reported	740	740	253	142	1,000
Total	*$2,270,996*	*$3,451,376*	*$4,273,439*	*$4,807,533*	*$5,939,236*
			Percentage distribution		
Inpatient hospital care	40.2%	39.4%	37.1%	39.3%	38.5%
Nursing home care	33.7	30.8	30.2	27.5	28.2
Physicians' services	9.9	11.0	12.1	12.0	12.1
Dental care	3.2	5.5	4.9	3.5	3.1
Prescribed drugs	7.9	6.8	7.1	8.2	8.0
Other services	5.1	6.4	8.6	9.5	10.2
Not reported	†	†	†	†	†
Total	*100.0%*	*100.0%*	*100.0%*	*100.0%*	*100.0%*

* Expenditures from Federal, State, and local funds under Medicaid. Excludes per capita payments for Part B of Medicare.

† Percent not computed.

SOURCE: United States Department of Health, Education, and Welfare.

Table 7. Medicaid Services, State by State, September 1, 1972[1]

• offered for people receiving federally supported financial assistance

\+ offered also for people in public assistance categories[2] who are financially eligible for medical but not for financial assistance

Additional services for which Federal financial participation is available to States under Medicaid.

FMAP[3]	BASIC REQUIRED MEDICAID SERVICES SEE BELOW*	State	Clinic services	Prescribed drugs	Dental services	Prosthetic devices	Eyeglasses	Private duty nursing	Physical therapy and related services	Other diagnostic, screening, preventive and rehabilitative services	Emergency hospital services	Family planning services	Skilled nursing home services for patients under 21	Optometrists' services	Podiatrists' services	Chiropractors' services	Care for patients 65 or older in institutions for mental diseases	Care for patients 65 or older in institutions for tuberculosis	Institutional services in intermediate care facilities	
78	•	Alabama		•			•				•			•				•	•	AL
50	•	Alaska									•	•								AK
64		Arizona																		AZ
79	•	Arkansas			•						•					•	•	•	•[4]	AR
50	+	California	+	+	+	+	+	+	+		+	+	+	+	+	+	+	+	+[4]	CA
58	•	Colorado		•		•					•	•	•		•		•		•[4]	CO
50	+	Connecticut	+	+	+	+	+	+	+	+		+	+	+	+	+	+			CT
50	•	Delaware	•	•		•			•	•		•			•		•	•		DE
50	+	D.C.	+	+		+	+		+		+	+	+	+	+		+	+	+[4]	DC
61	•	Florida		•							•	•					•	•	•[4]	FL
70	•	Georgia		•								•	•		•				•[4]	GA
50	+	Guam	+	+	+	+	+					+	+	+						GU
51	+	Hawaii	+	+	+	+	+		+	+	+	+	+	+					+	HI
72	•	Idaho		•							•	•	•	•	•	•	•		•[4]	ID
50	+	Illinois	+	+	+	+	+	+	+	+	+	+	+	+	+		+	+	+[4]	IL
55	•	Indiana	•	•	•	•	•	•	•	•	•	•	•	•	•	•			•	IN
58	•	Iowa		•	•	•	•		•		•	•	•	•	•	•				IA
59	+	Kansas	+	+	+	+	+	+	+	+	+	+	+	+	+	+	+	+	+[4]	KS
73	+	Kentucky		+	+				+	+		+	+				+	+	•	KY
73	•	Louisiana	•	•		•				•	•						•	•	•[4]	LA
69	•	Maine	•	•		•	•	•	•	•	•	•	•	•	•	•	•		•	ME
50	+	Maryland	+	+	+	+	+		+	+	+	+		+	+		+	+	+	MD
50	+	Massachusetts	+	+	+	+	+	+	+	+	+	+	+	+	+	+	+	+	+	MA
50	+	Michigan		+					+		+	+	+		+	+	+	+	+[4]	MI
57	+	Minnesota	+	+	+	+	+	+	+	+	+	+	+	+	+	+	+	+	+[4]	MN
83	•	Mississippi		•	•		•				•		•	•				•		MS
60	•	Missouri		•	•							•					•	•		MO
67	•	Montana	•	•	•	•	•	•	•		•	•	•	•			•	•	•[4]	MT

…mediate Care Facilities (ICF): P.L. 92-223 transferred the ICF program to …icaid (Title XIX) as an optional service, effective 1-1-72. States may at their …n include institutions for the mentally retarded, both public and private. …ootnote four.

73	●	New Mexico	●	●	●	●	●	●	●		●	●	●	●	●				●[4]	NM
50	+	New York	+	+	+	+	+	+	+	+	+	+	+	+	+	+	+	+	+[4]	NY
73	+	North Carolina		+	+	+	+				+	+		+	+	●	+	+		NC
71	+	North Dakota	+	+	+	+	+	+	+	+	+	+	+	+	+	+	+	+		ND
54	●	Ohio	●	●	●	●	●	●	●	●	●	●	●	●	●	●	●		●[4]	OH
69	+	Oklahoma			+								+				+		+[4]	OK
57	●	Oregon	●	●	●	●	●	●		●	●	●	●	●	●	●	●	●	●[4]	OR
55	+	Pennsylvania	+	●	●	●	+					●	+	+	●	+	+		●[4]	PA
50	+	Puerto Rico	+	+	+				+	+	+	+						+		PR
50	+	Rhode Island		+	+	+	+					+		+	+		+		●[4]	RI
78	●	South Carolina	●	●							●		●				●	●	●[4]	SC
70	●	South Dakota	●			●	●		●		●	●	●	●	●	●			●	SD
74	■	Tennessee		●							●	●					●	●	●[4]	TN
65	■	Texas		●							●			●	●	●	●	●	●[4]	TX
70	+	Utah	+	+	+	+	+	+	+	+	+	+	+	+	+	+	+		+[4]	UT
65	+	Vermont	+	+		+			+		+	+	+		+		+		+	VT
50	+	Virgin Islands	+	+	+	+	+		+			+								VI
64	+	Virginia	+	+		+	+		+		+	+	+	+	+		+	+	+[4]	VA
50	+	Washington	+	+	+	+	+	+	+	+	+	+	+	+	+	+	+	+	+[4]	WA
77	■	West Virginia	●	●	●	●	●	●	●	●		●	●	●	●	●	●	●		WV
56	+	Wisconsin	+	+	+	●	●	●	+	●	+		●	●	+		+		+[4]	WI
63	■	Wyoming																	●	WY
●	26	●	13	23	13	17	14	10	12	11	21	20	16	18	16	11	17	15	23	
+	27	+	22	25	22	20	21	11	21	14	20	24	21	20	20	13	22	16	17	
	53	Total	35	48	35	37	35	21	33	25	41	44	37	38	36	24	39	31	40	

* BASIC REQUIRED MEDICAID SERVICES: Every Medicaid program must cover at least these services for at least everyone receiving federally supported financial assistance: inpatient hospital care; outpatient hospital services; other laboratory and X-ray services; skilled nursing home services and home health services for individuals 21 and older; early and periodic screening, diagnosis, and treatment for individuals under 21; and physicians' services. Federal financial participation is also available to States electing to expand their Medicaid programs by covering additional services and/or by including people eligible for medical but not for financial assistance. For the latter group States may offer the services required for financial assistance recipients or may substitute a combination of seven services.

Services provided only under the Medicare buy-in or the screening and treatment program for individuals under 21 are not shown on this chart. Definitions and limitations vary from State to State. Details are available from local welfare offices and State Medicaid agencies.

[1] Data from Regional Office reports of characteristics of State programs.

[2] People qualifying as aged, blind, disabled, or members of families with dependent children (usually families with at least one parent absent or incapacitated).

[3] FMAP–Federal Medical Assistance Percentage: Rate of Federal financial participation in a State's medical vendor payment expenditures on behalf of individuals and families eligible under Title XIX of the Social Security Act. Percentages, effective from July 1, 1971, through June 30, 1973, are rounded.

[4] Including ICF services in institutions for the mentally retarded.

SOURCE: United States Department of Health, Education, and Welfare: Social and Rehabilitation Service, Medical Services Administration, Office of Program Planning and Evaluation, Public Information Office (SRS)-73-24801*

Index

Waterfowl and Wetlands

Toward Bioeconomic Analysis

Judd Hammack and Gardner Mallard Brown, Jr.

RFF PRESS
RESOURCES FOR THE FUTURE

First published in 1974
by Resources for the Future, Inc.

This edition first published in 2016 by Routledge
2 Park Square, Milton Park, Abingdon, Oxon, OX14 4RN
and by Routledge
711 Third Avenue, New York, NY 10017

Routledge is an imprint of the Taylor & Francis Group, an informa business

Publisher's Note
The publisher has gone to great lengths to ensure the quality of this reprint but points out that some imperfections in the original copies may be apparent.

Disclaimer
The publisher has made every effort to trace copyright holders and welcomes correspondence from those they have been unable to contact.

A Library of Congress record exists under LC control number: 74006815

ISBN 13: 978-1-138-96300-9 (hbk)
ISBN 13: 978-1-315-65903-9 (ebk)

WATERFOWL AND WETLANDS: TOWARD BIOECONOMIC ANALYSIS

The first of mankind had in common all those things which God had given to the human race. This community was not a positive community of interest, like that which exists between several persons who have the ownership of a thing in which each has his particular portion. It was a community, which those who have written on this subject have called a negative community, which resulted from the fact that those things which were common to all belonged no more to one than to the others, and hence no one could prevent another from taking of these common things that portion which he judged necessary in order to subserve his wants. Whilst he was using them others could not disturb him, but when he had ceased to use them, if they were not things which were consumed by the fact of use, the things immediately reentered into the negative community, and another could use them. The human race having multiplied, men partitioned among themselves the earth and the greater part of those things which were on its surface. That which fell to each one among them commenced to belong to him in private ownership, and this process is the origin of the right of property. Some things, however, did not enter into this division, and remain therefore to this day in the condition of the ancient and negative community.

Pothier, discussing the legal character of animals *ferae naturae*, in *Traité du Droit de Propriété* (No. 21), as quoted in Geer v. Connecticut, 161 U.S. 519 (1895)

WATERFOWL AND WETLANDS: toward bioeconomic analysis

Judd Hammack and
Gardner Mallard Brown, Jr.

Published by Resources for the Future, Inc.
Distributed by The Johns Hopkins University Press
Baltimore and London

Resources for the Future is a nonprofit corporation for research and education in the development, conservation, and use of natural resources and the improvement of the quality of the environment. It was established in 1952 with the cooperation of the Ford Foundation. Part of the work of Resources for the Future is carried out by its resident staff; part is supported by grants to universities and other nonprofit organizations. Unless otherwise stated, interpretations and conclusions in RFF publications are those of the authors; the organization takes responsibility for the selection of significant subjects for study, the competence of the researchers, and their freedom of inquiry.

This book is part of the RFF natural environments research program directed by John Krutilla. It was edited by Ruth Haas. Charts and maps were drawn by Federal Graphics. Judd Hammack is associate professor of economics and statistics at California State University, Los Angeles; Gardner M. Brown, Jr. is associate professor of economics at the University of Washington, Seattle.

RFF editors: Mark Reinsberg, Joan Tron, Ruth B. Haas, Margaret Ingram

Manufactured in the United States of America

The Johns Hopkins University Press, Baltimore, Maryland 21218
The Johns Hopkins University Press Ltd., London
Library of Congress Catalog Card Number 74-6815

ISBN 8018-1625-4

Library of Congress Cataloging in Publication data will be found on the last printed page of this book.

Acknowledgments

Our obligation to the late Gerald J. Paulik is singular and beyond measure, for without his aid on waterfowl biometrics, this book could not have been written.

Interdisciplinary work, drawing as it does upon persons in several fields, produces an indebtedness that cannot be given full expression here. We must ask forgiveness of many individuals for singling out only the relative few we mention.

The names and addresses of waterfowl hunters, provided by the Migratory Bird Populations Station, U.S. Bureau of Sport Fisheries and Wildlife, formed a critical part of our data-gathering process. We owe thanks to Walter F. Crissey, Aelred D. Geis, and Charles H. Lobdell for their part in furnishing the mailing list and for answering our many questions. John Chattin, the Bureau's Pacific flyway representative, patiently dealt with our queries and supplied literature on a wide variety of topics from his seemingly inexhaustible files.

Helpful and stimulating comments on our research were offered at one stage or another by David R. Anderson, Oscar R. Burt, James A. Crutchfield, Gregory Duncan, Anthony Fisher, Darius Gaskins, Jon H. Goldstein, and Michael F. Tillman. Lawrence E. Gales provided superb aid in communicating the stochastic model of chapter 4 to the computer. The Institute for Economic Research, University of Washington, was most generous in providing computer funds.

Resources for the Future provided financial support for the project throughout, and the organization, through John V. Krutilla, also provided constant intellectual and emotional support. We are most grateful.

February 1974

Judd Hammack

Gardner Mallard Brown, Jr.

Contents

Tables

Figures

WATERFOWL AND WETLANDS: TOWARD BIOECONOMIC ANALYSIS

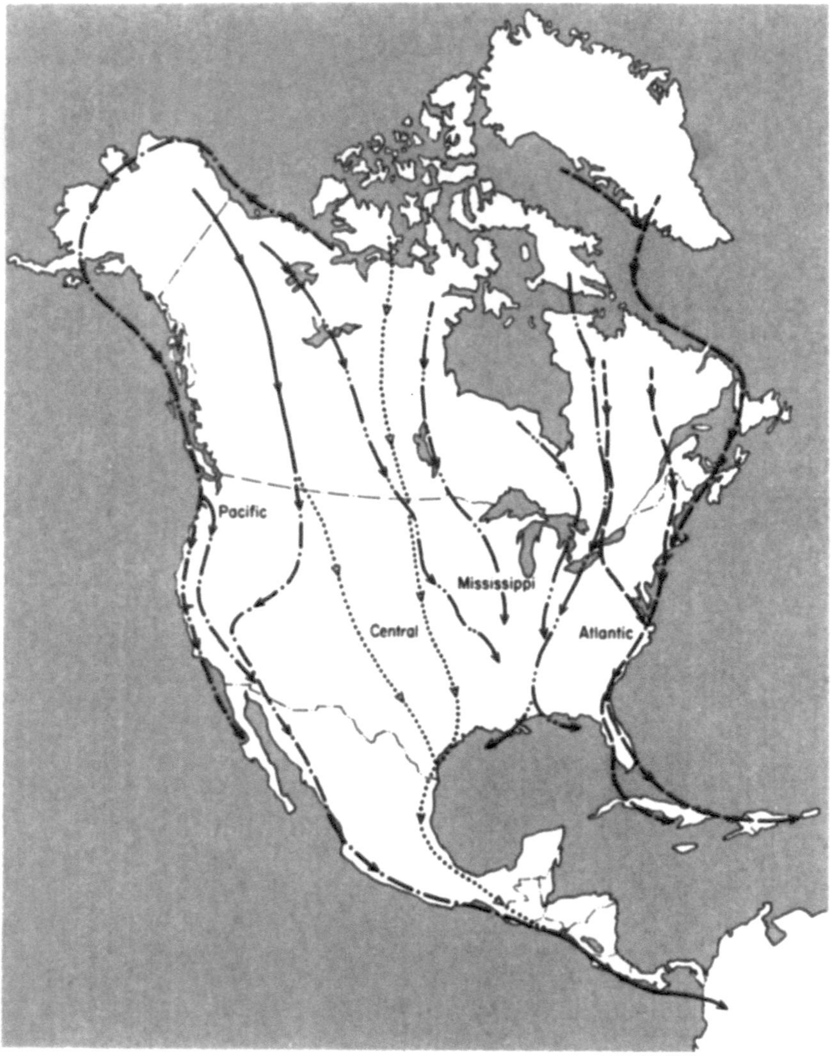

Major flyways of North America.

chapter one Introduction

Migratory waterfowl provide a basis for many recreational experiences. The birds may be hunted, or simply viewed and perhaps photographed. Unlike most consumer goods, waterfowl are not priced in a market, and so their value to humans generally goes unmeasured. And as a direct consequence, the value of wetlands used in supporting the birds also is not measured.

Society has at least one alternate and competing use for large amounts of wetlands: agricultural production. Farm commodities are conventionally priced, and the value of drained wetlands in agricultural use can be measured by conventional tools of analysis.

Deciding rationally whether wetlands should be drained, or whether new wetlands should be created, requires more information about waterfowl, including their value, than is casually available. Our goal is to redress the asymmetry of information, to help the waterfowl have their say.

THE GENERAL SETTING

Migratory waterfowl generally nest in the northern areas of the North American continent in the summer and fly south to open water in the fall and winter. Some species of teal have been known to migrate as far south as Peru, but most waterfowl winter in the United States, with some making a circuit through Mexico. Because of their migratory nature, the birds are under the jurisdiction of the central government when in Canada, the United States, or Mexico. North American waterfowl are an international resource in both a legal and a physical sense; the birds are as dependent upon their breeding grounds in the north as they are upon their wintering grounds in the south. In general, the quantity and quality of wintering grounds are believed to be adequate, and the critical factor in sustaining waterfowl populations is the amount of nesting ground.[1]

The rolling, pothole-pocked farmlands of central and southern Alberta, Saskatchewan, and Manitoba, together with parts of the neighboring states of North Dakota, South Dakota, and Minnesota, provide the prime duck-producing areas of the continent. The region comprises only 10 percent of the total continental breeding area, yet produces upwards of 55 percent of the total duck population in an average year.

The supply of superior nesting grounds has declined as farmers continue to drain the prairie wetlands to increase their arable land and eliminate the costs incurred in tilling around the potholes. Also, some wetlands have been claimed as refuse dumps for brush, and deeper ponds have been tapped for irrigation water.

Drainage of the more permanent wetlands has been particularly severe in the United States. According to a recent study, the average annual drainage rate since 1964 has averaged 1.9 percent of the total wetland acreage in the tri-state area of North Dakota, South Dakota, and Minnesota. In a 19-county area of Minnesota, 14 percent of the wetlands were drained in a recent 4-year period.[2] In the Canadian prairies, drainage appears to have proceeded at a considerably slower rate.

Drainage in the prairie pothole region is a matter of considerable concern since it threatens the nesting habitat of the dabbling ducks, which, with geese and diving ducks, are the waterfowl of major interest to hunters. Dabblers include mallards and pintails—two highly desired and relatively abundant species—and compose a larger percentage of the total hunter kill than either geese or diving ducks.

The actual and potential loss of habitat largely affects hunters, not viewers, of waterfowl. Walter F. Crissey has stated that even a 75 to 80

[1] Walter F. Crissey, "Prairie Potholes from a Continental Viewpoint," *Saskatoon Wetlands Seminar*, Canadian Wildlife Service Report Series No. 6 (Ottawa: The Queen's Printer, 1969), p. 167. Crissey's comment with respect to wintering grounds specifically referred to mallards. Generalization to other species, particularly dabbling ducks, seems reasonable.

[2] J. Larry Haddock and Lawrence W. DeBates, "Report on Drainage Trends in the Prairie Pothole Region of Minnesota, North Dakota and South Dakota" (Laurel, Md.: U.S. Bureau of Sport Fisheries and Wildlife, 1969), p. 7.